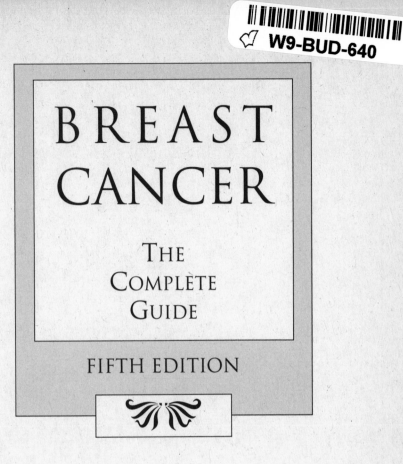

BREAST CANCER

The Complete Guide

FIFTH EDITION

BREAST CANCER

The
Complete
Guide

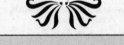

Yashar Hirshaut,
MD, FACP,
and
Peter I. Pressman,
MD, FACS

Fifth Edition

BANTAM BOOKS
NEW YORK TORONTO LONDON SYDNEY AUCKLAND

BREAST CANCER: THE COMPLETE GUIDE
A Bantam Book

PUBLISHING HISTORY
Bantam hardcover edition published October 1992
Bantam trade paperback edition published July 1993
Bantam revised trade paperback edition published May 1996
Bantam third trade paperback edition published September 2000
Bantam fourth trade paperback edition published September 2004
Bantam fifth trade paperback edition / October 2008

Published by
Bantam Dell
A Division of Random House, Inc.
New York, New York

Library of Congress Catalog Card Number: 2004052672

Bantam Books and the rooster colophon are registered trademarks of Random House, Inc.

ISBN 978-0-553-38591-5

Printed in the United States of America

Published simultaneously in Canada

www.bantamdell.com

BVG 10 9 8 7 6 5 4 3 2 1

To our patients, for their trust
and friendship

To our wives and families,
for their support and encouragement
in the writing of this book

To Ann Harris, our editor,
for her friendship and her
expert guidance

*We are grateful to our colleagues for their kindness
in reviewing portions of this book, with special thanks
to Doctors Mary K. Hayes, Clifford Hudis, Ruth Rosenblatt,
and Mark Sultan, and to Shivani Nazareth.*

*We wish to thank Charlotte Mayerson
for her invaluable help in the organizing
and writing of this book.*

CONTENTS

Foreword by Jane Brody, "Personal Health"
columnist for *The New York Times*   ix

BOOK I

FROM SUSPICION TO DIAGNOSIS

BOOK II

TREATMENT

Book III

After the Treatment

Book IV

Life After Cancer

FOREWORD

Jane Brody

"Personal Health" columnist for *The New York Times*

In early February 1999, a sonogram done as part of my annual mammogram and breast exam revealed a suspicious area in my left breast, which led to an ultrasound-guided needle biopsy and the diagnosis of an early and, I am happy to say, highly curable cancer. This was followed a week later by ambulatory surgery: a lumpectomy and sentinel node biopsy. I was in and out of the hospital and back home in just four hours.

I consider myself very lucky to have developed breast cancer when I did and to have a surgeon—Dr. Peter I. Pressman, coauthor of the book you now hold in your hands—who was one of the pioneers in surgical techniques that were no more aggressive than were needed for the disease being treated. I clearly remember writing in my first book, *You Can Fight Cancer and Win,* published in 1977, that if I ever developed breast cancer and had to lose my breast to live, then so be it. Those were the days of total or radical mastectomy for every woman treated for breast cancer. As I saw it, losing a breast was not nearly as bad as losing one's life.

How far we've come since then! No longer is mastectomy the most common approach to treating breast cancer, thanks to the devoted efforts of scores of researchers and clinicians such as Dr. Pressman and his coauthor Dr. Yashar Hirshaut who have greatly refined not only surgical techniques to minimize physical trauma, but diagnostic methods and postsurgical treatments. Together these have led to a steady increase in a woman's chances of surviving breast cancer while limiting the damage done to her physical and mental well-being. Even cancers that have already spread beyond the breast are now being managed as chronic illnesses rather than a quick and certain death sentence.

The authors were also pioneers in writing, for the benefit of all women and those who love them, a readily accessible and comprehensive guide to breast cancer diagnosis, treatment, and post-treatment: *Breast Cancer: The Complete Guide,* first published in 1992 and now appearing in a fully revised fifth edition. Through these five revisions, their book has stood the test of time and brought women and their loved ones the most up-to-date information available about managing this disease, the disease that for decades women have feared most.

But now it is time to replace fear with facts: More than 96 percent of women do not die of breast cancer and more than 70 percent of those who develop breast cancer do not die from it. Indeed, through an unending stream of improvements in diagnosis and treatment, each year the chances of surviving breast cancer have been rising by about 2 percent.

This book tells the story of this progress in full, yet easily understood, detail. In this new edition, you will find the most reliable information currently available on the role that diet and exercise can play in preventing breast cancer. You will find discussions of such important new developments as the use of breast MRIs as a diagnostic tool, especially for monitoring women who have already had cancer in one breast and for those with a defect in the genes BRCA1 and BRCA2 that renders them highly susceptible to developing breast cancer. For women at such high risk, there is now the option of skin-sparing and nipple-preserving mastectomy and breast reconstruction, which greatly reduces their risk of ever developing this disease.

You will also note that for most women with suspicious breast lesions on a mammogram or sonogram, much less invasive core needle biopsies are replacing surgical biopsies to determine whether a cancer is present. And you will find that, for seemingly early cancers, sentinel node biopsies are replacing removal of most or all of a woman's underarm lymph nodes, greatly reducing her risk of developing lymphedema, a chronic swelling of the arm.

Then there is the extraordinary progress being made in post-surgical treatments, both with radiation and chemotherapy. For some, partial radiation therapy and accelerated therapy that significantly shortens treatment time are being more widely used.

Hormonal therapies, especially postsurgical treatment with Arimidex, have significantly increased cancer-free survival in women with estrogen-receptor (ER)-positive breast cancers. And for women whose cancers are especially aggressive because they are positive for the gene HER-2/neu, treatment with the drug Herceptin has revolutionized their care, and now newer drugs like Avastin and Tykerb promise even better results.

Perhaps even more exciting, because it had long seemed so unlikely, is the progress being made in treating recurrent and metastatic breast cancer with a growing number of drugs and drug combinations that have added years of life worth living for many women I know.

But what excites me most is the promise held by modern genetics: the growing ability to determine on the basis of genetic tests not only who is at greater risk of developing breast cancer but also how an individual woman's breast cancer is best treated. No more "one size fits all." More and more treatments are being tailored to the genetic characteristics of a particular cancer, thus increasing the chances for long-lasting, disease-free survival and cure.

Of course, the many new diagnostic and therapeutic options also make matters more confusing for women, which is why a book like this one is so valuable. While I hope you have not had and will never get breast cancer, having available the information contained in this book and acting on it may one day help to save your life and preserve your physical and mental health.

So read on. Here's to your good health.

New York City
August 2008

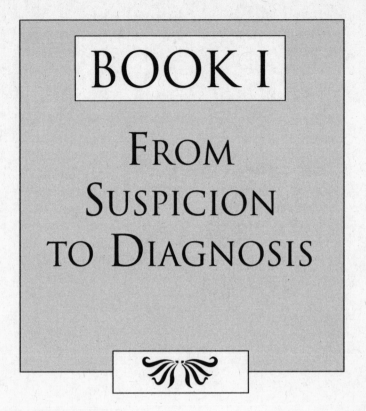

BOOK I

FROM SUSPICION TO DIAGNOSIS

CHAPTER

1

How Can a Book Help Me?

❧

The authors of this book are both physicians whose primary practices are in the field of breast cancer. Peter Pressman is a surgeon; Yashar Hirshaut, an oncologist. We share a philosophy about staying involved in all the phases of treating our patients, and in that sense we are both oncologists—one surgical, the other medical.

Both of us spend every day of our working lives with women who have breast cancer or fear that it lies before them. We have seen how they and their friends and families can sometimes be overwhelmed by this information, unclear as to how to proceed either in the practical matters or in the often devastating emotional ones.

The aim of this book is to provide you with a thorough, clear, step-by-step guide through the illness. More than that, we hope to act as "your brothers, the doctors," as people who care about you and want to share with you what we've learned from years of study and experience.

Why can't you get this kind of advice from your own physician? We certainly hope you can. But even the possibility of breast cancer poses problems so unusual that having an additional expert at your side may be of real help to you.

For example, if you've been told you have appendicitis, even though it's an emergency, the course of treatment is pretty straightforward. You should try to find a competent, well-trained, and experienced surgeon who will do the procedure at a good hospital. But you don't have to worry about the physician's philosophy toward appendectomy. You don't, in general, have to worry about which type of surgery he'll perform. There are not several possible postoperative treatments from which to choose.

More important, your survival chances after the removal of an unruptured appendix—unless there are unusual and unforeseen complications—are excellent. And unless you're a belly dancer or a bodybuilder, your concern about a small scar at the side of your abdomen is probably minimal. To put it another way, losing your appendix doesn't have much impact on your physical or social well-being, nor does it pose much of a threat to your self-image.

If, however, you've been told you may have breast cancer, you are facing all of those complexities—and more. It is our hope that this book will help women sort out such problems and approach them with as much confidence as possible.

As you may already have noticed, we are concentrating on breast cancer in women. We will not be addressing the illness in men, in whom it is rare, though the material on diagnosis and treatment would apply to them as well.

One other explanation: As a rule, we will use the first person singular "I" throughout the book, because that seems most comfortable for us. In fact, sometimes one of us will be the basic expert in a chapter, sometimes the other, and in some sections the material will be the result of a pretty evenhanded sharing of expertise and experience.

The book is sprinkled with stories about women (anonymous, of course) whom we have known in our daily work. We have used these anecdotes to help us explain the conditions we are describing, and also because we think it may be useful to you to read about other women who have "been there," to hear what they felt and experienced, and how they coped. Much of our own insight into the illness has come from them.

The best understanding of breast cancer and its treatment will probably come from reading this book straight through. Doing that will also guide you, step-by-step, through any experience you may confront. If, however, you have a particular question to which you want an immediate answer, you can refer to the table of contents or the index and go right to the section that concerns you. There, if they are necessary, you will find cross-references to other pertinent material in the book.

Book I takes you from the time you first suspect a problem through the diagnosis of what it is. It helps you put into place the best possible personal and professional support system, including a team of doctors. It explains what may have gone wrong in your breast, whether it is a type of cancer or some other condition. In addition to diagnosis, Book I also covers pathology and provides guidance in making the best preparations for treatment after you've found out what's wrong.

Book II has to do with genetics, with prognosis—the probable course of the illness—and with treatment: It describes the procedures and the side effects of surgery, radiation, hormone treatments, chemotherapy, and breast reconstruction.

Book III is a discussion of what happens after the initial course of treatment. It covers the appropriate medical follow-up as well as any recurrence of the illness. The last two chapters of this part describe what we know about the causes and prevention of breast cancer, the directions in which new research is pointing, and what future promise there may be for improving the treatment of breast cancer.

The final section, Book IV, relies heavily on the experiences of our patients in coping with the emotional impact of this disease, in understanding the reactions of others, and in the positive as well as the negative consequences of breast cancer that so many women have told us about.

*   *   *

While the continuing increase in the incidence of the disease during the previous two decades stopped in 2000, with the exception of skin cancer there are still more new cases of breast cancer among women than of any other cancer.

That is not good news. Clearly, we have to find out what is going on and why. But the fact is, we know more about the disease every day. The cure rate is definitely increasing; though 182,460 women a year continue to get breast cancer, a larger percentage of them are surviving.

We now know how to treat breast cancer without the devastation of women's lives that was the norm a few decades ago. We also know that getting the right treatment from the right physicians can make all the difference. To help you do that is the purpose of this book.

CHAPTER

2

GETTING STARTED

W hen you or someone you care about has or is facing the possibility of breast cancer, it is natural to feel many bewildering and frightening emotions. No one wants to get sick at all. Certainly no one wants to get cancer. And there are kinds of cancers that seem particularly terrible, not only because of their death-dealing potential but because they or their treatment hit us "where we live." Breast cancer, for most women, is one of those diseases.

The possibility that you may have breast cancer is made even more stressful because it is an illness in which you are going to be called upon to make several decisions that don't necessarily arise in other situations. As we'll see later in this chapter, it's important that along with a carefully chosen team of physicians, you and the people in your personal support system take a very active role in the management of your case. Though that may feel a little intimidating right now, it can make a real difference in your welfare.

There are people who, when they are ill, take the attitude "I'm going to find a good doctor and turn myself over to him. He knows better than I what should be done." Only to a certain extent is that a reasonable attitude in any medical situation. But breast cancer, with its many treatment possibilities, offers a special challenge to the patient.

WHAT DO I DO NOW?

For most of us, a serious threat to our health immediately takes center stage. Other concerns seem less important than they were before we learned of our illness. Though we may not articulate the thought, we understand that if we don't give first priority to taking care of the health crisis, there may not *be* any other concerns.

Even so, some women are so terrified of the thought of breast cancer that though they have found a lump or other abnormality in their breast, they suppress the knowledge, at least for a time. They may say to themselves, "That's nothing. I'm just imagining it," or "Next time I go to the doctor, I'll mention it," or "I've always had that. It's not worth worrying about."

Don't do this. We have seen too many women become the victims of their own fright and denial. Their illness, which would almost certainly have responded to treatment in its early stages, was so advanced by the time they finally sought help that it was too late.

So, the answer to the question "What do I do now?" is, first, get some perspective on what you are facing. Second, find good allies, the right doctors, to help you.

These are the concerns that women seem to worry about most:

WILL I SURVIVE?

Is the diagnosis of breast cancer a death sentence?

The answer isn't a simple yes or no but rather, in most

instances, an optimistic "probably not, and certainly not immediately."

Those answers were not always available to us. A couple of generations back, women did not talk about breast cancer, and there was not nearly as much public discussion of the illness or the almost overwhelming coverage in newspapers and magazines, on radio, television, and the Internet as occurs today. Self-examination was seldom done, and even when women did notice a small lump, they might have postponed taking any action out of a combination of ignorance and fear. Therefore, by the time they got to the doctor, they tended to be in later stages of the disease, and that very adversely affected their chances of beating it.

Moreover, in the past the medical profession was much less effective in dealing with the illness than it is now. The prevailing treatments were in general less successful, more disfiguring, and more seriously disruptive of the quality of the patient's life. Surgery was much more extensive, chemotherapy and radiation techniques were less refined, and we did not have as much experience with their use, their results, and their side effects as we now do.

WHAT IS TODAY'S SUCCESS RATE?

To understand the changes that have taken place, bear in mind that a five-year length of time is often used to express the success rate. And though we'll get into the stages of cancer (see pages 42–43), for the purposes of this comparison it is enough to say that generally speaking, cancers are classified mainly by how far they have spread. With those factors in mind, it is encouraging to see how much progress we have made.

Between 1960 and 1964, the five-year survival rate for all stages of breast cancer was 64 percent. For local cancers, it was 84 percent. For cancers that had spread to lymph nodes near the affected breast, the rate was 54 percent. Where the cancer had spread to a distant site, only 7 percent of the affected women survived.

From 1979 to 1984, the five-year survival rate for all stages was 75 percent; for local cancers, 90 percent; for those that had spread to nearby lymph nodes, 69 percent; and for distant cancer, 10 percent.

The most recent five-year figures show an overall survival rate of 88.5 percent and parallel improvements in the other stages. For local cancers it is 98.1 percent; for those involving the regional lymph nodes, 83.1 percent; and for distant cancer, 26.0 percent.

So, many more women are surviving. That doesn't mean that anyone can tell you definitively, without any doubt, that you are not going to be on the wrong side of the statistics. It does mean that your chances of conquering this condition are very good.

WILL I BE DISFIGURED?

Actually the question is often phrased more dramatically: Many women use the word *mutilated*. "Will I be mutilated?" The answer to that is a lot easier. It's a clear and unequivocal no.

In Chapter 8, we will discuss in detail the various types of surgery for breast cancer. The relevant thing to say now, however, is that what women quite rightly dread most—the disfiguring **radical mastectomy,** in which the entire breast and a lot of the surrounding tissue and musculature are removed—is not needed anymore.

The **modified radical mastectomy** removes the breast but leaves the muscles intact. The result is much less damage to the body by preserving the natural upper-body contours, and a much better situation for breast reconstruction.

Most women now are treated with what is commonly called a **lumpectomy,** a surgical procedure that is also referred to as a **wide excision.** In this technique for saving the breast, only the cancer, some surrounding tissue, and the nearby lymph nodes are removed. The remainder of the breast is then usually treated with radiation. These procedures will be discussed thoroughly in Chapters 8 and 9.

Most important to the concern of disfigurement is breast reconstruction. We will discuss this subject in detail in Chapter 12. When a mastectomy needs to be done, the techniques the plastic surgeon employs for reconstruction have been so improved that reconstruction is now usually carried out immediately after mastectomy, and a sense of wholeness almost completely retained. Most of my patients who have undergone reconstruction are pleased and relieved at the results.

THE QUESTION OF SEX

Because women themselves consider their breasts to be a central part of their sexuality, as well as because of the frequent emphasis on the breast in the media and in art, many of them fear that breast cancer means an end to their sexuality—that they will no longer be attractive, or ever again enjoy sexual experience.

Let's begin with what I think is the common happy ending to this part of the story: There is no doubt that women and their sex partners may have complex issues to work out after breast cancer treatment. But from what I have seen in my practice, breast cancer seldom has long-term or disastrous consequences on the personal lives of my patients. There is a period of adjustment, but it's my impression that it isn't very long and that most couples put their fears behind them and reestablish satisfying and loving relations.

Many single women who are not in a relationship at the time of their illness have great fear—even a sad certainty—that a "new" person will not want to take on as awkward a situation as this. They may worry that they won't be attractive to someone who has not lived through this experience with them. Again, though this evidence can't be statistical, I hear wonderful stories of strong and happy relationships built after breast cancer.

In fact, though it may be hard for you to imagine now, women often find that this experience takes its place in their history just as other difficult life experiences do. They surely would not have chosen it, but having had breast cancer has by no means ruined their lives.

Here's what one woman, now in her late forties, had to say at her five-year checkup:

"I had a mastectomy and at first I was in pretty bad emotional condition. Reconstruction wasn't advised at the time and I'm not sure I would have wanted to go through more surgery anyhow. I didn't have a man in my life at the time and I thought to myself, Okay, kid, you better fill up your life with other things because romance is out from now on. Well, then I met Michael and I have to tell you I was shaking like a leaf the first time he even stood close to me because I was afraid he'd feel how my breast was gone and be really repelled. But that's not the way it turned out at all. In fact, when I told him, I think it opened him up to a lot of tenderness that was good for both of us and that's stayed on in our relationship."

Another woman, trying to decide with her husband and her doctor what course of treatment was best for her, heard her husband ask incredulously, "What makes you think the only place you're sexy is in your right breast?"

A third patient, who was treated with only the removal of the cancerous lump and radiation, now says that aside from a thin scar, her appearance has hardly changed.

Indeed, there are so many happy endings after breast cancer treatment that it's hard to select among them.

The sum of these experiences? The majority of women who survive breast cancer make a good adjustment to any changes in their bodies that result from the illness or its treatment.

DEALING WITH YOUR EMOTIONS

I had a patient in the office recently to whom I had to explain that the small lump in her breast was indeed cancer. For the rest of the visit she shut out all the reassurances I could truthfully give her, as well as all the conversation we needed to have about treatment. "Am I going to die?" she kept asking. "Promise me that I'm not going to die."

No one can do that, as much as I wished I could. Yet this woman's fear is perfectly understandable. It is perfectly natural. It's a fear that everyone in these circumstances experiences. But to get the best treatment possible, to put together the best team of doctors, services, and loving support, you can't panic and let your fright overwhelm you.

"Easy for you to say" may be your reaction to that statement. But in reality, most women find that after the first shock of the threat of breast cancer, their own desire to survive soon pushes to the forefront. It overcomes any initial paralysis they may experience. They go ahead with what needs to be done to find expert help and to otherwise take care of themselves. (That patient I was describing came back a few days later, having absorbed the shock and far more ready to deal with her problem.)

Use whatever resources you can muster to support yourself

emotionally. Talk to your husband or partner, to trusted family members, or to friends. Think about earlier challenges in your life and how you overcame them. Deep-breathing exercises, meditation, and physical activity can be useful for some people during these first worrisome and uncertain days. That is especially true if you normally use such techniques for relaxation.

But whether or not you do these things, it seems to me that you'll get the most comfort and confidence when you begin to understand that though you are confronting a new and frightening adversary.

• You are not alone.

• There are competent and experienced specialists who can help you.

• Other people are beating this enemy every day.

There's more to take comfort from in what we've learned thus far:

• You are almost certainly not facing immediate death.

• You will almost certainly not be disfigured.

• You are almost certainly not going to be shut off from the physical side of your life.

A PERSONAL SUPPORT SYSTEM

Put out of your mind any idea that you should "keep a stiff upper lip" or suppress your anxiety. Don't do that. Talk as much as you need to, to whomever will be the most helpful. That may or may not be your husband or partner. If the person who is closest to you is likely to panic at the thought that you have breast cancer, or has a completely different approach to illness than you do, turn to a friend or a close relative to act as your sounding board. Or take into your confidence another woman who has had breast cancer in recent years. Don't use these people *instead* of a doctor; use them as companions on this journey you're setting out on.

Ask one of the people you most trust to act as your personal advocate in the period ahead. See if that friend, or relative, or husband or partner can accompany you to your medical appointments when you feel you need support or when you will be making treatment decisions. You may not want this personal ombudsman to take over for you, but it will be helpful if he or she keeps up with your case, knows your physicians, and understands you as a person. (For more detailed information on the use of a personal advocate, see pages 107–08.)

The emotional concerns we've been discussing are shared by most women who face the prospect of breast cancer. The first practical problem they encounter is finding a doctor. That is the task we'll consider next.

FINDING A DOCTOR

Why do you have to find one? A doctor may have been the one who first felt the lump in your breast or saw something suspicious on a mammogram. If you found a lump yourself, you may have gone to your own physician or to someone at a group practice. Isn't the doctor already found by now?

Maybe, but not necessarily. Probably, to get the very best diagnosis and care possible, you should look beyond the first person you've seen, even though you may decide in the end that she is the best person to treat you. No matter where you live, no matter what your experience with medical problems, no matter what access to specialists and medical centers you've had up to now, you want to find the very best physicians possible for each aspect of your diagnosis, treatment, and follow-up. That search for a team of doctors—usually beginning with a surgeon—is what you and the people who are supporting you must now undertake. And if you consider the factors below, one by one, the task can be accomplished without too much difficulty and your choices will fall into place.

WHAT KINDS OF DOCTORS TREAT BREAST CANCER?

The place most people start this search is at the office of the *radiologist* who takes their mammograms each year, their *gynecologist*, or their *family doctor,* who is sometimes an internist, a specialist in internal medicine.

You will have to ask yourself now whether you feel comfortable with the advice of this physician whom, up until now, you may have consulted only for fairly routine matters. Certainly you should consider the breast cancer specialist to whom she refers you, but you should also feel free to do a careful search of your own to be sure you are getting the best advice and care.

If, in other family health crises, you were pleased with your physician's referrals, you can proceed more confidently. Your doctor has probably already sent patients to this breast cancer specialist and has had a chance to see favorable results. If your own physician is a caring and intelligent human being, there's a good chance she will at least get you started on the right track.

Unless your illness is already in an extremely advanced stage, it is almost certainly to a *surgeon* that you will be sent next for the purpose of diagnosis. Why is that? Isn't a surgeon most likely to want to "cut"? As you will see in Chapter 4, an essential early step in finding out what's wrong is often a biopsy. It may be a needle biopsy. These procedures are reliable and are usually performed by a specially trained radiologist. Such biopsies may make it possible to avoid surgery when a cancer is not found. However, in many instances the final diagnosis still depends on a surgeon, who can remove suspicious tissue more completely for examination under the microscope. A surgeon is best suited to decide which forms of biopsy to use (see pages 75–89). This is not only because of his surgical skills but because he has unique training that makes his opinion at the diagnostic and treatment stages invaluable.

The surgeons who specialize in breast cancer have board certification in general surgery. They may have taken special training in breast surgery, and they have certainly devoted their practices primarily to this disorder.

An important member of the diagnostic team is the *radiologist,* a specialist who has been trained and certified in the use of X-rays and other forms of imaging that are used to look inside the body. This specialist has become an extremely important player in the diagnosis process, as we will see in Chapter 4. That is in part because of recent dramatic improvements in mammography, the X-ray procedure that produces mammograms—"pictures"—of the breast; in sonography, an imaging method that depends on the transmission of sound waves; in magnetic resonance imaging (MRI), a method that uses a magnetic field to produce images of the breast; and in needle biopsy techniques. Excellence in performing these examinations and in interpreting their results requires very special skills. It is therefore very important to consult a particularly expert radiologist.

The *radiation oncologist* uses radiation after a lumpectomy is performed and sometimes after a mastectomy. Radiation therapy may also be used locally to control advanced disease. The role of such treatment will be explored in detail in Chapter 9. (The radiation oncologist is usually not involved in the diagnostic process.) Since breast tissue is extremely sensitive to damage by radiation, it is crucial to find competent and experienced practitioners who have at their disposal the best (and usually, unfortunately, the most expensive) equipment possible for the planning and delivery of radiation treatment.

The *medical oncologist* generally sees breast cancer patients after the diagnosis and, usually, after any necessary surgery that follows. Medical oncologists are internists who specialize in the diagnosis and treatment of cancer. They most commonly use systemic therapy; that is, hormone therapy, chemotherapy, and more recently discovered biological therapies, which act *throughout* the body in the prevention of the recurrence of the disease as well as in long-term care. Briefly, chemotherapy is the use of special drugs that have a specific destructive effect on cancerous tissue. The hormones used in treatment also cause tumor shrinkage. (See Chapter 11.) Biological therapies are directed against specific molecules in the cancer cell or its blood vessels that control its growth and survival. This kind of treatment is often referred to as targeted therapy.

If a patient comes for treatment in a very advanced stage of breast cancer, the judgment may be made that surgery should not be used. (See page 153.) In that case, the oncologist will treat the patient from the start. I have in my own practice many women who came to me with advanced cancer but who nevertheless have done well. One woman came to my office eighteen years ago with a cancer so extensive that there seemed no reason to subject her to useless surgery. She has had a course of medical therapy and is not only still alive but seems fine.

Chemotherapy and hormone and biological therapies may also be used before surgery to reduce a tumor's size and prevent it from adhering to nearby normal tissues, enabling a mastectomy to remove the tumor more completely. In the case of a smaller tumor, shrinking it may make a mastectomy unnecessary because a lumpectomy may then be feasible.

A *plastic surgeon* repairs skin and tissue. After a mastectomy, he may be called upon to reconstruct a treated breast. In Chapter 12, we will explore the techniques of the surgeons who do breast reconstruction. Their results have become excellent, making it possible to produce a nearly normal appearance.

WHO'S IN CHARGE?

You are in charge, in the sense that you will have to get enough information to be able to put together the team of specialists that is required for the best treatment of breast cancer. You should choose the best person you can find in each specialty. Who becomes the leader of the team depends on the nature of the illness, which doctor you need to see most frequently, who knows you best, and who is willing to act as leader. Ideally, the treatment of breast cancer is a cooperative effort, with the command shifting as the need arises.

It is usually the surgeon who, at least initially, is the leader. It is he who must remove the tumor. Furthermore, as we will explore when we discuss the treatment of cancer in Book II, in most cases the other treatments of breast cancer are used to supplement the effects of surgery. Nevertheless, the radiologist, the radiation oncologist, the medical oncologist, the plastic surgeon, and the family doctor or gynecologist all play crucial roles, and each of these team members should be the very best physician available. What follows are guidelines to help you judge what "the very best" is, and then how to find it.

THE PERSONAL CHARACTERISTICS OF THE PHYSICIAN

THE DOCTOR AS ADVOCATE

I have to start by explaining my own attitudes and biases. When I look around me, I see two different kinds of physicians. There are those who view themselves as objective professionals, very much like judges. Their attitude is impartial; the patient and the cancer stand before them at the bar as equals. Such doctors go to great pains to explain to cancer patients the "reality" of the dangers of the disease and the difficulties in fighting it. They are certainly pleased if the patient "wins," and they take appropriate action in the treatment to try to achieve this end. But they don't seem to be passionately on the patient's side, a feisty adversary to the cancer.

Then there is the "defense attorney," the man or woman who gets in there—the tougher the case, the bigger the challenge—and fights for the client. That is the kind of doctor we all want: one who will not be intimidated by a grave illness, but who will fight it with all the vigor, skills, and techniques that can be mustered. Find that kind of doctor and you have a better chance to win your case.

THE INVOLVED HEALER

There is another, subtler question I want to get into, and that is to define for myself as a doctor how to be caring toward my patients and yet not be overwhelmed by my sympathy. Like anybody else, when a doctor is overwhelmed, he's not in very good shape to make the best decisions.

I see my patients as individuals I care about, and I want them to understand that. On the other hand, I want to be able to bring to their illness the kind of objectivity that good diagnosis and treatment require. It takes most doctors a long time to learn how to draw that fine line.

Once, many years ago, I was on my way home after a full day of tension and tragedy. In particular, one of my patients was doing very poorly, and I was lamenting the fates that had put her in such a position. And then I had an insight that has been a great help to me since then. I saw clearly that my role as a physician is not to lament but to find a way out—to look at the situation as it presents itself and to focus on finding constructive opportunities to make it better. It would not be helpful to the patient if I allowed myself to be paralyzed by anxiety. The patient needs a strong advocate, but one who can take an objective view of what is wrong and then, with a cool head, develop a strategy for overcoming it.

This does not mean your doctor should not be closely involved. It's very important to find a physician with whom you can have a personal relationship, to whom you can give your confidence, and from whom you feel a warm concern. Many doctors shun such a relationship. They try to stay emotionally detached. It's easy to understand why: They build a wall to protect themselves from getting hurt if the patient does not do well. But though this is not their intention, by reducing their vulnerability, it seems to me, they are also reducing their commitment. When the chips are down, such doctors may not fight as hard as they could. They may give up earlier than someone who has permitted himself to develop a warm, caring relationship with the patient.

And that is what you should look for: a doctor who will fight for you like a close friend. Avoid physicians who you think will insist on keeping their distance.

PATIENCE

When you first meet a doctor you are considering, make sure that she is patient in hearing your story and evaluating your condition. It is up to the doctor to establish the kind of atmosphere that allows you to feel that you are getting all the time you need.

Some medical offices are so busy, and the consulting rooms so tense, that you feel you are being rushed and that the doctor is anxious to get you moving through her "assembly line." If that is the feeling you get, trust it and look for someone else. Patience, the virtue our mothers talked about, is essential in a doctor who deals with breast cancer.

On the other hand, capable doctors are in demand, and their waiting rooms are often crowded. If there is a wait, you may want to take advantage of this opportunity. Talk to the women who are there. You are likely to learn a good deal about the doctor you are about to meet. I wish I could say that women never have to wait in my office, but they usually do. We try to schedule enough time for each patient, but emergencies arise, or somebody needs an especially long and painstaking explanation of her situation or extra time for comfort and reassurance. It can be difficult to balance giving the person before you all the time she needs and worrying about the patients you know are anxiously waiting outside.

Some of my patients handle the problem by calling ahead, before they leave for their appointment, to ask how we are doing, whether they should come right in or perhaps wait a half hour or so until the office traffic has eased.

THOROUGHNESS

This quality is closely related to patience. It takes a fair amount of time during the first visit to take a patient's history and to give her a complete physical examination. If the doctor isn't thorough, it is almost certain that important details will be missed. Note whether the physician gives you a chance to tell her everything that has happened since you discovered a lump or were told that your mammogram was suspicious.

She should also take a full history of past medical problems, allergies, drugs you take, and all relevant family and social details. These should include questions such as: When did you begin to menstruate? What was the date of your last period? How many pregnancies have you had? How many children? How old were you when you had your first child? Does anyone in your family have cancer? Breast or ovarian cancer? Your mother? Grandmother? Sisters? Cousins? Male relatives? Have any of them had genetic testing?

Watch to see whether the doctor takes her time during the physical examination. Does she examine both breasts? Does she carefully review the mammogram and any other test results you brought with you? Pay attention to these details and others like them to make sure that you are putting yourself in the hands of a meticulous person.

CAREFUL EXPLANATIONS

A good physician will encourage you to ask questions and will answer you thoughtfully and understandably. She will carefully explain to you the available options in your treatment and will ask what your feelings are about them. If a physician uses medical or technical terms that are not familiar to you, ask for a "translation" immediately. Do you understand what is wrong? What tests are needed? What treatment is planned? What alternative treatments may be available?

It is probably a good idea to bring someone with you to any early, exploratory appointments. Your companion can help you evaluate how the meeting went, and you will have someone to act as a sounding board in your later consideration of whether this particular doctor is the right person for you.

Your personal advocate can also help you remember the questions you should be asking, as well as the answers the physician gives to them. In that regard, it's a very good idea to take with you to the doctor's office a small pad on which you've written your questions and can record her answers. Even if you ordinarily have a good memory, you may find that under stress you "lose" some information you need.

You should not feel any embarrassment about asking questions, consulting your notes, or writing down what the doctor says. More and more patients follow this procedure and find it very helpful. In my own practice I don't mind if a patient asks to record the entire interview.

YOUR OWN DECISION

It is essential that you feel comfortable with the doctor who will be in charge of your care. It is equally important, as we will see on pages 28–29, that you be convinced that the particular approach to treatment that is being suggested is right for you.

These considerations are primary. If you are uncertain about any of them, you have every right to look further. This is much more important than worrying about hurting a doctor's feelings or being embarrassed about asking for your X-rays or records to take to another physician.

No one wants to be discourteous, and it's pretty safe to assume good intentions all around. But you have an absolute obligation to take the best care of yourself you can. That may mean "shopping around" and getting other opinions. It may mean insisting upon the release of the reports of the tests and diagnoses you have received (and paid for), taking your time in making decisions, and, if you like, having someone with you to consult with you and the physician.

TAKE YOUR TIME

Don't feel rushed to make a decision about a doctor. Breast cancer should be treated as soon as possible, but that does not mean within a day or two, and it certainly doesn't mean that speed is more important than making sound decisions.

The least satisfactory visits in my practice occur when a colleague calls and says, "There's a woman sitting across the desk from me whom I've known for years. She found a lump in her breast this morning, and I want you to see her right away," or a radiologist calls and says, "I just found something suspicious on a mammogram. I am sending the patient over to your office."

If I examine that woman immediately, tell her she probably has cancer, and outline a proposed plan of treatment, it's likely to be a disaster. Here is a person who woke up that morning, presumably healthy, and suddenly her world has caved in. There's someone talking to her about the loss of her breast or how to conserve it. A mammogram may not even have been done yet, and certainly has not been carefully studied. She's had no time to talk with her family or friends, to find out whom she really wants to consult with, or even to think about the questions she should be asking.

The first hours after you've been told that you may have breast cancer are bound to be upsetting. Anybody would feel, in those circumstances, as if the world had turned upside down. Give yourself time to talk to your family and friends and to compose yourself. Take your time.

Tell any doctor who may be urging great haste upon you that you'd rather go home now and that you'll call him tomorrow or the next day. You may decide in the end to go to the specialist he's recommending, but you'll get a lot more out of that relationship if you haven't hurtled into it.

SEARCHING FOR A DOCTOR

What is the best procedure to follow in finding these specialists? Even if the first doctor you see is someone you've known for years and whose good judgment has been proven to you repeatedly, give the matter some thought. Consider whether or not you want to seek other opinions. You are not "stuck" with the doctor who finds the lump, or the first doctor you consult. You do not have to choose or stay with the specialist to whom you've been referred.

In practical terms, that means that if your gynecologist or family physician has found a lump in a routine examination or your radiologist tells you of an abnormal finding on a routine mammogram, you may want to consult the breast specialists whom she usually deals with—or you may not. If you yourself have found the lump, you may want to go to your family doctor and have him manage your case—or you may not. If you go for an annual mammogram, you may want the results reported to the group practice you belong to—or you may not.

You should not prolong the search for a doctor as a way of avoiding timely action, nor should you keep "shopping" to the point of making yourself anxious and confusing the issue. But most insurance policies pay for—or even require—consultation at this point, so do get a second or even a third opinion until you like the physician you're dealing with and feel comfortable with her experience, training, hospital affiliation, and general approach to your particular situation. (We will discuss each of these factors later in this chapter.) You may get conflicting opinions that you will have to choose among. But until you feel comfortable with a particular plan of treatment, and confident in the abilities of each physician on the team, leave yourself open to other options.

"NETWORK"

How do you find a good cancer specialist? Try to investigate the problem through a variety of sources. Talk to friends, relatives, and colleagues about finding a doctor. You'll be amazed at how many people have had firsthand experience either as patients themselves or with people close to them.

Keep a list of those doctors women liked and those they didn't. Pretty soon you'll notice that one or two names keep cropping up on the "good" side of your list. Get a sense from the people who mentioned them of what those physicians are like, their hospital affiliation, and their general approach to the illness. Use these names to start your quest.

Breast cancer is, unfortunately, common enough in most cities that there are doctors, particularly surgeons, who treat only that condition. They are obviously experienced in most of its aspects. Experience is a valuable asset.

If you live in an area where there are no breast specialists, you should consider whether it is feasible to consult one in a nearby city. Even if in the long run you are going to have to rely on ongoing treatment from a doctor in your own area, I'd suggest that at the time of diagnosis, and of any surgery, you try to consult with such a breast cancer specialist.

OTHER WAYS TO SEARCH

What other steps can you take to find a good doctor?

• Consult the telephone book or search the Internet to see if there is a breast cancer hotline available in your area. Call the hotline for information about physicians in your community.

• Find out if there is a local women's health group or women's center. Such groups often know of doctors in the area who specialize in women's health problems. They sometimes keep records of women's experiences—good and bad—with local doctors.

• Call the best hospital in your region and ask for the names of breast cancer specialists. If there are several such people on staff, you may simply be given the names of the people next in order on the hospital's list. Still, this may be a useful place to start your search.

• Call your clergyman. He may know the names of good physicians in the community or may know other patients like yourself who have had the experience of looking for and finding a doctor.

Local, regional, and national cancer centers, organizations, and coalitions focused on the elimination of breast cancer and serving as advocates for those with this disease are listed in the appendix to this book (see page 379). Among the largest of these are:

• The National Cancer Institute (NCI)

• The American Cancer Society (ACS)

• The Susan G. Komen Breast Cancer Foundation

• Breast Cancer Network of Strength (formerly known as Y-Me National Breast Cancer Organization)

While none of these will provide you with the names of specific physicians, they may help you to network successfully so that you can learn more about the doctors who specialize in breast cancer in your community.

HOW DO YOU EVALUATE THE PHYSICIANS WHOSE NAMES YOU NOW HAVE?

One way to get started "checking out" a doctor is to consult the medical directories available at public libraries. State medical societies usually publish annual or biannual listings that describe a physician's training, specialty, and current hospital affiliation. There is also a directory of medical specialists that will give you such information.

A major source of data is the Internet. If the physician in question is associated with a university-affiliated or teaching hospital, it is likely that some information about his or her education, professional positions, and academic achievements will be posted on the websites of the institutions at which they work.

Specialized resources may be consulted, such as the National Library of Medicine, which lists all published research papers by author, and the National Cancer Institute "PDQ" list of physicians specializing in cancer surgery and medicine.

The first factor to consider is *training*. This is one of the simplest pieces of your detective work. If you are in the doctor's office, she may have her diplomas and degrees on the wall. Take note of what institutions they are from. If you don't see these documents, ask the doctor where she trained, or else consult one of the directories or listings described above. The medical school a physician attended is often less important than where she took her postgraduate or specialty training. The best training usually is at large, university-affiliated hospitals (often called teaching hospitals). Institutions like these treat many patients, and they also maintain high standards. There is usually additional training available specifically in cancer surgery and other cancer treatment.

The next factor to concern yourself with is *experience*. This is not to say that a smart young doctor fresh out of training at a great institution, very sharp about the latest techniques, can't do a good job. There is, however, for better or worse, a demonstrable correlation between, for example, the outcome of the surgery and the surgeon's experience in doing the procedure. The frequency of postoperative complications often is related to how many times the surgeon has performed a particular operation.

Hospital affiliation is another crucial issue. Make sure that the physician is on the staff of a hospital known to have both very high standards and good support services for the treatment of breast cancer patients. This is important not only because you want to be treated at the best possible institution but also because the fact that a physician practices at such a hospital shows that the best doctors in the community acknowledge his qualifications by accepting him as a colleague.

If you live in a very small community—without a hospital of this caliber and a pool of cancer specialists from whom to choose—you should seriously consider seeking diagnosis and treatment in a large regional hospital or in a nearby large city. Even if that won't be possible for the entire course of your treatment, it's what you should try for at the time of the diagnosis, surgery, and the planning of the treatment.

There are hospitals and medical centers that are specifically devoted to the treatment of cancer. The Dana-Farber Cancer Center in Boston, Memorial Sloan-Kettering Cancer Center in New York, and the M. D. Anderson Cancer Center in Houston are among these.

Some women so badly want to be treated at a hospital that is a cancer center that—if they don't already know an affiliated physician—they accept as their doctor anyone to whom the institution assigns them. There's little doubt that they'll get competent care, but that method of picking a doctor doesn't feel right to me. The most important consideration is to find a physician who is experienced, whose reputation among patients as well as other doctors is exemplary, whose approach to your case is carefully and thoughtfully arrived at, and who has your interests at heart.

Peer recognition—what his colleagues think of a doctor's abilities—is harder to find out but is a very useful piece of information. Doctors, as all nondoctors recognize, are reluctant to directly say unfavorable things about their colleagues. You may need to make such inquiries more subtly. For example, ask several doctors in the community who they think is the best breast surgeon in town. The same names will probably recur. If the physician you're investigating isn't mentioned, you already know a lot, but you might want to push this a little further by asking, "Do you think Dr. Jackson is in the same league?" You may have to watch closely here for the slight shake of the head, or put your ear tightly to the phone receiver to hear the meaningful pause or clearing of the throat. Though there aren't too many doctors who will be immediately forthcoming, responsible physicians will try to protect you from people, particularly surgeons, whose work is not first-rate.

As alluded to before, the opinions of *other women who have had breast cancer* are invaluable. This includes former patients of the physicians you are considering. Many of my patients point out that they often get phone calls from women who have heard through the grapevine that they had cancer. These people call and ask, "Whom did you go to?" "What kind of operation did you have?" and similar questions. A former patient's opinion should probably not be the only basis for making a decision to go to a particular doctor. If, however, a few women tell you of unpleasant or bad experiences with a doctor, that is a good reason not to go to him or, at the very least, to do a lot more investigation.

APPROACH TO THE DISEASE

One of the hardest judgments to make when you have breast cancer is whether the treatment that is being proposed is the right one for you. This is especially difficult because individual women may have specific goals of their own and may not know how to reconcile them with what they are being told is the proper course to follow.

A woman may say, "The most important thing for me is to preserve my breast." Another, perhaps expressing her hope for a normal, unimpaired life, will say, "I want to be able to go on playing tennis." Another will say, "The only thing that matters to me is survival. Cut off my breast tomorrow if that means I'll be safe."

These are important concerns, though obviously the primary factor that should determine treatment is the extent and nature of the illness. Given a particular patient's situation, however, there may be differences of opinion among physicians on what the treatment should be. A good doctor should be able to explain to you the principle on which he wishes to proceed and the interpretation that has led him to propose a course of action.

Why, given a certain condition, wouldn't every physician you see suggest the same treatment plan? Some women report running into doctors who seem to have a bias toward one treatment or the other; who, despite recent research and clinical experience, are slow to change; or who are especially cautious. Women have told me that such doctors have said, for example, "I never do lumpectomies. They're risky."

Nonetheless, there are genuine differences in how to "call" a case. Suppose removing the entire breast in one circumstance would result in a 100 percent chance of success, while doing a wide excision (lumpectomy) followed by radiation would yield a 97 percent success rate. In such a case, the advice of two different physicians might legitimately differ.

If an opinion does not seem reasonable to you or if you are particularly anxious about a recommended course of treatment, consult another doctor (as your insurance company may require you to do). The second physician may confirm that what is being planned is the only sound course of action; or you may have to choose between two conflicting opinions, or even seek a third specialist's advice. Even though this sounds troublesome, you owe it to yourself to be as sure as possible before you undergo an extensive procedure.

CHAPTER 3

WHAT'S GONE WRONG?

WHAT IS THE BREAST?

The breast is a gland, the mammary gland, designed by nature to produce milk so that a woman can feed her infant.

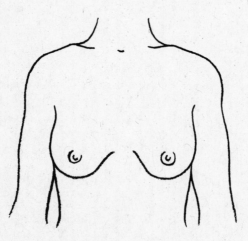

SIZE, SHAPE, AND POSITION

Though breasts come in a large variety of sizes and shapes, these differences have nothing to do with how much milk a woman can produce or how likely she will be to develop breast cancer.

The two breasts are seldom identical in size. In many women the left breast is slightly larger, though that is by no means the rule. The breasts of young women tend to be firmer and more conical in shape than those of older women. Except for those in the nipple, the breast has no muscles of its own, but rests on the muscles of the chest wall, the pectoral muscles. Breast tissue also extends toward the axilla (the underarm), the sternum (breastbone), and the clavicle (collarbone), down toward the lowest ribs, and back toward the latissimus dorsi (the muscle at the side).

NIPPLE

The nipple is slightly below the center point of the breast. Darker than the rest of the breast, its color varies from woman to woman. It becomes erect when it is stimulated, providing a firm protuberance for the baby to suck on. The nipple also becomes erect and may increase in size during lovemaking. Like the entire breast, the nipple changes considerably during pregnancy and lactation, becoming larger and darker in color.

AREOLA

The pigmented skin around the nipple is called the areola. It has tiny bumps on its surface, some of which are sweat glands, others the endings of the Montgomery's glands, which lubricate the nipple for breast-feeding. Like the nipple, the areola is darker than the rest of the breast and differs in color from woman to woman according to her complexion and during the various stages of life. A darkening of the areola is one of the earliest signs of pregnancy.

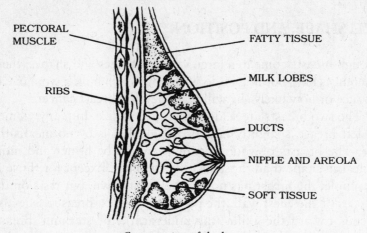

Cross section of the breast

ACINI, LOBULES, DUCTS, AND LOBES

An acinus is a sac lined with cells that can produce milk. The acini cluster together to form structures called lobules. The lobules empty into ducts that can carry milk to the nipple. The group of lobules that empty into any one duct is called a lobe. This milk-producing system is, of course, not normally activated until child-birth.

It is useful to think of this system as a tree: the major ducts that end in the nipple constitute the trunk; as the ducts become finer, they resemble branches that spread throughout the breast, back from the nipple, and end in the lobules, which are like the leaves of the tree.

FAT

The breast is cushioned with fat, which protects its important milk-producing organs. In fact, the breast is composed mainly of fat. In very small breasts there is so little fat that on examination you feel mainly glandular tissue, but the breast's composition is seldom less than one-third fat. As a woman ages, glandular tissue, no longer needed for infant feeding, is replaced by fat.

OTHER BREAST COMPONENTS

The breast is also composed of these elements:

- Connective tissue, called fascia, that encloses and supports it

- Nerves, which are necessary for appropriate responsiveness to breast-feeding and sex

- A large supply of blood vessels—arteries, veins, and capillaries

- The lymphatics, the veinlike vessels that drain lymph into the bloodstream (lymph is a fluid that transports lymphocytes, a type of white blood cell, as well as proteins and fat)

- A very small number of lymph nodes (only a few nodes are found in the breast itself, and these are on its periphery; most of the nodes that service the breast are in the adjacent tissue of the armpit)

Lymphatics are found throughout the body and serve to drain extracellular fluid from the tissue back into the bloodstream. The lymphatic system, and particularly the lymph nodes, play an important role in the body's defenses and in its immune system. In the area of the breast, the lymphatics go from the breast and nipple to the nodes in the armpit (axilla) and from there to the nodes above the collarbone (supraclavicular). The central and inner parts of the breast, however, can also drain to nodes under the breastbone (internal mammary).

WHAT IS BREAST CANCER?

As a way to get started, assume that you have been told that you have breast cancer, or that it is suspected, or that it must be ruled out. What does this mean? What *is* cancer?

CANCER

Cancer is not just one disease. It can appear in any part of the body and can take many forms. All of them involve the abnormal multiplication and spread of cells in the body. This unrestrained growth is caused by genetic changes in the cells that also empower them to move from their normal locale to other parts of the body.

The abnormal growth of cells often results in the formation of a tumor. Benign tumors, which are discussed on pages 43–48, can result from a limited loss of growth control of the cells. But when the growth is rampantly out of control, and when the cells have the ability to move from their original site and settle and grow in other tissues, the condition is cancer, a malignancy.

The term used for the most common types of cancer, and for most malignant tumors, is **carcinoma;** it arises from cells that line the organs of the body. A **sarcoma** is the term used to describe a tumor originating in bone, muscle, fat, or connective tissue.

Carcinoma of the breast occurs when this malignant change takes place in the cells that line the lobules that manufacture milk or, more commonly, in the ducts that carry it to the nipple. Since most of these cells are found in the upper part of the breast, in the outer quadrant, or in the area around the center of the breast, these are the locations in which most cancers occur. It is rare for tumors to originate in the fat or nonglandular tissues of the breast. When they do, they are called sarcomas.

PHYSICAL CHARACTERISTICS

Any lump is first examined physically with the physician's fingers (palpation) in order to decide whether it is "likely" to be cancer. What is its shape? Terms such as *well-delineated, irregular,* and *diffuse* are used to describe the contours of the tumor. Is it *hard* or *soft? Movable* or *fixed?*

In general, a tumor is more likely to be malignant if it is firm and irregular in shape. Those factors do not always mean that cancer is present, but they do make us suspect this, and they lead us to the final step in our investigation, an examination of the cells under a microscope by a pathologist (see Chapter 5). These cells are obtained from a biopsy, which is discussed on pages 75–89.

From the pathological examination, the cancer is classified by such characteristics as the pattern in which it grows, the arrangement of the cells, their variety in size and shape, the frequency with which they divide, and the presence on their surface of receptors for the hormones estrogen and progesterone. (See Chapter 5.)

KINDS OF BREAST CANCER

As noted, most cancers in the breast originate in the ducts, and are called ductal or duct cell carcinoma. A much smaller number originate in the lobules: lobular carcinoma. When we look at the cancer cells through a microscope, we usually can identify them as either ductal or lobular, although sometimes both types may be present.

A few ductal tumors have a specific appearance or pattern that can be identified under a microscope. These tumors have been named and grouped into subcategories that include *tubular, medullary, mucinous, papillary,* and *adenoid cystic.* You may hear these terms in the doctor's office, but the percentage of women who have any particular one of these cancers is relatively small. It should also be said that the prognosis for women with these cancers is excellent.

IN SITU CANCERS

If the cancer cells remain within the confines of the duct or lobule, within what you may hear referred to as the basement membrane, it is called an **in situ cancer,** meaning it is confined "in that site." These cancers rarely form a tumor mass and therefore cannot be felt during a physical examination. They are detected by mammography (see page 59).

In situ cancers are sometimes referred to as precancerous. This is not an accurate term, and I consider its use dangerous. In situ cancer cells multiply like other malignancies, though they may be slower-growing. They are not life-threatening if they are treated promptly, but *they are cancer.* They must get prompt attention—or the advantage of early detection will be lost and a more serious illness may result.

In situ cancers of the duct, often referred to as DCIS (ductal carcinoma in situ), were rarely seen until mammography screening has become much more common in recent years and mammography techniques have been refined. The result is that we are able to find tiny, very early cancers of this type and to treat them very successfully.

In situ cancers of the lobules, also called LCIS (lobular carcinoma in situ, or lobular neoplasia), are often discovered incidentally during a biopsy when we are investigating a minimal thickening or a subtle abnormality. LCIS may show the same abnormality on mammograms as does DCIS. This type of in situ cancer is most common in premenopausal women, and there is some likelihood that if this cancer appears in one breast, it may also occur in the other. For that reason, if a lobular carcinoma in situ is found, the second breast should be watched particularly carefully.

INFILTRATING CANCERS

If the cancer cells have penetrated the membrane that surrounds the duct or lobule, they are said to be **infiltrating,** or **invasive,** and they eventually form a lump that can be felt on physical examination. The smallest infiltrating cancers, however, can be detected only on a mammogram, a sonogram, or an MRI. (The term *invasive* does not imply that the cancer has spread to any other part of the body. It is used interchangeably with the term *infiltrating.*)

Infiltrating Cancer of the Duct

This cancer, which you may hear referred to as infiltrating ductal carcinoma, is the most common type of breast cancer and is the cause of many of the signs we normally associate with breast cancer.

As the cancer cells invade the fatty tissue around the duct, they may stimulate the growth of fibrous, scarlike tissue that surrounds the cancer. Thus, the actual size of the cancer is often smaller than the size of the lump may suggest. A welcome result of this thickening is that it makes the mass easier to find during physical examination as well as on a mammogram.

Depending on the location of the ductal cancer, it may cause the nipple to retract, or it may result in a nipple discharge or skin changes such as puckering or dimpling. These signs may also be caused by benign conditions (see below), but they are a signal that warrants prompt investigation.

Infiltrating Cancer of the Lobules

This condition, also called infiltrating lobular carcinoma, occurs when cells stream out in single file into the surrounding breast tissue. About 15 percent of breast cancers originate in the lobules.

Because it does not provoke the kind of fibrous growth we see in ductal cancer, and so may be harder to detect on a mammogram, cancer of the lobule is likely to be larger than ductal cancer when it is first detected. It also feels softer and is likely to be described as a thickening rather than as a lump.

As we have discussed, if we find a lobular cancer in one breast, it may be present in the other breast as well. For this reason, the second breast should be watched, and a biopsy performed if a mammogram, sonogram, or MRI reveals any suspicious findings or if a lump develops. You should discuss this with your surgeon if a lobular cancer is found.

PAGET'S DISEASE

A tumor close to the nipple will sometimes be detected because of scaliness, oozing, or hardening of the skin of the areola or the nipple itself, or because of an ulcer on the nipple's surface. Though the problem may prove to be a simple eczema that responds to local treatment, a biopsy must be performed to rule out the presence of the malignant cells that are characteristic of this relatively rare cancer. If these so-called Paget cells are found, it usually indicates that there is an underlying in situ or invasive ductal cancer in the breast.

CYSTOSARCOMA PHYLLODES

This rare malignant breast tumor usually appears in women in their forties, often after a history of rapidly recurring fibroadenomas, benign lumps discussed on page 46. The tumor seems very much like a fibroadenoma when it is excised, but when it is examined under a microscope, we see many elongated cells that originate in the fibrous tissue of the breast and resemble a sarcoma.

Though cystosarcomas rarely spread to other parts of the body, their edges tend to invade the adjacent breast tissue, and these tumors tend to recur locally. For these reasons, when we remove the tumor, we also remove a rim of normal tissue around it. If a cystosarcoma is large or if it recurs, a mastectomy may be necessary.

INFLAMMATORY CANCER

This uncommon condition accounts for fewer than 1 percent of all breast cancers and usually presents itself as a swollen and reddened breast that may look as if there is an infection present. There is usually no lump, and the condition does not respond to antibiotics. When a biopsy is performed, cancer cells are found. The breast is inflamed because this aggressive cancer has spread to the lymphatics in the skin, where it induces a pink discoloration. (See page 153 for a discussion of the treatment of inflammatory cancer.)

BREAST CANCER DURING PREGNANCY

Unfortunately, we are now seeing more breast cancer in pregnant women than we did in the past. That is probably because many women are delaying their pregnancies until ages when breast cancer begins to become more common.

Pregnancy is usually a happy time in a woman's life. She's not thinking about breast cancer; she's also not examining her breasts to look for it. Nor, probably, is her doctor. Moreover, her breasts are swelling and changing in contour in the normal course of the pregnancy. For that reason, breast cancer in pregnant women tends to be found at a relatively later stage.

We used to think that pregnant women did more poorly than other women with breast cancer because of the increased hormonal activity of pregnancy. Now we have learned that if compared stage by stage, the results are about the same for pregnant women as for others with breast cancer. The problem, as we have noted, is that in pregnant women treatment is initiated at a later stage of the disease. (For a discussion of the treatment of breast cancer during pregnancy, see pages 153–54.)

SIZE AND SPREAD

Among the most crucial considerations of a cancerous tumor have to do with how big it is and how much it has spread. Here, the commonsense conclusion is the right one: We hope for a small tumor, under 2 centimeters in size (about 3/4 inch), that has not spread to the lymph nodes or to a distant site (has not metastasized). The smallest tumors are detected by the radiologist at the time of screening; they cannot be felt in a manual examination.

Having said that, it is important to note that it isn't until a tumor is over 5 centimeters (about 2 inches) or more in size that it gets to be called large, and also that some women with long-standing large lesions do well.

The spread of breast cancer is usually referred to in the following ways:

- *Local,* meaning it is confined within the breast, though it may be in several locations there

- *Regional,* meaning that the lymph nodes, primarily those in the armpit, are involved

- *Distant,* meaning the cancer is found in other parts of the body as well

THE CLASSIFICATION OF CANCER

Why do these classifications and fine distinctions matter? Why, if you have cancer, don't we just get on with the treatment? To a woman facing breast cancer, this certainly feels like the first priority.

Patience is important here, for both the woman and her physician. This is true even though diagnosis may take longer than we would like. The reason as precise an identification as possible is important—of the cell type, its differentiation, tumor size, the relationship to adjacent breast tissue, and the spread to adjacent or distant places in the body—is that these are the factors that affect risk and that make it possible to determine what ought to be done to treat the patient most effectively.

The system of classifying cancer is complicated, and the methods and criteria vary from country to country, region to region, and sometimes even from medical center to medical center. The explanations that follow, drawn from the American Joint Committee on Cancer (AJCC) staging system, have been limited to what you may hear in the doctor's office or read about, as well as what you need to know in order to join your physician in assessing your risk and in choosing the treatment that is appropriate for you.

TUMORS

Tumors are classified primarily by certain standard characteristics:

A. Have the cancer cells demonstrated the ability to leave their site of origin? In situ cancer cells, which have multiplied within a duct or lobule but remain confined to that site, are less likely to metastasize than cells that have begun to infiltrate normal breast tissue.

B. How big is the tumor? When the cells have invaded the breast fat and formed a tumor, we consider the size.

C. What is the condition of the skin over the tumor site? Is it broken? Retracted? Swollen?

D. Has the nipple retracted into the breast, or does it still protrude?

E. Is the tumor attached to the pectoral muscle or the chest wall?

You also may hear of the designations Tis, T1, T2, T3, or T4 in connection with tumors. These simply mean the tumor is being

rated according to the criteria described above. The simplified list
that follows will help us begin to examine this rating system.

Tis is an in situ ductal or lobular carcinoma or Paget's disease of
the nipple with no associated invasion of normal tissue.

T1 is a tumor under 2 centimeters in size. Such tumors are
further subdivided into:

> **T1mic** with "microinvasion"—that is, extending less than
> 0.1 centimeter beyond its ducts or lobules of origin
>
> **T1a,** an invasive tumor that extends 0.1 to 0.5 centimeter
> from its source into surrounding breast tissue
>
> **T1b,** invading 0.5 to 1 centimeter
>
> **T1c,** invading more than 1 centimeter but less than
> 2 centimeters

T2 is a tumor 2 to 5 centimeters.

T3 is a tumor over 5 centimeters.

T4 is a tumor of *any size* that is accompanied by any of the
following characteristics:

> **T4a,** extension to chest wall, not including the major
> (pectoralis) muscle
>
> **T4b,** edema (swelling) or breakdown (ulceration) of the skin
> or nodules on the skin (satellites)
>
> **T4c** characteristics of both T4a and T4b, extending to the
> chest wall and skin
>
> **T4d** inflammatory cancer (having the appearance of
> inflammation of the skin)

LYMPH NODES

After biopsy, the lymph nodes in the armpit (axilla) are classified:

NX means that involvement of the lymph nodes cannot be
determined—for instance, in situations where they have been
previously removed.

N0 means there is no cancer present.

N1 means there is cancer involvement, but the nodes are movable, not fixed in place by the spread of cancer.

N2 means the nodes are attached to one another or to adjacent blood vessels, or on X-ray studies there is evidence of the involvement of the lymph nodes behind the sternum (internal mammary).

N3 means there is spread to the nodes just below or above the collarbone. It is also N3 if enlarged nodes behind the sternum can be seen pushing up the bone and are accompanied by enlarged lymph nodes in the left armpit (axilla).

METASTASIS

Metastasis, or spreading, must be evaluated next. Has the cancer spread from the breast to the underarm lymph nodes? Is it now present elsewhere in the body? The cancer is said to have metastasized if it has spread beyond the area of the breast and the axillary lymph nodes into other parts of the body.

THE STAGES

The conditions we've been describing—of the *T*umor, the lymph *N*odes, and *M*etastasis—are taken into account in order to determine the stage at which the cancer has been found. This is called the **TNM system** of staging. Staging is a vital tool in measuring risk and in choosing treatment.

When the tumor is small, the lymph nodes are not involved, and there is no metastasis, the cancer is considered Stage I. The other end of the scale, Stage IV, describes the situation where the cancer has spread to a site far from the original tumor. Stage II and Stage III fall between those two ends.

Classifying into these stages means evaluating all factors related to TNM. A woman might have a quite small tumor but also involvement of the lymph nodes. Conversely, the tumor may be large but confined to one area, with no evidence of spread. The various combinations of these factors are considered together to determine the extent and stage of the disease.

The chart on the next page very neatly sets out the combinations of characteristics of the tumor (T), the nodes (N), and the metastasis (M) that make up the stages. N0, for example, means there is no node involvement. M1 means that there is metastasis to a distant site. Note that Stages II and III on this chart have been further broken down into subcategories. After the pathologist examines the tissues removed during surgery the staging system becomes more precise and stages are then given the prefix "p."

This material is the stuff of the cancer specialist: When the stage of the cancer is precisely determined, we can assess the risk and choose the appropriate treatment.

You should know the terminology not only because you may hear or read about it but because it will help you understand and evaluate the reasons for the treatment that is being suggested for you.

IT MAY NOT BE CANCER AFTER ALL

Not every breast problem is cancer, nor is every lump. In fact, about 90 percent of lumps or other suspicious breast changes turn out to be benign tumors or cysts. You should carefully investigate each abnormality, as we will see in Chapter 4, Diagnosis, but in most instances these conditions will prove not to be serious enough to be a source of worry.

Cancer is only one of several causes of lumps or other irregularities of breast shape. The other common conditions that may account for such problems follow.

Stage Groupings*

Stage	Classification		
	T	N	M
0	Tis	N0	M0
I	T1	N0	M0
IIA	T0	N1	M0
	T1	N1	M0
	T2	N0	M0
IIB	T2	N1	M0
	T3	N0	M0
IIIA	T0	N2	M0
	T1	N2	M0
	T2	N2	M0
	T3	N1	M0
	T3	N2	M0
IIIB	T4	N0	M0
	T4	N1	M0
	T4	N2	M0
IIIC	Any T	N3	M0
IV	Any T	Any N	M1

*Used with the permission of the American Joint Committee on Cancer (AJCC), Chicago, Illinois. The original source for this material is the *AJCC Cancer Staging Manual, Sixth Edition* (2002) published by Springer-Verlag, New York, www.springer-ny.com.

BREAST CYSTS OR GROSS CYSTIC DISEASE

A cyst is a sac filled with fluid. You or someone you know has probably had a cyst sometime, perhaps on the eyelid or the gum. Such cysts are lined with cells that produce secretions. They are usually surgically removed.

Breast cysts are different. They are really dilated, pinched-off sections of ducts that "passively" fill up with fluid rather than manufacturing it themselves. They do not ordinarily have to be surgically removed.

Breast cysts are usually first observed in women in their late twenties and thirties. They rarely develop in women past menopause. The chances are that if you develop one cyst, you're likely to develop more. Women prone to cysts will find that the cysts tend to shrink or disappear after menopause.

Typically round and evenly contoured, breast cysts may also be movable. They may change quite dramatically in size during the menstrual cycle. They can be extremely small or quite large, as much as 5 centimeters or more in diameter.

Though some women experience pain or tenderness with breast cysts, particularly around the time they menstruate, most often there are no accompanying symptoms. You usually find out you have a cyst because you or your doctor discovers a lump in your breast. A lump must be investigated. It shouldn't be there.

The doctor will aspirate the lump by injecting a small amount of anesthetic into the skin, inserting a hollow needle, and drawing out the fluid. The mass should disappear. If it does, it was a cyst. If it doesn't, or if fluid cannot be withdrawn, the lump should be surgically removed and examined. That does *not* mean that it is cancer. It may only mean that it is a cyst that for reason of its position or other factors could not be successfully aspirated.

Any fluid that is aspirated from the cyst is examined by the doctor. If it is tan or greenish in color, which is considered typical of cyst fluid, there is nothing more to be learned from it and the doctor can simply throw it away.

If, however, the fluid is golden-colored or tinged with blood, it should be examined by a pathologist, because it may indicate the presence of a rare cystic cancer.

If cysts, after they are aspirated, tend to recur in the same place over a period of years, they should probably be surgically removed. There is some evidence that women with recurrent cysts are at a slightly higher risk of developing breast cancer after menopause.

There remains a fair amount of controversy about whether the repeated appearance of large cysts places a woman at higher risk for getting cancer. At this moment, no one knows for sure. We do know, however, that the converse isn't true—that is, many women who do get breast cancer have never had such cysts.

In my opinion the question should be put slightly differently.

There is the very practical problem that in women who have fairly lumpy breasts, it may be hard to distinguish *new* lumps or distinguish between cysts and cancerous tumors. And a cyst, by its position or size, may "hide" a malignancy.

FIBROCYSTIC DISEASE (FORMERLY CALLED CYSTIC MASTITIS)

Sometimes used when a woman is prone to small cysts, the terms *fibrocystic disease* and *cystic mastitis* would best be put to rest. They are "nondiseases." In the monthly changes that take place in the breasts as they prepare for pregnancy and then "turn off," ducts may pinch off, inflammations may come and go. Very rarely do these changes result in the risk of cancer.

Physicians often tell women they are "cystic" because they have painful or lumpy breasts. Having a lot of cysts or "lumpiness" in the breast can be uncomfortable and cause concern. The lumps may swell and become tender before menstruation and then shrink or even seem to disappear once the period begins. But these are not indications of malignancy or of life-threatening disease.

There is, however, one caution to be mentioned here: Sometimes a lumpy area is surgically removed and the pathologist's conclusion from his postsurgery examination (see pages 91–94) is "fibrocystic disease." He may tell us that he has seen under a microscope a condition called **hyperplasia** (meaning there are too many cells in the tissue he's examining) or **atypia** (meaning that the appearance of the cells is unusual, or "atypical"). While hyperplasia alone is not associated with an increased risk of breast cancer, women with extensive atypical ductal hyperplasia (ADH) are more likely to develop breast cancer. How such risk may be reduced is discussed on pages 313–16.

FIBROADENOMAS

The term *fibroadenoma* is used to describe an orderly growth of cells, confined to the breast, that results in benign, movable, and rounded lumps. Rounded lumps in teenagers and young women are almost always fibroadenomas. Because these lumps tend to grow, they are usually removed. Since the risk of breast cancer increases with age, any such breast masses definitely should be removed and examined through biopsy in women over twenty.

INFECTIONS

Various infections, several of them associated with pregnancy and nursing, occur in the breast and can be successfully treated with antibiotics. These disorders include bacterial mastitis and abscesses.

A more persistent problem, called chronic subareolar infection, is found just around the areola, in the central part of the breast. It tends to be recurrent, and treatment with antibiotics should begin as soon as possible. As with any abscess, the site may need to be surgically opened and drained.

FAT NECROSIS

When, for any of a variety of reasons, the cells of an area of the breast die, a small, hard, flat lump may appear. This condition, called fat necrosis, may follow an injury. It is usually seen in women over fifty and is benign; but because we also see an increase in breast cancer in women of this age, a biopsy should be performed. Obviously, a diagnosis of fat necrosis, or "destruction" of some fat cells, comes as a great relief. The condition does not cause any problems and requires no further treatment.

INTRADUCTAL PAPILLOMA

Intraductal papillomas are tiny, polyplike, benign growths that occur, frequently several at a time, in the ducts behind the nipple. Intraductal papilloma is the usual cause of a watery or bloody discharge from the nipple. Because such a discharge may also be a warning sign of cancer, it should be investigated by biopsy as soon as possible. To do that, the affected ducts are removed, commonly during an outpatient procedure in the hospital.

MAMMARY DUCT ECTASIA

Mammary duct ectasia is a benign condition in the ductal system in which the ducts become distended and clogged. Usually occurring in women in their forties, the problem may present itself as a lump, there may be swelling and a nipple discharge, and an area of the breast may become inflamed. Because this disorder can look so much like cancer, you must make sure that a biopsy is performed so that on the one hand, it is confirmed that you do not have cancer, and on the other hand, you are not treated as if you did, with more heroic measures than are necessary. Sometimes the inflammation caused by this disorder will go away on its own. If it is troublesome, or if the symptoms keep recurring, you and your doctor may want to discuss the advisability of localized surgery to correct the problem.

MONDOR'S DISEASE

An inflamed vein or phlebitis of the breast can cause a fairly superficial, flat lump and a drawing sensation that sometimes radiates down toward the abdomen. This condition, called Mondor's disease, usually appears without warning and is treated with heat and mild pain medication to relieve the discomfort. It is self-limiting and may take a few weeks to go away. The same type of superficial phlebitis, also called phlebothrombosis, can occur next to a surgical biopsy either in the breast or the adjacent armpit, and may extend down the arm.

CHAPTER

4

DIAGNOSIS

W e've now considered the normal breast and the various things that can go wrong with it. How do you use that information to ascertain what is going on in your own body when you suspect there may be a problem or when a lump has been found?

Breast tumors are usually discovered in one of five ways: women find a lump themselves, they are discovered by a doctor during a physical examination, or they are detected on a mammogram, sonogram, or MRI (see page 73). If all women were having mammography of good quality, 90 percent of all breast cancers would be found by X-ray (see page 59).

If you have found a lump yourself, you're in good company. It may seem startling, but most malignant lumps are still found by women themselves, either through self-examination or by chance. This observation is a humbling one for doctors.

Why are women such experts? Because they know how their own bodies normally feel at various times during the month. They know the contours of their own breasts, and they are therefore in the best position to notice any changes. It naturally follows that the more familiar you are with your breasts, the better prepared you are to detect any changes.

The first step in identifying potential problems is to learn as much about your own breasts as you can. Breast self-examination (sometimes referred to as BSE) is the best way to do that, though being alert to your breast contours even when you're not specifically examining your breasts can be extremely useful. Many women have found a suspicious lump when they were washing themselves in the shower or scratching a mosquito bite. Even "accidental" discoveries such as these, however, are much more likely if you have already learned the topography of your breasts through self-examination.

Sometimes, either accidentally or in deliberately examining your breasts, you may notice that there is a painful spot. This is not at all uncommon. There is an old saying, "If it hurts, it's not cancer." That's usually true, but in a very small percentage of cases, cancerous lumps do hurt. You should call the painful place to your physician's attention.

BREAST SELF-EXAMINATION

A reminder of a fact already stated is useful here: About 90 percent of all breast lumps turn out to be benign. By learning the techniques of self-examination, you are not specifically learning how to discover a cancer. You are learning to spot changes in your breasts that may or may not mean trouble—mostly "not."

Another comforting fact: Describing this monthly procedure may make it sound more complicated and time-consuming than it actually is. After all, most people in our society have a daily routine that, if it were outlined in detail, would sound as if we had no time during the day to do more than our morning and evening toilet. Think of all the separate steps involved in flossing and brushing our teeth, taking a bath, combing our hair, keeping our fingernails trimmed, taking vitamins, shaving, putting our contact lenses in and taking them out, and so on.

This list sounds ludicrous, because we've done all these things so often that they are built into our daily schedule. We don't have to mark on our calendar, "7:30, brush teeth." The aim now should be to make breast self-examination as much a part of your life routine as brushing your teeth—except that you have to do it only once a month, not twice a day.

When it is done properly, breast self-examination can significantly reduce a woman's risk of advanced-stage cancer. Unfortunately, most women do not know the proper technique. Learning it could greatly increase the possibility of detecting a cancer in its early stages.

A TIME SCHEDULE FOR BREAST SELF-EXAMINATION

AT WHAT AGE SHOULD I BEGIN?

A good time to start is in the late teens or early twenties. That's usually when women first visit a gynecologist or a women's health facility, and this is a convenient opportunity to begin to learn how to perform self-examination and to incorporate the habit into your life.

WHEN CAN I STOP SELF-EXAMINATION?

Never. It is, as we'll see, an easy thing to do, and you should continue the procedure throughout your life, especially since breast cancer becomes more common as you get older.

HOW OFTEN SHOULD I EXAMINE MY BREASTS?

You must examine your breasts, carefully and thoroughly, once a month. In addition to this scheduled, thorough examination, however, you'll find that as you become familiar with the appearance and contours of your breasts, you'll also be a more alert observer of any changes that may take place between examinations.

WHEN DURING THE MONTH SHOULD I DO MY EXAM?

We tie the timing of self-examination to the menstrual cycle, because the breast's texture and contour often change during the month. You may have noticed that a few days before you get your period, your breasts become firmer and fuller. They also can become tender—in some women slightly so, in others quite painfully. The breasts may feel lumpy at that time of the month— "nodular," your doctor may call it.

This is a natural result of premenstrual engorgement. It does not indicate a cyst or a cancerous lump. The swelling, tenderness, and lumpiness will almost certainly disappear after you menstruate. For these reasons, you should not perform your regular breast self-examination just before your menstrual period.

Examine your breasts every month, ten days after the start of your period. If you miss the tenth day, do your examination as soon afterward as you can. Do not wait until the next month to "catch up."

Postmenopausal women should examine their breasts on the first day of every month; this makes it easy to remember.

Some women who are not yet of menopause age have had a hysterectomy, with their uterus removed but one or both ovaries retained. If you are in that situation, you may feel your body going through the various stages of the menstrual cycle even though you don't actually menstruate. Choose a regular time each month when your breasts are not swollen for your self-examination.

THE ELEMENTS OF BREAST SELF-EXAMINATION

There are two general aspects of examining your breasts: what you see and what you feel.

VISUAL OBSERVATION

Remember: You are not looking for cancer. You are studying your breasts, first, to observe their *normal* appearance so that you will have a reference point in the future from which you can spot something new. You are also looking for changes from what you may only casually have observed in the past or for conditions that seem to you unusual for your normal breast.

What is "normal" differs from person to person. As we have noted, in many women the breasts are of slightly different size. The nipple may be at a different level on each breast. One or both nipples may be somewhat retracted—that is, pulled inside. In order to identify changes, you would need to have noted such normal details of the appearance of your breasts.

THE STEPS

1. Take off your blouse and bra and stand about 2 feet in front of a mirror that has a good, clear image.

2. Put your hands at your sides and observe the general contour of each breast.

   • Is the shape of the breast even, without any visible swelling or distortion?

   • Are both breasts their usual size?

   • Is the nipple in the same position on each breast?

   • Do the nipples protrude, or is one or both of them retracted?

   • Do your breasts appear different in any way from the last time you looked at them?

3. Now raise your arms above your head.

   • Do you see any dimpling of the skin?

   • Is there a rash of any type?

   • Are there other changes in the skin's surface?

4. Place your hands on your hips and, flexing your shoulders forward, continue to visually observe the surface of the skin as described above.

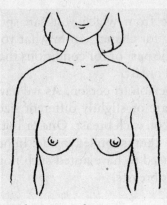

[1] Observe your breasts in a mirror.

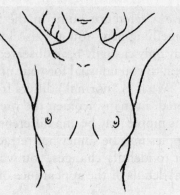

[2] Raise your arms above your head.

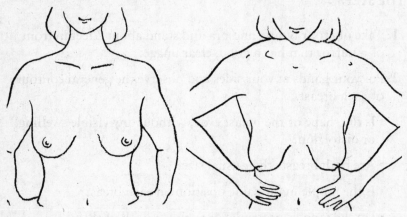

[3] Place your hands on your hips.   *[4] Flex your shoulders forward.*

Breast self-examination

PALPATION

Palpation is the technical term for examining by touch—in this case, feeling your breasts with your fingers and hand.

1. Still standing in front of the mirror, cradle the left breast with the left hand beneath it. With the right hand, feel the breast carefully with the tips of your three longest fingers.

   • Is one area more lumpy than any other?

   • Are there any changes from your last examination?

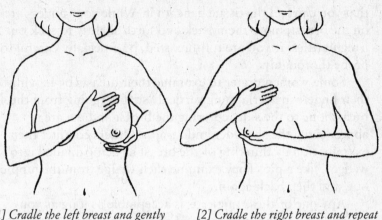

[1] *Cradle the left breast and gently feel it with the fingers of your right hand.*

[2] *Cradle the right breast and repeat this palpation.*

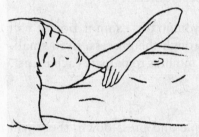
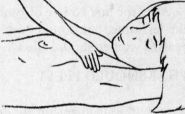

[3] *Lying down with your right hand behind your head, palpate the right breast with the fingers of your left hand.*

[4] *Repeat this procedure with the left breast.*

2. Now cradle the right breast and repeat this palpation.

3. Lie down, flat on your back, with a pillow under your right shoulder. Stretch your right arm behind you, bend your elbow, and put your hand behind your head.

Again using the pads of the three longest fingers of your left hand, examine your right breast from the edge of the nipple out to the rim of your breast and then up your chest toward the shoulder and armpit.

Keep pressing the tissue, going clockwise in circles that spiral from the areola out. Use enough pressure on the skin so that you can feel the tissue beneath it. While your fingers are on the breast, move them back and forth slightly to seek out irregularities. If you are full-breasted, be especially careful to probe thoroughly.

Some women prefer to examine their breasts by moving their fingers in overlapping vertical "strips," going from the breastbone to the side, covering the breast and the area approaching the shoulder and armpit. Others conduct their examination by thinking of the breast as being divided into wedges, like a pie. They examine each wedge from the nipple out, and then back again.

Any one of these methods is acceptable as long as you carefully cover the entire area of the breast and the chest as it approaches the shoulder and the armpit.

4. Now repeat the palpation of the left breast.

After the first couple of times you do this examination, it will take less time, but do not rush through the process. Even small-breasted women should allow two minutes to palpate each breast.

WHAT SHOULD I FEEL?

If you put your finger on the nipple and press down, there will be little resistance, because the ducts between the nipple and the chest wall are very fine. When you get to the areola, you will be able to feel more definitely the ridge beneath it. This is the start of the firmer tissue—primarily the ducts and lobules of which the breast is composed. This part of the breast—from the areola to the outer edge—is shaped almost like an inverted plate.

What else will you feel? Soft fat, of course. If you are rather thin or are of childbearing age, you will feel proportionately less fat and more breast tissue.

Some women will feel a lump or the kind of nodularity described earlier. *This should be checked by a physician the first time you feel it*. However, after you have had a professional examination of your lump or "lumpiness" and have been told the condition is not a cause for concern, you will learn to differentiate between irregularities that are simply part of your own physiology and those that are new.

As we have seen, if you examine your breasts close to the time of your menstrual period, you may very well find an unfamiliar thickening. The changes in texture that accompany the menstrual cycle are to be expected and are of no concern. It is only a fresh lump that persists during the month that needs to be investigated.

Nipple Discharge

Though some physicians suggest it, I don't really think it's necessary during your regular self-examination to squeeze your nipple to look for a discharge.

If, however, you observe a discharge in the course of your examination, or if a discharge is apparent at other times during the month, *then* squeeze the nipple. Do this a few times over the course of several days. If the discharge continues, consult a doctor.

The Armpit

If you have a cold or other infection, the glands under your arm may be slightly tender. This may also happen if you have a blocked sweat gland under your arm that becomes irritated. Sometimes there is breast tissue in the armpit, and it may swell during the menstrual cycle or during pregnancy, like other breast tissue. Very rarely, however, an enlarged lymph node is the first sign of breast cancer. If you notice a lump in this area, have a physician look at it just to be sure that nothing is amiss.

TRAINING IN BREAST SELF-EXAMINATION

It would be ideal to have a doctor go through the breast self-examination process with you in her office so that you could see for yourself exactly what is involved and she could check to see that you are applying the right amount of pressure for a thorough examination. Unfortunately, few doctors take the time for a careful training session, and the truth is, many of them may not be as expert in the procedure as you need them to be.

The steps we've just gone through should serve you well, but if you feel uncertain about performing them, try to go to a breast specialist to learn self-examination. Either the physician or a well-trained nurse at such offices will be able to get you started. The American Cancer Society provides free information on breast self-examination. Please consult the Resources at the back of the book for a list of some of these sources.

A FINAL—FOR THE MOMENT—WORD ON SELF-EXAMINATION

There is no way that we can statistically evaluate the benefits of breast self-examination, but we do know the following:

• The procedure is simple.

• It is free.

• It can be done on a regular basis.

• It is not dangerous.

• It is the way most breast lumps are found.

PHYSICAL EXAMINATION BY A PHYSICIAN

If you are doing regular breast examinations of your own, why do you need a doctor's input, especially when the record of women finding breast lumps is so good?

The reason is that breast self-examination *plus* professional examination will improve your chances for successful treatment if you do get breast cancer, because it will improve the chance of early detection. Even if there is nothing suspicious in your breasts, you should have an annual professional physical examination, because a skilled doctor may find a lump you missed.

One of my patients came to me after her gynecologist, in a routine annual checkup, found a tiny lump that turned out to be a very early stage cancer. The woman said, just before we performed a lumpectomy (see pages 138–140), "I'm glad you've drawn a line on my breast where you're going to operate. It's the first time I've been able to feel the lump myself."

Why does this happen?

EXPERIENCE

The abnormality may be so tiny or ill-defined that only someone with a great deal of experience can feel it. Almost every day of my own life I examine women and feel certain tissue alterations. I think: "There's a lump." "Here's a thickening." "This spot feels different." "There's an asymmetry here." "Here's a place that's a little harder than the rest of the breast."

When a breast surgeon, in particular, feels a lump or a firm area, he is much more likely than a layperson to know what's going on, to be able to predict with a fair amount of accuracy the significance of any abnormality. Over the years, experience has taught breast surgeons how to interpret what we are feeling, because over those same years the findings from biopsies have illuminated what we've discerned during palpation. Many, many times, we have felt a lump, removed it in a biopsy, and then have learned, firsthand and from the pathologist's examination, what it was. It is not surprising, therefore, that breast specialists can tell so much by palpation.

MAMMOGRAPHY

A **mammogram** is an X-ray of the breast, taken with special equipment, that pictures the fat, the fibrous tissues, the lobes, the ducts, the blood vessels, and the other tissues of the breast. Mammography is performed by an X-ray technologist under the supervision of a radiologist. The interpretation of the mammogram is performed by a radiologist.

During a mammography, an X-ray beam is passed through the breast to produce a black-and-white picture called a film-screen mammogram. Like other "flat" pictures—paintings, maps, ordinary photographs—the mammogram gives us a two-dimensional view of a three-dimensional object.

Digital mammography is a technique that has advantages over standard mammography. Since it is a digital image it can be more easily stored and readily transmitted for review by others. It can be converted to a standard format for comparison with previous mammograms. Because the digital picture can be manipulated after it is taken, with regard to brightness and magnification it may have advantages for dense breast tissue. *No other screening method approaches the sensitivity of mammography in detecting the earliest and most curable tumors. Only the mammogram can pick up other important abnormalities, such as microcalcifications.* (See page 86.)

WHEN SHOULD I HAVE A MAMMOGRAM?

Guidelines for a mammography schedule differ depending on the purposes for which it is used and how various risks and benefits are interpreted. Mammography is used for **screening,** to monitor the breasts of apparently healthy women to make sure no abnormalities are present. It is also used for **diagnosis,** to investigate a lump or other problem of the breast.

The following mammography schedule reflects the recommendations of both the American Cancer Society and the National Cancer Institute.

1. If a lump has been found during self-examination or by a physician, the next step in the investigation is a mammogram, whether or not the patient has had one in the preceding year.

2. Younger women who are symptom-free but who have a very strong family history of breast cancer (see page 298) should start having annual mammograms at an age ten years earlier than that of the youngest first-degree relative to have breast cancer.

3. All women over forty—whether or not they are symptom-free—should have a mammogram every year. This includes women over seventy, provided they are in good health.

4. All women, whatever their age, who have had *any* type of breast cancer or a previous biopsy demonstrating a high-risk benign condition should have an annual mammogram.

WHERE DO I GO FOR A MAMMOGRAM?

This is a particularly important consideration, since the following factors can vary tremendously, depending on who does the X-ray: the quality of the picture itself, the accuracy with which it is interpreted, the comfort of the patient during the procedure. In Chapter 2, we discussed some of the methods you can use to find a good doctor. Review those before you go for your mammogram. Bear in mind that mammography is one of the instances talked about earlier where, if there is not an excellent facility and an excellent radiologist nearby, you may want to go out of your community to find them.

Most important: Under the Mammography Quality Standards Act of 1992, all mammography facilities must be certified by the Food and Drug Administration. In most states, the accreditation that is the basis for the government certification is provided by the American College of Radiology, which takes into account the quality of the machine as well as the training and experience of the physician, who must submit samples of mammograms of different types of tissue and other evidence of the quality of her X-rays as well as of her interpretations. Most mammography facilities in the United States have been certified as of this writing. On the Internet the Food and Drug Administration has a list of certified mammography facilities which is updated weekly. Go to www.fda.gov/CDRH/ MAMMOGRAPHY/certified.html and search under your zip code or state. If no certificate has been issued, do not use the facility for your mammogram. Following this advice may cause you problems and inconvenience, but nothing like the problems that can arise from using a substandard mammography facility.

There is one peculiar but valuable test of whether you are making a good decision: If a radiologist's office is not busy, if you can walk right in and not wait ... probably you'd do best to walk right out again. The ironic fact is that though it can be annoying to have to wait for an appointment and then wait in a doctor's office, heavy traffic is almost inevitable in an excellent mammographer's office.

Also consider the following factors that are specific to this test:

1. Find out whether the doctor you are considering is a general radiologist or whether she specializes in mammography. You want someone who is an expert in this field.

2. Ask what mammography technique she uses. Film-screen mammography continues to be an accurate method of breast X-ray examination. As noted above (see page 59), digital mammography has advantages and is therefore becoming more widely used. It is particularly useful for dense breasts.

3. Mammography studies are not easy to read. They should be interpreted by skilled, specifically trained, experienced specialists. One way to identify such experts is to ask the advice of a breast surgeon. Surgeons are in a good position to make this judgment, because they must rely on mammographers for specific information on matters such as the precise location of the tumor, its shape, and its probable nature. If the person who performs and interprets the mammogram makes a mistake, the surgeon will know it all too soon and his own job will be a lot harder. It is crucial to good surgeons that they work with good mammographers. Use that fact to help yourself.

4. Mammography studies are done in several kinds of facilities and by several different kinds of doctors and technologists. A radiologist's office may do only mammography, or it may be a general radiology office where one radiologist has a special expertise in mammography. Mammography may also be done in a breast screening center, in a hospital, or in a physician's group practice.
    Whichever of these you are considering, the basic questions to ask are:

• Who is taking the picture?

• Who is interpreting it?

• Who is controlling the quality of equipment, technique, and the "reading" of the results?

5. Mammograms vary in price according to individual characteristics of a facility, such as affiliation and location, and may be expensive. Nearly all health plans now pay for screening mammograms. In fact, the majority of states now require that health insurance policies cover screening mammograms. Self-insured corporations are exempt from this requirement, although many offer coverage anyway. Be sure to check your health plan. In addition, many centers around the country will provide mammograms to women who need them based on what they can afford to pay. Call the American Cancer Society at (800) ACS-2345, for help in finding such a facility. For free screening mammography, call your State Department of Health (check your phone book). Every state now has a Breast and Cervical Cancer Early Detection Program, funded by the U.S. Centers for Disease Control and Prevention, which offers free screening to women unable to pay. You can also look for a community women's health center in the phone book, or ask your company's nurse if she knows where you can get a good screening mammogram you can afford.

It is important to stress that the recommended schedule of mammography we have reviewed be followed by all women. When you have selected a good facility, it is desirable to have your yearly study performed at the same place so that the past and current X-rays can be easily compared. Mammograms cost anywhere from $90 to $400, with an average of about $250. Digital mammograms cost more, from $350 to $425. Medicare pays for yearly mammograms for women over sixty-five and for those with disabilities. Some radiologists will accept your insurance as full payment for an annual screening mammography if they are in the "network" of your health insurance.

HOW IS A MAMMOGRAM DONE?

1. You will be asked to remove all clothing from the waist up and any necklaces or jewelry you may be wearing. For this reason, you may find it more convenient to go for this procedure wearing a skirt or pants and a top. Avoid wearing

deodorant and powder, because they may produce little spots that look like calcifications.

You should be given a paper gown or a clean cloth gown to wear when you walk from the place you change your clothes to the room in which the mammography machine is located. Fasten the gown front or back, however you are instructed.

2. The machine that is used for mammography is a vertical structure. That means that you do not have to lie down for this X-ray. Instead, you will stand, or sit on a chair, and will be helped to prop your breast on the small protruding platform, first facing front and then to the side.

You will be asked to lean forward and to raise your arms to very specific positions so as to open a clear view of the breast. The machine will then be adjusted so that your breast is firmly compressed between two surfaces referred to as a platform and a compression plate. An X-ray plate will be positioned under your breast for the first pictures, then at its side for the next. You will be asked to stay perfectly still and to hold your breath while the picture is taken. The procedure is then repeated for the second breast.

3. The mammogram is read by the radiologist, and a report is sent to the physician who requested the study or to the physician you designate. This usually takes only a day or two.

Under the Mammography Quality Standards Reauthorization Act of 2003, a summary of the written mammography report must be sent by the mammography facility to the patient in terms easily understood by a layperson. This refers to every patient who has a mammogram, not only self-referred patients.

WHOM WILL I DEAL WITH?

Screening mammography does not require that a physician actually examine you. Most of the data that show that screening can reduce the rate of death from cancer come from trials in which the patients underwent mammography without any contact with the radiologist. It does depend on highly skilled technologists and, optimally, "double reading" (in which two radiologists review all films), which has been shown to reduce the error rate (missed cancers) by 5 to 15 percent. The addition of a breast examination by a physician can provide a more complete screening and a sense of security, but it is more expensive and is usually not included. You may wish to schedule your visit to the gynecologist to take place before your annual mammography so that any questions raised at a breast examination can be considered at the time your mammography is completed. Make sure to tell the technologist if you know of any abnormality. If you are menstruating, it is preferable to schedule your mammogram for the first part of your cycle. Breast tissue is less dense in appearance on X-ray at this time.

Several women have told me that they ask the person scheduling appointments whether the radiologist will be in the office at the time of their mammograms so that there can be a preliminary reading of the X-rays. If an abnormality is then seen that requires additional X-rays or a sonogram, these can be done during the same visit. Whether or not you have seen the radiologist, it is still not uncommon for patients to be asked to return for additional studies to clarify a possible problem. There is no way to avoid the anxiety this creates.

When abnormalities are found on mammograms, radiologists are becoming increasingly involved in the diagnostic process, using various types of refined equipment and techniques to perform procedures. They may recommend sonography, an MRI, or needle biopsies, all of which may be performed in their offices.

DOES A MAMMOGRAM HURT?

To obtain the best pictures of breast tissue, which is necessary to detect the earliest signs of cancer, your breast must be brought as far as possible onto the platform under which the X-ray film is placed, and held firmly in place by a plastic compression plate, or paddle, pressing against it from above. This is the only way to produce clear pictures. This pressure may be uncomfortable but should not be painful. If you are premenopausal, scheduling your mammogram in the first part of your menstrual month—when your breasts are less tender and dense—will reduce the discomfort. If the pressure placed on your breast is painful, you should ask the technologist to stop and try to reposition you. It is by working with the technologist that the best results can be assured.

WHAT ARE THE LIMITATIONS OF THE MAMMOGRAM?

Though mammography is very sensitive tool for detecting early cancers, about 10 to 15 percent of the time a malignant lump will not show up on a mammogram. Why is that?

1. A mammogram depicts only the breast itself. There are areas close to the chest wall and at the periphery of the breast that may not actually show up on the film.

2. Even a slight shift in the position of the breast on the X-ray plate can mean that an abnormality is missed.

3. Mammograms, like other X-rays, show soft tissue as gray. Hard or dense tissue appears as whitish. This means that the fat of the breast is gray on the mammogram; the lobes, the ducts, and other breast tissue are white. Tumors, because they are dense, will also be white. For this reason, tumors in the dense or fibrous tissue of the breast are harder to spot (white against white) than tumors in the fat (white against gray). Infiltrating lobular carcinomas are more likely to avoid detection than duct carcinomas, because of the way they grow (see page 37).

   Since women of childbearing age have breasts that are dense with the components needed for nursing, it may be somewhat harder to read their mammograms than those of older women, whose breasts are composed primarily of fat and are thus less dense.

4. An important caution is necessary here: Even if the mammography report does not seem to indicate any abnormality, if you or your doctor felt something unusual, or if you have the sense that something is not quite right in your breast, additional investigation with other imaging studies needs to be done, this time using sonography and/or an MRI.

A negative mammogram does not rule out the presence of cancer, and a persistent lump should always be investigated. The track record of women and their physicians in detecting cancer is too strong to be ignored, even in the presence of a negative mammogram.

IS THERE ANY WAY TO MINIMIZE THESE LIMITATIONS?

Though there are limitations inherent in the technique, the best way to avoid problems in mammography is to go to an excellent radiologist in an excellent facility. Make sure the equipment has been certified by the Food and Drug Administration. Refer to the section above on choosing a radiologist and to the material in Chapter 2 on choosing a physician.

If you know you may have a lump:

- Ask the doctor who examined you to mark it with a spot or circle of ink before you go for your mammogram.

- If for any reason that is not possible, make sure to explain to the person doing your mammogram that you are there because there is something suspicious in your breast. Show the responsible technologist the place where you think it is.

- If you have had implants to enlarge your breasts, special positioning by the X-ray technologist is needed so that all the breast tissue is examined. MRI is particularly useful when there are implants.

- Whether or not the area in question is marked, look for yourself; make sure that it is positioned on the film plate. If you think it isn't, don't be shy about pointing that out. If it turns out you were wrong and the breast is positioned properly—well, great! You've lost nothing.

HOW ARE MAMMOGRAMS READ?

Accurate reading of mammograms, even those of the highest technical quality, requires an expert, experienced radiologist who has the time to observe often minute abnormalities among large numbers of normal X-rays he or she reviews. Sometimes this means finding tiny areas of calcification (microcalcifications) at their earliest stage of development within ducts, when they are still faint shadows. Often only a careful comparison of new with prior films will show a change that arouses the suspicion of the radiologist. To increase accuracy, magnifying lenses are regularly used. The mammography machine itself may be used to provide magnification. Sometimes the patient has to be called back for additional X-rays of a particular region of a breast, taken at different angles. Although these maneuvers are helpful and permit adequate interpretation of most mammograms, as noted earlier, some offices have two radiologists read the same films (double reading) to improve reliability, while *computer-assisted* interpretation of digital images (CAD) continues to be studied as another way to get maximum information from each X-ray.

Expressing the degree of uncertainty in a mammogram interpretation has long been a problem. It has become an even more important issue now that the law has mandated that every patient have access to the results of her mammography studies. The American College of Radiology has developed a uniform nomenclature for reporting mammography findings. Most reports now conclude with a BIRADS (Breast Imaging Reporting and Data System) assessment. The seven BIRAD categories have the following meanings:

BIRADS 0
Incomplete because more information is needed; often occurs when previous films are not available. When films become available the BIRADS category changes.

BIRADS 1   Negative (N).
There is nothing to comment on. The breasts are completely normal.

BIRADS 2   Benign Finding—Negative (B).
Also a negative mammogram, but the radiologist may wish to describe the presence of a benign finding, such as a fibroadenoma, a lymph node within the breast, scattered calcifications, or even a breast implant.

BIRADS 3   Probably Benign Finding (P)
                    Short-Interval Follow-Up Suggested.
A finding is present on a mammogram that is almost certainly benign but may need another evaluation shortly to be sure it is not changing.

BIRADS 4   Suspicious Abnormality (S)
                    Biopsy Should Be Considered.
There are lesions found that do not have the characteristic appearance of breast cancer, but there is a possibility of their being malignant. The radiologist, therefore, is sufficiently concerned to advise a biopsy.

BIRADS 5   Highly Suggestive of Malignancy (M).
The lesions seen have a high probability of being cancer. Appropriate action should be taken.

BIRADS 6
Known malignancy established by biopsy but additional information is needed.

HOW DO I GET THE RESULTS OF MY MAMMOGRAPHY?

Food and Drug Administration regulations require that every facility performing screening mammography provide a woman with a report of her mammography results in clear, everyday language. In addition, a report is sent to your physician. If you do not understand the report, ask for an explanation.

IS A MAMMOGRAM DANGEROUS?

If there is something suspicious in your breast, the crucial thing is to find out what, if anything, is wrong. There is no significant radiation risk from investigative mammograms.

This question does arise, however, when we are considering this procedure for annual screening purposes. In that case, the most important reservation people have about mammography has to do with its safety. What is the risk that the exposure to radiation during the procedure—and from repeated mammograms over the years—will itself cause cancer?

The risk has been greatly reduced in recent years as mammography techniques have been improved. Much less exposure is now required than in the past. Strict guidelines are in place for the use of mammography equipment.

Still, you can't reduce the risk to zero. Anyone who tells you there is no risk is oversimplifying. Nevertheless, it is clear that at this time the benefits of mammography far outweigh its possible problems. There are several compelling reasons for this belief:

- Mammography is at this time the best screening tool we have to detect very early cancers. MRI can be more sensitive, but used alone it has not yet been shown to be as valuable as mammography for screening purposes.

- The probability of danger from radiation seems to be a great deal smaller than the probability of danger from an undetected cancer.

- The breast tissue of women in their teens and early twenties is more sensitive to low-level radiation than it is when they get older. For this reason, unless there are especially suspicious circumstances (see page 60), we advise women under thirty-five not to have routine screening mammograms.

- Conversely, we feel fairly confident that the radiation risk to women over thirty-five is very, very small.

At the moment, there are no known problems from high-quality mammography, and it does seem to be doing a good job.

WHY IS MAMMOGRAPHY IMPORTANT?

Mammography is essential as a diagnostic tool if there is any abnormality of the breast. It is also the *only* proven screening tool for finding early cancers in seemingly healthy women.

When an annual mammogram is combined with physical examination by a doctor, there is more than a one-third reduction in mortality from breast cancer. We have established this figure on the basis of an over-forty-five-year ongoing randomized study of the incidence of breast cancer among a population of about 62,000 women, some of whom had regular mammograms and physical exams and others of whom did not. The data from this screening project by the Health Insurance Plan (HIP) of Greater New York have been confirmed in a variety of ways in other studies in the United States, Sweden, Holland, Denmark, and England.

When we combine mammography with professional physical examination and self-examination, we have a powerful early-warning system against breast cancer. And the earlier that cancers are found, the better the chance for survival and for breast preservation.

SONOGRAPHY

There may yet be another way to add to our ability to detect breast cancer early. As technology improves, sonography is beginning to supplement the benefits of mammography. Also called ultrasound (and used during pregnancy to view the fetus), sonography uses high-frequency sound waves to examine the breast. A small amount of gel is applied to the breast and an instrument called a transducer is moved across its surface. The transducer emits short pulses that either pass through the tissue or—if the tissue is solid—bounce back. The results of this sound wave interaction are recorded on a screen and photographed. No radiation is used.

Because it cannot find microcalcifications or provide an overall picture of the breast, and because its findings are not always reproducible, sonography has not been considered a good general screening tool. However, new, better-designed sonography machines and better-trained radiologists have significantly improved the quality of sonograms in recent years. Using the sonogram for guidance, experienced radiologists can readily biopsy suspicious areas found during physical examination, mammography, and sonography. The result of these advances is that more women, particularly younger women with dense breasts, are having sonograms at the same intervals as mammography. The technique is very useful for studying a specific density that was previously seen on a mammogram or MRI, or a lump that has been felt but is not seen on X-ray. If the density is a liquid-filled cyst, the sound waves will go through it. If it is a solid mass—a fibroadenoma (see page 46) or a cancer—the sound waves will bounce back.

WHEN SHOULD I HAVE A SONOGRAM?

Increasingly, sonography is being employed to complement mammography for the screening of apparently normal women for breast cancer. While the guidelines for mammography have received a great deal of consideration and are by now fairly well-established, there are no universally accepted guidelines for sonography.

The following reflects my own views on when sonography is indicated:

1. When lumps that are felt on breast examination are not seen on a mammogram. Sonography is used to investigate their nature.

2. When densities are seen on mammography. Sonography can disclose whether they are benign cysts, which may be allowed to remain, or solid tumors, which might need to be biopsied.

3. As a monitoring procedure for women who have multiple breast cysts.

4. When a patient's breast tissue is extremely dense on mammography, as in young women, and there is concern that a tumor may be missed.

5. To investigate or biopsy an abnormality seen on MRI.

6. In the follow-up of women who have had breast cancer, as an additional way to find small cancers. Sonography can also be added between annual mammograms as an independent annual screening procedure.

WHERE DO I GO FOR A SONOGRAM?

Radiologists who specialize in mammography are often skilled in sonography as well and can discuss whether it would be a useful procedure for you. It does add expense, and may almost double the cost of the visit.

MAGNETIC RESONANCE IMAGING

Magnetic resonance imaging (MRI) is an imaging method that is routinely used to diagnose conditions in other parts of the body. It is increasingly being used in conjunction with mammography for the diagnosis of breast cancer. An MRI image is created with the use of a magnetic field rather than with radiation. Before the procedure a contrast material, gandolinium, will be injected into a vein. You will then be placed in a face-down (prone) position with both breasts hanging through an opening in a specialized table. Very little breast compression is needed for this study. An MRI identifies tumors by locating their increased blood supply. MRI of the breast has been found useful in the following circumstances:

1. To determine the extent of cancer in a breast where a newly diagnosed cancer has already been detected by mammography, and in order to see whether the tumor can be safely removed by lumpectomy and a mastectomy can be avoided. It is also a useful way to make certain that there are no areas of concern in the other breast.

2. To search for the source of breast cancer in women who have developed enlarged axillary lymph nodes that on testing prove to contain cancer. If physical examination, mammography, and sonography are all negative, an MRI may be able to detect a hidden tumor in the breast.

3. To preoperatively search for an unsuspected cancer when a prophylactic mastectomy is planned.

4. In women who have breast implants, particularly those filled with liquid silicone, to determine whether the implants remain intact or are leaking.

5. For screening the breasts of women who are known or suspected to have mutations of the BRCA1-2 genes (see page 114).

6. For screening the breasts of women who have a strong family history of breast cancer but are not known to be carriers of a recognized mutation.

MRI of the breast is more sensitive than a regular mammogram but is not used in routine screening because it may show many abnormalities which—while they are not likely to represent cancer—must be biopsied to make certain this is the case. These are known as false positives. Suspicious areas are biopsied by core needle biopsy techniques similar to those described on page 79. They may be performed using ultrasound or MRI as a guide.

BREAST-SPECIFIC GAMMA IMAGING (BSGI)

Breast-specific gamma imaging is a technology being developed as an alternative to MRI. A radioisotope, Tc-Sestamibi, is injected into a vein. The isotope concentrates in tumor tissues. A gamma camera highly sensitive to the very small doses of radioactivity emitted by the isotope scans the breasts and shows whether there are any areas where an increased amount of isotope has collected. BSGI appears to be as sensitive as an MRI but is more specific—it produces fewer false positives, so that fewer biopsies are needed. The procedure takes less time than an MRI and is less expensive and more comfortable. It is performed in a sitting position with the breast on a platform, as in a mammogram, but compression is not used.

THERMOGRAPHY

Thermography is a procedure that uses a special camera to measure and record the heat pattern of the breast, on the premise that tumors emit more heat than does the normal surrounding tissue. Though this method has been used and investigated for over forty years, clinical trials have thus far not demonstrated its effectiveness in detecting early breast cancer. There is no reason to undergo this examination unless you want to participate in an experimental study. (Nor is there any reason to wear a bra with a built-in heat-measuring device as a form of self-examination.

Stick to the palpation techniques for self-examination we've already discussed.)

TRANSILLUMINATION

Sometimes called diaphanography, transillumination is based on the observation that cancerous tissue absorbs more infrared radiation than benign tissue. The breast is lit—"transilluminated"—and its image recorded onto special film or, through another process, viewed on a television monitor. There is no reliable evidence that transillumination is useful in detecting breast cancer.

XEROMAMMOGRAPHY

A technique developed by the Xerox company, xeromammography is a form of mammographic examination that results in a blue image on white paper, a "positive" rather than a negative image. It does not have the accuracy of film X-ray, and the machine used for conducting this examination is no longer being manufactured.

BIOPSY

WHAT IS IT?

Biopsy is a procedure that removes a sample of tissue from the body so that it can be examined under a microscope. In a breast biopsy, the tumor and surrounding tissue are removed and examined under a microscope so that the pathologist can identify the cells that are present, characterize them, and determine whether they are malignant. The details of the pathologist's examination can be found in Chapter 5.

Even the word *biopsy* can have frightening associations for many patients. For that reason, it is important to bear one fact in mind: Most biopsies of breast lumps are needle biopsies and reveal no malignancy. For the majority of women, therefore, biopsy is a reliable tool for establishing that they do *not* have cancer.

WHY DO I NEED A BIOPSY?

As we've discussed before, an experienced doctor often knows by its "feel" what a lump is, and after a mammogram—often accompanied by a sonogram or even an MRI—he may be able to quite accurately predict whether a tumor or thickening in the breast is malignant or not.

That educated hunch, however, is not enough to go on. The final diagnosis of breast cancer depends on an examination of the suspicious tissue under a microscope.

WHO PERFORMS BIOPSIES?

Depending on the nature of the biopsy, the procedure is performed by a radiologist or surgeon who is experienced in breast cancer diagnosis. The tissue that is removed during the biopsy is examined by a pathologist, a physician who specializes in identifying disease by microscopic examination.

WHAT ARE THE TYPES OF BIOPSY?

Several kinds of biopsy are used to examine breast tissue. These are called fine-needle aspiration, core biopsy, mammotome biopsy, and two forms of formal (open) biopsy: incisional biopsy and excisional biopsy.

FINE-NEEDLE ASPIRATION (FNA)

WHERE?

The procedure is usually done in the office of a surgeon or radiologist.

HOW?

The skin of the breast around the lump or thickening is cleaned with an antiseptic solution, usually alcohol or Betadine. A small amount of local anesthetic is injected into the skin. A thin, hollow

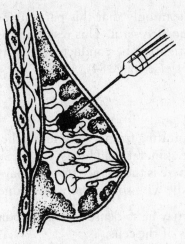

Needle aspiration biopsy

needle, often called a fine needle, is inserted into the lump, and any fluid that is present is drawn into a syringe.

If the lump is a solid (not fluid-filled) mass, we push the needle back and forth through the tissue to free some cells, aspirate them into the syringe, and then smear them on a glass slide. The slide is then treated with a preservative and sent to a laboratory for microscopic analysis by a pathologist.

PAIN?

Aspiration may be a little uncomfortable, but it should not cause you any serious pain. Most of the nerves of the breast are in the skin, which has been anesthetized.

FINDINGS

If the lump is a cyst, as breast masses most often are, needle aspiration turns out to be the treatment as well as the diagnosis. When the doctor withdraws the fluid, he not only identifies what's wrong; he also cures it.

When the fine-needle aspiration reveals a solid mass, and the sample is sent for analysis, a pathologist's report of "no malignant cells seen" does not necessarily mean that no cancer is present. It may mean only that this particular attempt to find a malignancy was unsuccessful. This result almost *always* requires that further investigation be conducted, usually by an incisional or excisional biopsy (see page 84).

LIMITATIONS

• When we are aspirating from a solid mass, the needle has to pass through the skin, fat, and breast tissue. Since we can't actually see it, there is the chance that we may miss the tumor. Guiding the needle with sonography can reduce this risk.

• A breast tumor may be so dense that the needle is unable to dislodge samples of the cells.

• Even if a cell sample is obtained, it may be so small that the pathologist can't depend on it for reliable answers.

WHY BOTHER?

Even though the results of this procedure sometimes mean only that a surgical biopsy is needed, there are several circumstances in which a fine-needle aspiration is particularly helpful:

• When we have strong reason to suspect a malignancy. The aspiration may confirm the cancer's presence, and surgical biopsy will not be needed.

• When several areas in the breast need to be evaluated.

• When we are sure that there is a malignancy and that a mastectomy will be needed. We will often know from the aspiration what kind of cells we are dealing with, and will thus be able to skip the step of an open biopsy (see pages 83–89) to provide that information.

• It is much less expensive than an operation and can be done at the time of mammography or an examination by a surgeon.

• Best of all, needle aspiration is a wonderful method if it yields the happy ending that there was a cyst that now is gone.

CORE BIOPSY

WHERE?

This procedure is done in the surgeon's or radiologist's office.

HOW?

The skin is cleaned, usually with an antiseptic solution called Betadine, and a local anesthetic is injected.

A large-caliber needle within a spring-loaded device is inserted into the lump to obtain a sliver of tissue, which is then sent to a laboratory for microscopic examination.

PAIN?

Because the needle is large and more manipulation is required, even though you have been given a local anesthetic you may feel pain. If you do, immediately tell the doctor and ask for more anesthetic.

FINDINGS

Because actual tissue is removed with the core biopsy, more detailed information can be obtained than with a fine-needle aspiration biopsy.

LIMITATIONS

• Though the cell sample is larger than the one we get with fine-needle aspiration, it is still quite small. Therefore, if cancer or a definitively benign condition is not found, we still have to investigate further with a formal biopsy.

• When a well-defined, solid mass is present, highly accurate information can be obtained, permitting diagnoses of benign or malignant conditions. However, with more subtle and less distinct "thickenings" of the breast, the sampling may be incomplete and a surgical biopsy may still be needed even if no evidence of malignancy is found.

WHY BOTHER?

The larger sample obtained by core biopsy permits the pathologist to view suspicious cells in the setting of the normal breast structures from which they arise.

MAMMOTOME BIOPSY

WHERE?

This procedure is done in a radiology facility by a radiologist or a surgeon.

HOW?

The skin is cleaned, usually with Betadine, a local anesthetic is injected, and a nick is made in the skin. A large-caliber needle is advanced into the breast by a suction-type mechanical device to obtain several slivers of tissue, which are sent to the pathology laboratory for microscopic examination. If microcalcifications are being biopsied (see page 86), the tissue removed is X-rayed to see whether it contains the microcalcifications seen on the mammogram, and a tiny metallic clip is placed at the site of biopsy before the needle is removed. This makes it possible to locate this site again if surgical removal of additional tissue becomes necessary.

PAIN?

Because the needle is large and manipulation is required, even though you have been given a local anesthetic, you may feel pain. If you do, immediately tell the doctor and ask for more anesthetic.

FINDINGS

Since more tissue can be removed, more information can be obtained than with a fine-needle or core biopsy.

LIMITATIONS

• Though a significant amount of tissue can be obtained, if cancer is found, it is still necessary to investigate further with a surgical biopsy in order to determine the extent of the malignancy.

• If a malignancy is likely and an open biopsy will be needed anyway, this procedure may prove to be unnecessary, as well as an extra expense.

WHY BOTHER?

Mammograms often show groups of microcalcifications (see page 86) whose nature needs to be investigated. Fine-needle aspirations and core biopsies usually do not provide enough information. Mammotome biopsy is an effective way to find out whether such microcalcifications are associated with benign or malignant tissue changes. If no cancer is found, it may be possible to avoid an operation.

STEREOTATIC BIOPSY

WHERE?

The procedure is carried out in a radiologist's office or in the radiology department of a hospital.

HOW?

It is usually performed with the woman in a face-down (prone) position, with the breast hanging through an opening in a specialized table and the X-ray equipment below. It is less commonly carried out in a sitting position. After a mammogram is taken, a needle is placed directly into the lump being tested with the aid of a computer, and its position is verified. Depending on the caliber of the needle, either a fine-needle aspiration, core biopsy, or mammotome biopsy is done.

PAIN?

Depending on the size of the needle, you may feel some pain despite having been given a local anesthetic. If you do, ask the doctor for more anesthetic.

FINDINGS

It is a highly accurate procedure.

LIMITATIONS

• If microcalcifications need to be investigated, this procedure cannot be done if these calcifications seen on the mammogram are too faint or if the breast is too thin.

• When used to diagnose very small tumors, a stereotatic biopsy may not provide a large enough sample to make it possible to tell the difference between premalignant changes and true cancers.

WHY BOTHER?

This procedure is needed when a lump is seen in a mammogram or by sonography, and where calcifications have been detected.

• If the tumor is benign, it may be possible to avoid a formal biopsy.

• If the tumor or calcifications are malignant, it may be possible to carry out a one-stage instead of a two-stage procedure (see page 89).

• It is less expensive than a surgical biopsy.

SONOGRAPHIC BIOPSIES

Sonography may also be used to guide a small needle into a solid mass in order to remove cells. This procedure is called a fine-needle aspiration biopsy under ultrasound guidance. Similarly, a core biopsy can also be performed under ultrasound guidance.

MRI BIOPSIES

When a suspicious area is found on an MRI of the breasts, the biopsies performed are completed in the same way as in the stereotatic biopsies for mammography described above. If the abnormality can also be identified by sonography, core biopsies under sonographic guidance are sometimes done. Such biopsies are easier for the patient and also less expensive.

SURGICAL (OPEN) BIOPSY

WHERE IS SURGICAL BIOPSY DONE?

This procedure should always be performed by a surgeon in a facility where the tissue can be examined by a pathologist as soon as it is removed. This is possible only in a hospital or in an ambulatory facility with an excellent laboratory and a pathologist on the premises prepared to handle the tissue. If a surgeon insists that he can do the biopsy in his office, unless that office is located right in a hospital, you should go to a different surgeon.

Biopsies are performed on an outpatient basis. You are not assigned a room or a bed; you do not have to stay overnight. The hospital department is often called the ambulatory center or day surgery. You should call your insurance company in advance to request authorization for the biopsy, making sure to ask whether your policy requires a second opinion.

On arrival at the facility, you will be asked to fill out forms that give personal, medical, and insurance information. You will be assigned a hospital identification number if you have not been a patient in this institution before. The admitting officer may fasten a plastic identification bracelet to your wrist.

Next, you will be asked to change into a hospital gown. A nurse will interview you, take your blood pressure and pulse (vital signs), and make certain that all your preoperative tests and operative permits are in order and in the chart. Your anesthesiologist will review your chart. An attendant will walk you to the operating room, where you will meet the anesthesiologist. An intravenous (IV) is started, anesthesia is administered, and the biopsy is performed by your surgeon.

After the biopsy, you will be wheeled to a recovery room, where your condition will be monitored by a nurse. When you are fully awake, you will be given something to eat, and you will then be free to change back into your street clothes and leave. You must arrange to have someone pick you up and take you home because you will not be allowed to leave unescorted.

HOW?

A cut or incision is made in the skin as deep as is necessary to reveal the suspected tissue. This is called an open, or formal, biopsy.

There are two basic types of open biopsy:

• If a tumor is large and only a small piece of it is removed for examination, the surgery is called an **incisional biopsy.**

• If a tumor is small and the biopsy removes it completely, the surgery is called an **excisional biopsy.**

Much of the surgical procedure is the same for both types of biopsy:

1. The surgeon will scrub his hands and will put on sterile gown, gloves, cap, and mask.

2. The skin of the affected breast is cleaned, usually with the antiseptic Betadine.

3. The upper part of the patient's body is covered with a sterile drape, except for the breast that is to be biopsied. Part of this drape is arranged so that the patient's head is separated from

.the site of the surgery. As a result, the patient is not able to watch the procedure.

4. Because an electrical instrument called a cautery may be used (see below), a grounding pad is placed under the buttocks.

5. Anesthesia is administered.

6. A cut is made in the skin over the tumor. The cut goes through the fat and breast tissue until the tumor is reached.

7. The surrounding tissues are removed, with the tumor in the center. This is called an excisional biopsy. In an incisional biopsy only a segment of the tumor is cut out.

8. To control bleeding, the surgeon may use a cautery and/or clamps or sutures.

9. When the tumor or segment of the tumor has been removed, the surgeon stitches the tissue, the fat, and the skin to close the incision and then carefully bandages the site of the biopsy.

NEEDLE LOCALIZATION

The sophistication of mammography technique alerts us to the presence of tiny tumors, some of which it may not be possible to see or feel without X-ray. In some instances such tumors may also not be visible on mammograms, and are only discovered by sonography or MRI. Most of these tumors turn out to be benign, but they do have to be removed for microscopic examination. To accomplish this, just before the surgery a technique called needle localization is employed.

1. Either in the hospital's radiology department or in the radiologist's office, she X-rays the breast, locates the suspicious area, and inserts a needle into the breast so that its tip is at the site of the tumor. The needle has a tiny hook at its end that fixes it in place. The needle is sometimes placed under the guidance of sonography. In some cases, more than one area may need to be localized or more than one imaging technique—such as mammography *and* sonography—may be needed to identify all areas of the breast requiring biopsy.

2. The patient immediately goes to the location where the biopsy will be performed and is prepared for surgery. The surgeon makes an incision and follows the needle's course to the site of the tumor.

3. The tumor is removed in a standard biopsy procedure.

SPECIMEN RADIOGRAPHY

Mammography may reveal the presence in the breast of **microcalcifications,** tiny flecks of calcium that sometimes can indicate the presence of an early breast cancer.

Microcalcifications are suspect if they are clustered in one area of the breast or are branching in appearance. In most instances, scattered specks of calcium are no problem. Microcalcifications ought to be investigated by biopsy if they are clustered or if they have appeared since the last mammogram. In fact, the investigation of microcalcifications is one of the most common reasons that breast biopsies are done.

The problem is that though the microcalcifications are picked up by the mammogram, we are not able to see them during surgery. Under these circumstances, we probably have to take out a larger section of breast tissue than we would if there were a visible tumor. Therefore:

• We use needle localization to target the questionable area.

• We X-ray the excised section before the surgery is complete to make absolutely sure that we've adequately removed the tissue containing the calcifications.

• Both the X-rays and the tissue are sent to the pathologist.

ANESTHESIA

Anytime a doctor makes a cut in the body, an anesthetic is needed to eliminate pain. Generally speaking, the type of anesthesia—as well as the type of biopsy—is determined by the size and location of the tumor.

- If the tumor or other abnormality is small, well-defined, and near the skin's surface, the surgeon will probably use local anesthesia, a medication that is injected into the site of the procedure to make it insensible to pain. (Local anesthesia may also be used after the incision is closed to minimize postoperative discomfort.)

- The skin's surface will be cleaned, usually with the antiseptic Betadine. The anesthetic is then injected into the skin and into the tissues surrounding the tumor.

- You will be awake and able to respond, though there will be no sensation in the area that has been anesthetized. The surgeon will pinch the skin or touch you with a surgical instrument to make sure the anesthetic is working. If you feel anything, by all means tell him.

- In addition to the local anesthesia, you may be given an intravenous medication, one that is injected into a vein. It will further reduce the pain and will relax you or put you briefly to sleep. This is called monitored anesthesia care (MAC), and is the type of anesthesia most frequently used in ambulatory surgical procedures.

- A general anesthetic is a medication, usually in the form of inhaled gas, that causes a loss of sensation and of consciousness. It may be used for a large excision, particularly in cases where cancer is strongly suspected or where there are other circumstances—such as a small but deep tumor—that may cause the patient to feel some pain. Using this type of anesthesia allows the surgeon to excise enough tissue to get information not only about the tumor but also about the surrounding tissue. Often this is not possible with local anesthesia.

- In addition, there may be circumstances when the patient herself, for personal reasons, does not want to be awake during the procedure.

Before the biopsy, make sure to carefully discuss with the surgeon which anesthetic he plans to use, what the alternatives are, and under what circumstances he may decide to administer another drug during the course of the procedure. Talk it over thoroughly until you understand and are comfortable with the plan.

PAIN?

You should feel no serious pain during a biopsy. If you do, tell the surgeon at once so that he can remedy the situation. You may feel some sensation of the tugging of skin or tissue. Women report that this feels peculiar or unpleasant but that it does not hurt.

After the biopsy you may feel the mild discomfort that can occur when any cut or wound is healing. Most women don't seem to need much medication to deal with this discomfort.

ONE-STAGE OR TWO-STAGE PROCEDURES?

It used to be that before a patient had a breast biopsy, she was asked to sign a statement that gave the surgeon permission to perform a mastectomy immediately if he found cancer. This was based in part on the erroneous theory that introducing a needle or other instrument into the tumor or operating a second time would "spread" the cancer. Often, therefore, a woman would go in for a biopsy and would learn only when she woke up in the recovery room with a radical mastectomy that she had breast cancer.

Women's advocacy groups very properly worked to eliminate this often traumatic surrender of control. The result is that the one-stage procedure has almost been eliminated. Most patients now have a biopsy, frequently a needle biopsy, wait for the results, and then, if cancer is found, give themselves time to get used to the idea. The biopsy will provide the information necessary to explore treatment options with the surgeon as well as with other specialists. The definitive breast surgery is usually done later.

There are, however, some circumstances in which this "rule" of the two-stage procedure doesn't serve the patient best. In such instances, and with her understanding and consent, the biopsy and the surgery are performed in the course of the same operation.

- The cancer may have been found at a stage when breast conservation is no longer feasible, and a one-stage procedure will spare the patient the ordeal of two separate procedures. A needle biopsy has already been done and the diagnosis is known.

• Similarly, where breast cancer is strongly suspected, the patient and the doctor may have thoroughly discussed in advance breast conservation through a wide-excision removal of the tumor and surrounding tissue (lumpectomy), as well as the lymph nodes. In such instances, unless there are unanticipated findings, many women prefer to have the biopsy and surgery done in one stage.

• You should review the biopsy plans carefully with your surgeon before the procedure and jointly arrive at a plan for your biopsy and any surgery that subsequently may be necessary. Also check with your insurance company to make sure that a second opinion is not required before a one-stage procedure.

RESULTS

We will discuss in the following chapter the procedure the pathologist follows to examine the tissue that has been surgically removed from the breast. We will also review the points that the pathologist's report will cover. This report will tell us definitively whether or not cancer cells are present.

If you are going to have a biopsy with a local anesthetic, it is a good idea to make a pact with your surgeon beforehand that even though you will be awake while the procedure is taking place, you won't ask him—and he won't tell you—how things look to him or what he thinks the percentages are. Most of the time he won't really know, and it is certainly not in your best interest to distract him during the procedure. He is busy and needs to give his full attention to the surgery.

Hard though it is to wait for the results, it is worse to be given information that turns out to be inaccurate, or to receive important news while you are on the operating table, under partial sedation and not truly alert. It isn't until the pathologist's report is available (see pages 91–94) that the results can be certain.

CHAPTER

5

PATHOLOGY

❦

The pathologist, the medical specialist who examines and analyzes the tissue removed during the biopsy, provides the key not only to finding out whether cancer is present but also to the subsequent treatment. We have been more successful in helping people with breast cancer in recent years largely because we've been able to better tailor the treatment specifically to what the pathologist has discovered.

In the following sections we will look at how the pathologist works and how he arrives at his conclusions. It is not possible for the nonspecialist to absorb all the technical details of a pathologist's report, but some understanding of the process may help you to understand what your physician tells you after the biopsy, and may also help you to formulate important questions about the treatment that will be planned if cancer is found.

Labeling and Transporting the Specimen

As soon as the biopsy is performed, the following steps are taken:

1. Each tissue sample is immediately placed in a plastic container.

2. The patient's name, her hospital identification number, the date of the biopsy, and a number or letter designated for the particular sample are marked directly on each container.

3. A requisition form is completed that gives the patient's name, the surgeon's name, specific details about the tumor and the specimen, a summary of the patient's related medical history, and a list of all the tissue samples that have been submitted.

4. The specimen containers, together with the form, are carried by an attendant or sent through a pneumatic tube carrier directly from the operating room to the pathology department.

5. In most hospitals, the pathology department has a direct intercom connection with the operating room. This is especially important if a quick, preliminary examination, called a frozen section (see page 92), is required by the surgeon before he completes the surgery.

Patients sometimes worry that there will be a mix-up and that the tissue the pathologist examines and reports on will not really be theirs. It is impossible to say, "No way. That could never happen." On the other hand, there are so many controls and identifying safeguards along the way that the chances of a mistake of this sort occurring at a reputable hospital are practically nil.

The Pathologist's Examination and Report

When the specimen arrives at the pathology laboratory, the process of examination immediately begins. The date and time the specimen arrives are recorded, a pathology number is assigned, and government-required formal documents are filled out to ensure that specimens are properly identified. All this information is usually entered into a computer.

1. The pathologist first performs a *gross examination*, in which he reads the surgeon's description on the pathology requisition of each specimen he receives, and then inspects and notes on his own report its physical characteristics, including weight, dimensions (width, height, and breadth), contour and shape, and texture. The pathologist may also comment on the specimen's color. (The fat of the breast is yellow; the ducts and other vessels are white.) When a malignancy is visible to the eye, it may appear as an irregular patch of white discoloration.

2. The surgeon may have placed sutures on the sides of the specimen in order to orient the edges as superior, inferior, anterior, medial, and posterior. In that case the pathologist will apply different colors of ink to each of them so as to be able to identify these margins accurately.

3. The specimen will next be cut, or *sectioned*, first for the *frozen section* and then for the *permanent section*.

4. A sample is taken from a few areas of the tumor or suspicious tissue, as well as from the edges (margins) of the total specimen.

5. A frozen section may then be performed. (See below for a fuller explanation.) The results of this examination will be available in a matter of a few minutes.

   • A very small piece is cut from the excised tissue, and liquid nitrogen is used to instantly harden it by freezing. A specially refrigerated instrument, called a cryostat, is then used to cut this tissue so it can be examined under the microscope. This is the frozen section.

6. A permanent section is then prepared. It will take several days for the results to be obtained. The tissue that remains after the frozen section is placed in a preservative called formalin,

which fixes it in much the same way that boiling an egg hardens its contents.

7. Any water remaining in the tissue sample is removed and replaced with paraffin.

8. After twenty-four hours, the permanent section is firm enough to be prepared for microscopic analysis. Very much the same analysis is done on the frozen section as well:

   • The specimen is cut into slices that measure 1/50,000 inch, thinner than tissue paper, less than one cell thick.

   • The slices are mounted on glass slides and stained with chemical dyes that will present different shades of red and blue when placed on different types of tissue.

   • The pathologist then reads the slides under his microscope and issues a report on what he sees.

   • Additional preserved tissue is carefully stored so that if questions arise in the future, it can be retrieved for study.

People sometimes ask why we bother with the time and trouble of a permanent section if we've already done a frozen section. We use a frozen section only if we need a quick answer during an operation to determine how to proceed with surgery (see "Sentinel Lymph Node Biopsy," page 133). This is possible because the slides prepared from a frozen section can be just as accurate as those from a permanent section if there is a positive diagnosis of cancer.

The problem lies with the opposite result: Even if no cancer cells are found, we cannot be satisfied with the results of a frozen section because it is not as comprehensive as permanent sections. These are its limitations:

• Since only a minute part of the tumor is taken for examination, we cannot be certain that the unanalyzed portion doesn't contain malignant cells.

• If the original tumor is quite small, we don't really want to "waste" tissue on a frozen section, since its results may not be definitive. We would rather use the complete specimen for the more reliable results of the permanent section.

• Where an area of microcalcifications is removed, there is usually no tumor, so a frozen section should not be requested. The pathologist needs to prepare multiple permanent slides to provide a complete answer.

Tumors may also be described in terms of "grade." You may hear about different grading systems, which are used to describe how active the tumor cells appear to be. The system developed by Bloom and Richardson, which is the most widely used, assigns a score of 1, 2, or 3 to nuclear grade (explained in the next section), the number of cells dividing, and how closely the tumor resembles normal breast tissue. The scores are then added to determine the grade. However, such grading provides a rough approximation at best, and is seldom used to determine the nature of treatment you will receive.

WHAT DOES THE PATHOLOGIST OBSERVE?

THE CELLS

You may hear the terms *differentiated* and *undifferentiated* in reference to cancer cells. These terms describe the degree to which the cells seen under a microscope resemble normal cells. While differentiated cells are close to normal cells in appearance, undifferentiated cells have an abnormal appearance.

Except for red blood cells, all cells have a central dense portion, or nucleus, that contains the chromosomes and controls most of the cell's functions. The rest of the cell, called the cytoplasm, is engaged primarily in manufacturing proteins and processing glucose. *Nuclear grade* is the term used to describe the extent to which the nuclei of breast cancer cells are altered from their normal counterparts.

Normal ducts and lobules are lined around their periphery with a single or double layer of cells arranged in an orderly pattern. When cancer develops, the proliferating cells do not present

themselves in orderly rows but are randomly dispersed, sometimes forming a complete blockage of the duct. This is an *in situ*
cancer. If these cells break through the basement membrane of
the duct or lobule, it is an *infiltrating* cancer.

Normal breast cells are under strict growth control and have a
rigorously programmed, very limited ability, to divide. Malignant
cells grow and divide rapidly.

In normal cells and in some cancer cells, the genetic material
DNA appears within two sets of chromosomes. This normal state
is called *diploid*. Malignant cells may have either fewer or more
chromosomes, in which case they are referred to as *aneuploid*.
The presence of abnormal genes and their protein products, such
as HER-2/neu and p53 (see pages 182–83), are tested for.

THE LOCATION AND PATTERNS OF THE CANCER

As we discussed in Chapter 3, though the breast contains fat and
blood vessels and other components, most breast cancers originate in the ducts and lobules. About 85 percent of all breast
cancer occurs in the ducts, and the remaining 15 percent in the

Breast carcinoma

INTACT BASEMENT MEMBRANE

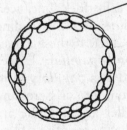 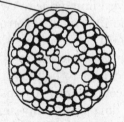 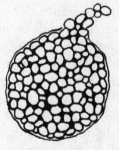

Normal duct or lobule
One to two layers of
normal cells.

In situ cancer
Duct or lobule filled
with cancer cells.

Infiltrating carcinoma
Cancer cells break
through the basement
membrane into the
fatty tissue of the
breast.

lobules. The pathologist will tell us whether the cancer is ductal or lobular.

The pathologist examines samples from the edge, or margin, of the piece of tissue that was removed during the biopsy in order to determine whether there is a clear border of normal tissue around the specimen. If there isn't—if the cancer goes right up to the inked edge—it may indicate that there may be more cancer in the adjacent tissue remaining in the breast. Where there are several ducts or lobules involved, if confined to the same quadrant of the breast it is called *multifocal*. When the cancer is found in more than one quadrant it is called *multicentric*.

The pathologist will examine the tumor and the surrounding tissue to see whether cancer is present in the fat of the breast, the blood vessels, or the lymphatics, or whether it is in situ—that is, confined to its site of origin.

The pathologist will report the type of cancer: whether it is confined to the ducts, ductal carcinoma in situ (DCIS), or whether it originates in the lobules, lobular carcinoma in situ (LCIS). He will also note whether there is only a single duct or lobule with an in situ cancer, or more than one, and whether it is widespread throughout the tissues examined.

Lobular carcinoma in situ is not usually described as having special subtypes.

When ductal carcinoma in situ is discovered by the pathologist, the pattern of cells within the ducts is described. As we have seen, normal ducts have a lining one to two cells thick. In cancer, cells pile up along the duct wall. Protrusions form, extending out from the wall toward the center of the duct. If these extensions are small, the tumor is referred to as *micropapillary*. Larger protrusions cause the cancer to be identified as a *papillary* form of DCIS. In some cancers the protrusions join into crisscrossing walls that divide the duct into many smaller areas. These are called *cribriform* types of DCIS. When the ducts are entirely filled with cancer cells, they are called a *solid* form of DCIS. At times so many cells are growing into the duct that those in the center begin to die (necrosis), leaving only a residue of debris. This is *comedo* DCIS. The virulence of tumors is reflected in the degree to which the ducts are filled. Those most likely to lead to recurrences are comedo carcinomas. Some pathologists simply segregate the different patterns of DCIS into comedo and noncomedo types.

Once the cells have broken through the basement membrane of the duct or lobule, they invade, or infiltrate, the surrounding tissue. Depending on the site of origin, the pathologist will report whether the cancer is an infiltrating ductal carcinoma or an infiltrating lobular carcinoma.

Sometimes even the most expert pathologists will have difficulty deciding whether tiny in situ and microinvasive cancers are of the ductal or lobular type. Since the type of treatment sometimes depends on knowing this information, permanent sections can be prepared and stained with the E-cadherin immunostatin, which has proven to be highly specific for telling these types apart. Lobular carcinomas typically do not stain with this agent, while ductal cancers do.

Ductal carcinoma in situ

NONCOMEDO TYPE

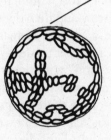 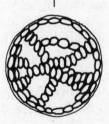 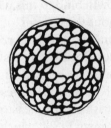

Papillary and micropapillary   *Cribriform*   *Solid*

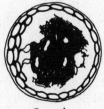

Comedo

THE HORMONE RECEPTOR ASSAY

In addition to performing the gross and microscopic analyses of the tissue, the pathologist sends unstained routine paraffin section slides to test for the presence of estrogen and progesterone receptors in the tumor cells. Because this test takes time, the results will rarely be ready at the time of the pathologist's report on the permanent section, but they will usually be available in about one week.

If these receptors are present, the tumor is said to be estrogen receptor-positive or progesterone receptor-positive. However, if there are two separate tumors in the same breast, we may find upon examination that one is receptor-positive, the other negative. These findings have an impact on the planning of postsurgical treatment, since receptor-positive cells are more likely to respond to hormonal therapy.

TESTING FOR HER-2

All breast cells have a growth factor receptor called HER-2 on their surface. Under appropriate conditions, when factors stimulating growth bind to this receptor, the cell begins to grow and then divide. About 25 percent of breast cancer cells have a greatly increased number of HER-2 receptors. Such tumors have a greater tendency to recur. Tumors are tested for HER-2 "overexpression" with the antibodies to HER-2, using a method called immunohistochemistry (IHC). When IHC results are not conclusive, another, more sensitive test is used to measure HER-2 levels. This test is referred to by the acronym FISH, which is short for fluorescence in situ-hybridization. Tumors that overexpress HER-2 are referred to as HER-2 positive.

THE FINAL DIAGNOSIS

The final pathology report is the place in which the pathologist summarizes his findings and establishes the diagnosis. It should be noted that reports prepared by pathologists working at different institutions vary and may not include everything listed below. Results of other tests may also be added.

The final diagnosis may conclude that the condition is benign, in which case the patient is home free. If malignancy is present, the cancer cells may be described with regard to the following characteristics:

- Tumor size

- Tumor type—ductal or lobular

- Presence of invasion—noninfiltrating (in situ) or infiltrating

- Cell differentiation—well to poorly differentiated

- Nuclear differentiation—nuclear grade

- Tumor grade—numerical evaluation of tumor structure

- Vascular invasion—the presence or absence of tumor cells in blood vessels or lymphatics

- Extent of tumor—multifocal or multicentric

- Margins of removed tissue—negative or involved by tumor

- Hormone receptors—present or absent

- HER 2/neu—overexpressed, present, or absent

- Proliferation index—the percent of cells dividing or preparing to divide

As we will see, these conclusions will help determine the course of treatment.

The pathology report may be available two or three days after the biopsy, though in some pathology departments it can take as long as a week. Before the biopsy, you should ask your surgeon how long the hospital laboratory usually takes to issue the pathology report. Having that information in advance will help make the waiting easier, since you will know that the amount of time is routine for this laboratory and not an indication that something is wrong or that information is being withheld.

THE MEANING OF THE DIAGNOSIS

If the pathologist's report concludes that only a benign condition is present, you can feel both relieved and reassured. You have had a physical examination, a mammogram, and a biopsy. You have done everything possible, with the very best techniques now available, to make sure there are no malignant cells present. That exercise wasn't a waste of time or money—it provided you with invaluable information.

Though rare, a biopsy may show changes in breast tissue that imply a higher risk of developing malignancy, such as extensive and severe atypia of cells or multiple intraductal papillomas. While no additional surgery is needed, such findings may alert you to carefully adhere to your schedule of mammograms and yearly breast examinations. Preventive treatments may also be considered (see pages 313–16).

If the biopsy reveals the presence of cancer, the pathologist's findings will help point the way to the best treatment. Yet the pathologist can describe only what has been removed from the breast and examined in the laboratory. His findings are crucial, but they are not the whole story. They must be interpreted jointly with those of the surgeon, who performed the biopsy and actually saw the tissue in its natural setting. If any uncertainty regarding the nature of the tumor remains, you or your surgeon may want to get a second pathologist's opinion on the findings.

The surgeon should share the pathologist's report with you and interpret for you its detailed findings and the treatment he recommends based on those findings. How to act on that information is the subject of the next chapter.

CHAPTER

6

AFTER THE DIAGNOSIS

T here's almost no need to describe the relief and joy everyone feels when the news is good, when no malignancy is found. One of my patients recently said, "Each day I waited seemed like an eternity. I thought Tuesday would never pass, and then, even though I went to work on Wednesday, the whole office seemed to be like a slowed-down movie projection. Then when we found out—well, my boyfriend and I were both crying and laughing at the same time. There's no way to tell you how I felt, as if I had entered real life again."

The story is obviously different when a malignancy is found. This is a moment that for most people becomes frozen in time. Women can recall the date and the exact circumstances under which they heard the news that they had cancer. The scene is etched vividly in their minds: They see where they were, hear the voice and the words again and again.

It is information that does not go down easily. Patients who ordinarily have perfectly good memories call a few hours after they have learned that they have breast cancer to ask me to repeat what I said, because "it did not sink in."

This is the most normal and human of reactions. It is very hard to absorb everything you are told under such circumstances. If you want to make such a telephone call, your doctor should be sympathetic and tell you again what you need to know.

THE PHYSICIAN'S ROLE

In many instances, the doctor who on the basis of a physical examination, a mammogram, or a pathologist's report is the first to say "I think it's cancer" can seem to the patient to be the villain. When the very person to whom you have turned for help becomes the bearer of horrible news, it is hard to imagine that that same human being can be your advocate, and it's easy to feel distrustful.

It is also true that women are sometimes upset about the way in which the news of their breast cancer was broken to them. Their complaints are often justified, but speaking as a doctor, I have to say that there is no good way to tell someone she has cancer. There is no good time or place to convey this news.

This is not a book whose theme is to explain how difficult life is for physicians. It is not "harder for me than it is for you," and I have little patience for physicians who equate their own strong feelings of sympathy with the real thing—the pain and shock their patients are experiencing. Nevertheless, having to tell a patient she has cancer is a very hard thing to do. The sadness and stress that are involved can take their toll on any compassionate person. Sometimes a doctor will draw back and seem to remove himself from the patient because he cannot cope with the powerful emotion of this encounter. Understandable though such an attitude may be, it is not what the patient needs at this moment, when reassurance and clarity are required.

Receiving the News

All of us have our own ways of dealing with what we see as a threat to our lives, and that is how most people perceive a diagnosis of cancer. But there does seem to be a general pattern in these reactions: First we are shocked and frightened; then we confront the danger. We prepare ourselves to face it by completely focusing on the problem itself.

The first reaction of a woman in my office recently was to put her hand up protectively and say in an anguished voice, "Don't say that. Don't talk about it. There's no way it can happen to me."

Other women have a delayed reaction. They tune out and need to call or come back again to actually register what they have been told. Still others don't seem particularly distressed at the moment. They throw themselves into a conversation about treatment and prognosis, and it is only later, usually on that same day, that the news really hits them.

An Approach to the Diagnosis

As a patient, you don't have any control over how you will be presented with the facts of your illness. But for me as a cancer specialist and for you as a patient, there is an approach to the diagnosis that is most desirable and, ultimately, most beneficial, no matter how the diagnosis has been conveyed. Remember:

- Something *can* be done. This is a difficult problem, but it is possible to deal with it. A program can be devised that will help.

- Breast cancer is certainly not an illness one would choose to have, but it does respond to treatment.

- The most productive attitude for both the doctor and the patient is to approach the illness with a determined and optimistic pragmatism.

ACTING ON THE DIAGNOSIS

After the shock, faced with the knowledge that you have breast cancer, you have to be as smart as you can be.

First, consider again whether the doctor who has presented you with the diagnosis is the right one to continue taking care of you. Refer to the section on pages 14–29 on finding and choosing a doctor. Many insurance companies require a second opinion at this point, before you undergo any further surgery. Even if your policy does not have that restriction, you should consider whether you want to seek that second opinion (see Chapter 2).

Find someone whose attitude, skill, and compassion allow him to say to you, verbally or through his reputation and demeanor, "I care about you. I am here to help you. I can do it well. There is hope." You should feel, after your search, your consultation, and your deliberation, "You are the one I have decided to trust. I will participate in all decisions, but I want you to be my ombudsman, an expert with whom I can share the responsibility for evaluating and treating my illness."

If you cannot enter into a relationship with a doctor feeling confident about both those declarations, look elsewhere.

HOW FAST DO I HAVE TO ACT?

Some of the considerations here are psychological, some medically significant. Whichever factors you want to assess, you should move with all deliberate speed—but you should not, even at this point, rush into a hasty decision.

A sensible goal is to have treatment under way within three to four weeks after diagnosis. Is it dangerous to wait that long? The answer is straightforward: Though growth rates for different types of breast cancer can vary, there is no evidence of a measurable change for any of them in a period of three or four weeks.

If you have selected a surgeon and then are told he cannot operate for a week or two, that is probably fine. Most surgeons will try to schedule your procedure as soon as possible. As with mammographers, excellent surgeons are bound to be busy, but it is almost certainly worth waiting a short time for a surgeon who has both superior technical skill and sound judgment.

In fact, there is a tricky point to consider: If a breast specialist can take you right away, it is legitimate to wonder whether he is busy enough to be the right person for you. Surgeons who have excellent track records, judgment, and experience are almost certain to have crowded schedules, and will rarely be able to operate immediately. Under most circumstances, they are also worth waiting for—not only because, in the language of our trade, they know "how to cut" but also because they know "what to cut." Scheduling an operation may also take a little longer if two surgeons are needed, as when reconstruction is done immediately after a mastectomy (see Chapter 12, Breast Reconstruction).

Nonetheless, getting through the waiting period, or the period in which you are making your choices and decisions, can be very difficult. Some women rush to action. They want to get the whole thing over with, to get the cancer out of their bodies as quickly and thoroughly as possible.

Other women can get stuck in conflicting advice, collecting so much information that they unnecessarily complicate what might otherwise be a fairly simple procedure. Reread Chapter 2 now if you feel you need help in the process of selecting a surgeon. Read the material that follows, in Book II, in order to understand and evaluate the types of treatment that are being offered to you.

ALTERNATIVE TREATMENTS

When you go through Book II, you will notice that there is no chapter on what are popularly called alternative treatments for breast cancer. That is because I consider reliance on such treatments a prescription for tragedy. The only time I ever see what I call nineteenth-century cancers—those that are large and have spread extensively by the time of the first visit—is when a woman comes to me after being treated with unconventional treatments or when she has relied on the curing techniques of disciplines such as Christian Science.

What we are seeing under such circumstances is a missed

opportunity to cure a now-uncontrolled cancer. Standard treatment, as we will see, works to a very large degree. As far as my own and other research has shown, nontraditional treatments do *not* work. If they did, they would certainly be used by many doctors. I honestly do not believe it is the resistance of the medical establishment to unusual techniques that accounts for the fact that most physicians do not rely entirely on dietary or psychological or other unproven modes of treatment.

Physicians want to help people, both for their patients' sakes and for their own. Particularly when we are dealing with people with cancer, we are willing to stretch the boundaries of what may or may not help.

There is generally no harm in vitamin supplements, high-carbohydrate diets, and such, *unless* they delay, interfere with, or replace other proven treatments or cause health problems of their own. Good nutrition, especially when you are sick, is important for your well-being, but it is not a substitute for vigorous, effective treatment. On the other hand, some supplements may actually interfere with the function of established drugs; therefore, your oncologist should know what you are taking to prevent this possibility.

A patient with seriously advanced disease recently told me that she watched the tumor on her breast grow for several months because every time she mentioned it to her "alternative physician," he would tell her that the symptom was unimportant, that "local disease" was the last to respond to his treatment, and that the tumor growth was therefore of no significance!

In Chapter 15, Prevention, we will discuss the question of psychological attitude and cancer. Actually, we will discuss my own strong feeling that you don't get cancer because of your psyche. To intimate that psychological attitude does play such a role unfairly increases the burden on those who are ill. It is the worst instance I know of laying a guilt trip on someone. The same may be said about treating breast cancer with psychological methods.

Certainly you should do everything you can to help yourself approach your illness in a positive, constructive way. You should do everything you can to make yourself feel comfortable emotionally. We don't know everything about the mysterious factors that govern why it is that under similar medical circumstances one patient survives and another does not. We *do* know that enemas, macrobiotic diets, relaxation techniques, deep massage, group healing, and the like are *not* a substitute for good medical treatment.

YOUR PERSONAL ADVOCATE

Though we talked about this earlier, in Chapter 2, it is worth repeating what I think may be a crucial part of your treatment and recovery: The way to be a "good patient" is not to be a docile, obedient one.

Some interesting research has been done that seems to indicate that patients who take an active part in the management of their own illnesses—not just breast cancer—do better than those who passively accept what is prescribed for them. I know that the call to be an active participant in your own treatment can sound intimidating. There may in fact be times when you will be tired or discouraged or frightened, or will simply need help in understanding what is being told to you.

"I've got a really good memory," one of my patients told me. "Part of my job is to store away in my brain all sorts of facts. But after I sat in your office that day and listened to you tell me about my cancer and what you recommended—well, by the time I got home, I couldn't remember anything. I couldn't tell my husband one clear fact—except that I had it."

• You need someone to help you remember.

• You need someone to help you evaluate what is being recommended.

• You need someone whose shoulder you can lean on.

If you have not already done so, by all means try to get yourself a personal advocate, someone who understands that you want his or her presence when you deal with breast cancer. For some women, that person will be their husband or partner. Other women, even if they are part of a couple, will feel that an adult child, or a sister or other relative or a friend, has the steadiness and sympathy and good sense they need.

And those *are* the qualities you want. Someone who has had breast cancer may be the right choice. Someone close to you who is a health worker or doctor may be suitable. But the main ingredients are these three: steadiness, sense, and sympathy.

Talk directly to the person you choose. Don't assume, just because you ask him or her to accompany you to one doctor's visit or a test, that the person realizes you want a continued presence. Explain that you are not asking your advocate to make decisions for you and that you are not going to require a constant babysitter. Do spell out exactly what you have decided you're going to need. Consider the following issues:

• Do you want her to sit in with you during medical consultations?

• Do you want her to participate in conversations with the physicians you consult?

• Do you want her to meet with you before your appointments to help you formulate the questions you should ask?

• Do you want her to take notes?

• Is she someone who will understand if you change your mind? You may decide along the way that you prefer to proceed on your own, or to find a new person to help you. That is perfectly fine. Your first priority is to feel confident in what you are doing, as well as in the people who constitute your support system.

YOUR FEELINGS ABOUT YOUR DIAGNOSIS

WHY ME?

At one time or another during our lives we have all heard the phrase "Why me?" and to a certain extent, at one time or another during our lives, we have all asked that question or shared the feeling it expresses. It is human nature to look around us and wonder why, out of all the people we know, this particular misfortune is being meted out to us.

We will talk in Chapter 15 about the scientific risk factors of any particular woman's getting breast cancer, but it is important to understand that breast cancer is not a punishment for bad or imprudent behavior. Escaping it is not a reward. Despite what you may have read in the popular press, *there is no such thing as a cancer personality*.

As to the philosophical question raised here, I think of the response of one of my patients who asked, "Why *not* me? So many women get breast cancer these days that it's no big surprise any one person gets hit with it."

In fact, after the initial reaction to a positive diagnosis, the question "Why me?" seems to disappear, and most women get on with what they have to do to take care of themselves.

BUT I FEEL FINE

One of the reasons the diagnosis of breast cancer comes as such a shock to many women is that usually they have no symptoms. They aren't short of breath, they don't have any pain, their kidneys are fine, their digestion is normal. They may not even feel a lump. Many patients say they have "never felt better."

And yet they have been told that they have cancer, a grave disease. One woman, in trying to explain this dichotomy to me, held up a strand of her hair. She said, "It's as if someone told me that at the end of this piece of hair there is a knot that can kill me. I would find that very hard to believe, because it isn't causing me the slightest trouble."

All I could think to tell her was that the best thing she could do, if that were the case, would be to get rid of the knot. And that—getting rid of the knot—is what we must turn to next: the treatment of breast cancer.

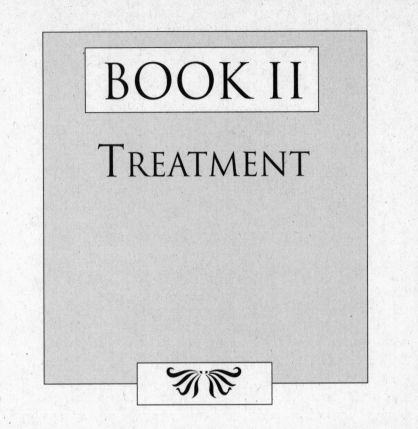

BOOK II

TREATMENT

CHAPTER

7

GENETICS

❦

We do not know why breast cancer is such a common disease, but we do know that some women are at high risk of developing breast cancer because they have an abnormal gene.

This is the fifth edition of this book. A rewarding aspect of each revision has been our ability to report the major ongoing advances that are being made in treatment. Since the fourth edition, the knowledge of the genetics of breast cancer has grown to the point where an understanding of the issues involved may be of significant benefit to you in planning your treatment. This new chapter introduces you to this important, rapidly advancing field.

We inherit genes in pairs, one from each parent. A defective gene has a change in its structure, called a mutation, which interferes with its function. There is an equal chance that a mutated gene can be inherited from your mother or from your father. A person who has a mutated gene is called a carrier. In 1994 and 1995, BRCA1 and BRCA2, two genes related to breast cancer, were cloned—replicated exactly. The procedure of cloning permits large amounts of purified genetic material to be produced so that the structure and function of each gene can be closely studied.

Women who carry the BRCA1 and BRCA2 genes with specific mutations have an increased risk of developing both breast and ovarian cancers. The level of the risk depends on which of the two genes has the mutation. Of all breast cancers, only about 7 percent can be attributed each year to genetic causes (see page 298). Of these hereditary cancers, 45 percent are attributed to BRCA1 and 35 percent to BRCA2. The genetic causes of the remaining 20 percent have not yet been identified. Although these are called breast cancer genes, they are also associated with other tumors. Among them, as noted, is ovarian cancer, although this risk, while substantial, is less than that for breast cancer. Men who are BRCA carriers have an increased incidence of both breast and prostate cancers. There is also evidence that BRCA2 carriers, both female and male, may have an increased risk for pancreatic cancer.

Both BRCA genes are very large molecules that can undergo mutations along their entire length. The nature and the frequency of BRCA mutations vary among national groups. Among Ashkenazi Jews, who are of eastern European origin, two mutations in BRCA1 and one mutation in BRCA2 account for most abnormalities. This is called a "founder's effect." It occurs in isolated homogeneous communities whose populations tend to intermarry, increasing the probability that any who carry a genetic mutation will transmit it to their offspring. (A similar founder's effect also appears in a BRCA2 mutation in Iceland.)

For women with BRCA1 or BRCA2 mutations the lifetime risk of developing breast cancer is 85 percent. For ovarian cancer the risk with BRCA1 is 62 percent and for BRCA2 18 to 27 percent.(See pages 310–13.)

HOW DO I PROCEED?

Tests for the breast cancer genes are now widely available. As a result, more women who have had breast cancer, and their relatives who may not have had breast cancer, will be learning whether they carry a mutation. But gene testing should not be considered the kind of test that provides yes-or-no answers to those who are tested. The results are not always straightforward and if a mutation is found, there are implications of increased risk not only for the person tested but for other family members as well—male and female. Moreover, each of their children has a 50/50 chance of inheriting the gene.

A genetics counselor is uniquely qualified to help you through the testing process. She has had specialized training and can explain to you all aspects of testing, its interpretation and implications, before the test is done.

WHO DOES THE TESTING?

Testing is usually done in hospital-affiliated facilities where a team consisting of a physician and a genetics counselor is available. There are some private physicians who are trained in genetics and conduct testing and counseling in their offices. In general, it is not wise to have the test done in the office of a provider who does not have special expertise in genetics and uses a prepared sheet to outline benefits and risks of testing to you.

WHAT CAN I EXPECT?

You will initially meet with the genetics counselor. She will take a detailed family history, and ask you about any cases of cancer or known hereditary diseases in your family. On the basis of the information you have given her, she will create a "family tree," a diagram that shows whether you truly are at risk for hereditary breast cancer and whether testing is actually indicated. When there has been breast or ovarian cancer in the family, or you are under the age of forty and have a cancer—particularly if you are of Ashkenazi Jewish background—testing is advised. In some cases, a pattern of cancers other than breast-ovarian may exist and point toward a different gene, such as abnormal pTEN or Chek 2. A blood sample is then drawn.

It may take several weeks for the results of testing to be known. Once this happens, you may be reassured—or you may be asked to meet with the physician and genetics counselor team to discuss what precautions, if any, you will be advised to take.

PRIVACY MATTERS

Most of the time women are referred for testing after they have already had some form of cancer treated, either recently or years ago. Later, their relatives who have not had cancer may be tested. BRCA1 and BRCA2 are *susceptibility genes*. A woman who is healthy but carries one of them faces the statistical risks cited earlier, but many such women never develop either breast or ovarian cancer. Knowledge of being a carrier, however, can play an important role in prevention, as discussed in Chapter 15. If you have breast cancer and carry a breast cancer gene, that knowledge may affect your treatment (see below).

If you have breast cancer, this information is already known to your doctors and often to health insurance companies. What if the companies find out that you carry a mutation, regardless of whether you have or haven't had cancer? Will there be discrimination? Will you be less likely to get insurance?

Most insurance companies will cover the costs of testing and genetic consultations if you meet the risk criteria that justify testing. There are laws that protect the privacy of your medical information. Such information can usually be shared only if you sign a permission form for its transmittal—including transmittal to insurance companies. While you may choose not to inform your insurance company and pay for the genetic testing yourself, you should know that many states have laws prohibiting insurance companies from determining your health insurance rates on the basis of genetic information. This year Congress has enacted legislation—the Genetic Information Non-Discrimination Act (GINA) which applies to health insurance and job discrimination. Unfortunately, however, similar assurance cannot be given about how this information will affect your life insurance policy.

HOW MAY KNOWING YOU HAVE A MUTATION AFFECT YOUR TREATMENT?

If you are a carrier, both breasts are at risk for the future development of cancer. If you already have a cancer you will be asked to consider whether mastectomy or even bilateral mastectomy may be more advisable than lumpectomy because of a greater risk that a new tumor will develop in either breast. However, mastectomy is not mandatory in this setting if you are willing to accept future close monitoring of the breasts by imaging techniques such as mammography and MRI.

TIMING

As women and their physicians are becoming more aware of the benefits of knowing genetic information, testing is more frequently being recommended after an initial diagnostic breast biopsy or following lumpectomy and axillary lymph node surgery. The results can be expedited so they can be available in two to three weeks. During this time, systemic therapy can be started and completed. When the results are available, a decision can be made either to follow through with radiation therapy as planned or to have mastectomies and consider reconstructive breast surgery.

CHAPTER

8

SURGERY

S urgery is the first line of defense against most breast cancers, and for most patients it is the primary means by which
a cure can be achieved. That is not a new piece of information. Surgery—cutting the cancer out of the body—has
been the basic treatment for many years. What has changed
are the kinds of treatment that now supplement breast surgery
and the kinds of surgery performed.

It used to be thought "the more the better"—the more tissue
you removed, the better the chance of getting all traces of cancer
and therefore preventing a recurrence. Because of what we have
learned in recent years, less radical surgery has become common.
At the present time, most women whose cancers are detected early
can be treated without breast removal—with the excision of the

cancerous lump, a margin of normal tissue, and some of the underarm lymph nodes, followed by treatment with radiation.

Thirty years ago radical mastectomy—an extensive procedure we will examine in the following pages—was the only treatment for breast cancer. When modified radical mastectomies became more common and a woman asked a surgeon about them, she might be told, "Sure, have a modified radical if you want to play Russian roulette with your life." When, several years later, lumpectomy—which is a partial mastectomy—was developed, the same surgeon might have told an inquiring patient, "Sure, have a lumpectomy if you want to play Russian roulette with your life."

There are people in all walks of life who like doing things the "same old way." They tend to stick with the ideas and methods they are familiar with. Don't choose such a person as your surgeon. Find a surgeon with good judgment, who is open to new ideas, and whose techniques are not limited to what *used to be* standard. To put it plainly, do not choose a surgeon who hasn't changed his ways in twenty years. You should be told of all the options available to you.

The treatment of breast cancer is less standardized than that of many other illnesses. Because they know this, some patients believe that there are many different surgical procedures to choose from. In fact, there are only two:

- The breast is conserved in a procedure commonly known as lumpectomy; this is almost always followed by radiation therapy and sometimes by hormone therapy and/or chemotherapy.

- The breast is removed in an operation called mastectomy. Breast reconstruction may be used after mastectomy, either immediately or at a later date, and systemic treatment may also be used. (Systemic treatment refers to treatment with drugs that travel through the bloodstream, thus circulating throughout the body.)

In both of these approaches, lymph nodes under the arm are always removed if any of the nodes contain malignancy. These surgical procedures and the circumstances under which what kind of surgery is to be done depends on what seems correct for the pathology that was found, the size of the tumor and breast, and what is known about the genetic background of the patient and her family, as well as what is acceptable to the patient.

BEFORE THE SURGERY

DRUGS AND ALLERGIES

If you have been having any discomfort, such as headaches, and have been using any pain medication containing aspirin, you should stop taking it a week or two before surgery, because aspirin may interfere with blood clotting. Blood thinners such as Lovenox, Plavix, and Coumadin need to be discontinued under the direction of your physician. Nonsteroidal anti-inflammatory medications (NSAIDs) also need to be stopped. Prepare a list ahead of time of all medications you are taking, as well as the dosages, and take it with you to the hospital. Be precise in informing the resident or nurse who takes your medical history of these medications. If you have taken aspirin or any other prescription or over-the-counter drug in the past few days, mention it. Also be sure to tell the resident or nurse of any allergies you have, particularly to medications, even though your own physician may already have this information on record.

The use of monoamine oxidase inhibitors (MAOIs), such as Nardil or Parnate, is particularly problematic, and these should be stopped two weeks before surgery. These are antidepressive medicines, and you should check with your physician for possible temporary alternative therapy. It is advisable to stop drinking alcohol and smoking at least two weeks before surgery as well.

HOSPITAL ARRANGEMENTS

Nowadays breast surgery is usually done in an outpatient setting. However, you are likely to be admitted to the hospital if you require an extended period of observation, if a mastectomy is carried out, and, in particular, if breast reconstruction is done. Even if you do enter and leave the hospital on the same day, arrangements have to be made for your admission. Someone in the surgeon's office will make these arrangements. This procedure is necessary to ensure that an operating room and an anesthesiologist are available on the day you are scheduled to have surgery. If necessary, a bed will be reserved in the hospital. In that case, you probably will be asked whether you want a private or semiprivate room, although the hospital often will not be able to accommodate your wishes because of overcrowding. Bear in mind that most hospital insurance covers only semiprivate rooms, so you will have to pay the difference in the daily rate if you choose a private room. Also, remember that even if you are admitted as an inpatient, it will be on the day of surgery.

ADMISSION

Procedures for admission can differ a great deal from hospital to hospital, as do the amount of time you have to wait and the atmosphere of the admitting office. It is a very good idea, if possible, to have someone accompany you. You should also bring something to read, or a crossword puzzle, or anything else that will divert you in case there is a delay.

You will need your insurance card and any other health insurance or relevant Medicare/Medicaid information. The hospital may clear your admission with your insurance carrier. You will be interviewed by an admissions officer and asked for the name of the person who should be notified in case of an emergency.

PREADMISSION TESTING

During the week before surgery, you will have an appointment at the hospital for routine blood tests and an electrocardiogram. Chest X-rays and additional studies may also be ordered. A history and physical examination may be performed as part of this testing or by your own physician.

YOUR GENERAL MEDICAL CONDITION

Because you will not be in the hospital for a medical workup, you should make sure that you report to the anesthesiologist and the surgeon such matters as heart, lung, or circulatory disease; diabetes; or any other current medical conditions you may have. Tell them if you have a cold or an upset stomach, or if you drink, smoke, or use drugs. If you have a defibrillator for your heart you should have clearance from your cardiologist before surgery. Automatic implantable cardioverter defibrillators (AICDs) have to be turned off prior to surgery and it is necessary to know the name of the manufacturer and the model number.

Don't dismiss any detail as too insignificant or embarrassing to mention. It is better for the medical team to be aware of *all* this information than to be surprised by some complication. If you are under the care of a cardiologist or internist, you should also inform that doctor about your surgery. These specialists and your surgeon should communicate with one another so that any appropriate care will be available if you need it.

BLOOD TRANSFUSIONS

Blood transfusions are not used during biopsies or lumpectomies and are rarely needed during most mastectomies. Certain types of breast reconstruction, however, may require transfusion. You should discuss this possibility with your physician and consider whether you want to donate blood yourself before your surgery, to be stored so that it will be on hand should you need it. As far as we know, monitoring for the AIDS virus and other contamination of our stored blood supply is now effective; but many people are understandably concerned about this problem, given the gravity and extent of the AIDS epidemic. You can donate up to two units of your blood at one-week intervals, and if there is enough lead time before your surgery, you may want to do that. As we have said, you probably won't need blood, but there is no harm in discussing the possibility of transfusion with your surgeon.

TALK TO THE SURGEON

You should have a clear understanding of what is going to be done, and the reasons for any particular procedure. You should also be aware of any risks of the surgery, which leads to a pre-surgery formality, the informed consent form, that many patients find quite troubling.

INFORMED CONSENT

After you have been admitted to the hospital, the usual procedure is that before your surgery, you will be asked to sign an **informed consent** form. Your doctor or a staff resident with whom he works should present this form to you. It should be given to you prior to any sedation, which can affect your alertness, and enough in advance of the surgery so you can read it carefully without feeling pressured. The form usually will specify:

• The name of the surgical procedure

• Which breast is being operated on, right or left

• The doctor's name

• That the risks of the surgery and the anesthetic have been explained to you

• That intravenous medication, including drugs, anesthesia, and blood transfusions, may be administered

• That any tissue or parts that are removed during the surgery may be examined and disposed of

• That you understand all of the foregoing and that you consent

Some forms ask a lot more. They may ask for consent to videotape or televise the procedure. They may ask you to consent in advance should the surgeon decide during the course of the operation that other measures are necessary.

These forms are so broadly drawn because they were designed to cover many types of surgery. In abdominal surgery, for example, there is a strong possibility that unforeseen complications may arise. Breast surgery, on the other hand, is a fairly straightforward operation, and there are rarely any complications.

If the procedure specified on the form has a different name than that which you and the surgeon agreed upon, ask that it be changed. The form should very explicitly state the surgery you have consented to undergo. If there is anything else on the form that worries you, ask to see your doctor. Make sure you understand and feel comfortable with what you are signing. Cross out and initial anything you don't agree to. You should not be going into surgery worried about the fine print on a consent form. You might even want to ask your surgeon whether you can have the form to study a few days in advance so you can make sure you are comfortable with it.

Informed consent forms were designed to make sure that doctors tell patients precisely what is planned for them as well as the risks involved. The form obviously also protects the doctor, in that it spells out what he has told the patient he plans to do. In a sense, however, the form is less important than it looks. The physician is responsible for what he does, whatever the form says. And, from another perspective, the best insurance against mishap in surgery is not informed consent but an excellent doctor.

A COMPANION

If you are going to have ambulatory surgery (see page 120), you are required to have someone with you to help you get home. Your relative or friend will be asked to wait in the waiting room until you recover from the immediate effects of surgery and anesthesia. If your surgery is more complex—for instance, if it includes breast reconstruction—you will be admitted to the hospital after surgery is completed. If that is to happen, ask the surgeon in advance how long it will take before you will be brought to your room after surgery. He may then be able to arrange for your companion, whether a family member or friend, to wait for you in your room. Of course, any estimate of time should include possible delays before the procedure and should take into account the time of the surgery and the time afterward in the recovery room. Make a definite arrangement about when and where the surgeon will meet with your friend or relative to report on how the surgery went. After surgery, there is often needless confusion and anxiety for the family and the physician because they have trouble finding each other.

Remind your family or friends that the surgeon will be able to tell them whether the operation went well, whether there were any complications, and what your general condition is. Remember, however, that he will not be able to give them the kind of detailed information about your condition that will be available only after the pathologist's report, nor will he be able to say exactly how long you will be in the hospital or what the next step in your treatment will be.

NURSING

Many of my patients ask whether, if they are admitted, they should hire a private-duty nurse to be with them after the surgery. If you can afford it, or if your insurance covers the cost, do it. Make the arrangement before your surgery so that the nurse will be there when you are brought back to your room. Hospital nursing staffs are very lean in these economically difficult times, and your own nurse, for at least the first two shifts after your surgery, can be enormously helpful in doing such things as monitoring your blood pressure, giving you a bedpan or taking you to the bathroom, administering your medications, and keeping you comfortable. Particularly if you are having a complicated breast reconstruction, well-trained private-duty nurses are a necessity. If your insurance company is reluctant to pay for private-duty nurses, ask your surgeon whether he can write a note explaining why such nursing is essential.

If it is not possible for you to manage the cost of private-duty nursing, ask a competent friend or family member to stay with you, if possible, for the remainder of the day and the night following your surgery.

FOOD AND DRINK

You will be instructed not to eat or drink anything after midnight of the night before the surgery is scheduled.

OTHER PREPARATIONS

Your armpit may be shaved in preparation for lymph node surgery (see pages 133–35).

You will be asked to remove all jewelry (including watches, chains, and rings), as well as any eyeglasses, contact lenses, hearing aids, or dental bridges. Give these things to your companion to keep for you. Metallic body piercings should be removed, if possible.

Because electrical instruments used during surgery may react with synthetic fabrics, any underpants you wear must be cotton.

GETTING READY FOR THE SURGERY

As we saw when we discussed surgical biopsy:

1. The surgeon will put on a scrub suit, cap, and mask. He will scrub his hands and then be helped into a sterile gown and sterile gloves.

2. The patient's skin in the area to be operated upon will be cleaned, usually with an antiseptic solution called Betadine.

3. The patient's body will be covered with a sterile drape, leaving uncovered only the area to be operated upon.

MONITORING DEVICES AND OTHER AUXILIARY EQUIPMENT

You will be very carefully watched all during the surgery:

• A cuff will be placed on your arm to measure your blood pressure.

• An electrocardiograph machine will monitor your heart rate.

• A clip will be placed on your fingertip to measure blood oxygen and to monitor the conduct of the anesthesia.

- If you require full anesthesia, a tube may be placed in your throat to help you breathe after you are asleep.

- A grounding pad will be placed on the thigh, because an electric cautery may be used.

- Stockings that prevent clotting through compression will be placed on your lower legs.

- Sometimes during an extended operation, a kind of boot that provides intermittent pressure to the lower legs may also be used to prevent clots from forming in your legs.

- For an extended operation a tube (catheter) will be placed in your bladder to measure urine output during surgery.

In sum, the latest technical equipment will be brought into play in the operating room to make the surgery as risk-free as possible. Much of this equipment will be hooked up while you're still awake, and there may be conversations going on among a fair number of doctors, nurses, and technicians. There may also be a lot of noise as equipment is put into place.

Patients sometimes say that they feel as if they are being completely ignored during what one woman described as "all that frenzied activity." The fact is, people are preparing for the surgery about to be performed and are getting you ready to receive its benefits. That is what most of the bustle is about. It is, however, inexcusable for medical personnel to alarm the patient by thoughtless comments. The anesthesiologist and the surgeon should take a few minutes to talk to you in as reassuring a manner as possible, but it is also wise to remember that this is a very busy time for everyone in the operating room.

ANESTHESIA

An anesthesiologist is a specialist who, after receiving a medical degree, went through several years of training in anesthesiology, the science of administering drugs that induce a loss of sensation and of consciousness.

The first thing to say about anesthesia is that you should meet the anesthesiologist yourself and talk to her, person to person, before your surgery.

• She should take your medical history and ask you, among other details, about any problems with the functioning of your heart, your lungs, or your circulation.

• Any allergies should be carefully reviewed, as well as any prior experiences you have had with anesthesia.

• Tell the anesthesiologist anything you think may be relevant. If you have a cold, tell her. This is not a time for secrets. It's another chance to make sure that all the details of your condition are known. Remind the anesthesiologist if you are a heavy smoker or drink a lot or use drugs or other substances. If a nurse asks you the same questions, answer her as well. It is in your own interest to be frank.

The type of surgery as well as the patient's medical history determine what anesthesia will be used. However, since breast surgery is a fairly superficial procedure, on the "outside" of the body, it does not require the deep anesthesia necessary for abdominal or chest surgery.

In general, for most breast surgery the following sequence will be followed:

1. When you get to the operating room or just before you are brought there, an intravenous infusion, an IV, will be started. A fine catheter, which is connected by tubing to a plastic container through which fluids and any intravenous anesthesia will be administered, will be placed in your arm.

2. You will be given an intravenous medication such as Versed. This drug is a sedative that makes you drowsy. Another medication, such as Diprivan (propofol), will put you to sleep instantly, though its effects last for a relatively short time.

3. If only a limited surgical procedure is planned, pain will be controlled with a local anesthetic, such as Xylocaine, which is

injected into the skin of the breast. The combination of intravenous sedation and pain control by local infiltration (injection) is known as "monitored anesthesia care" or MAC.

4. Should deeper anesthesia be needed, once you are asleep this can be accomplished by administering an intravenous agent such as Diprivan (propofol).

5. Anesthesia will continue to be administered as long as the surgery is in progress.

6. Throughout the surgery the anesthesiologist will carefully monitor your vital signs (heart rate, blood pressure, respiration, and blood oxygen content), making sure that your body's systems are functioning well.

THE SURGICAL PROCEDURES

MASTECTOMY

WHAT IS A MASTECTOMY?

Mastectomy is the surgical removal of the breast.

WHAT ARE THE TYPES OF MASTECTOMIES?

Modified radical, radical, total, and partial mastectomies are the general categories. As we have seen, *lumpectomy* is the term commonly used when only a limited portion of the entire breast is removed. *Breast conservation* is another way of expressing it. You may hear the term *Halstead* used to describe a radical mastectomy, and *simple* used in place of *total*. The circumstances under which each type of surgery is appropriate are discussed below.

MODIFIED RADICAL MASTECTOMY

We begin with the modified radical mastectomy, because it is the mastectomy most commonly performed in the treatment of

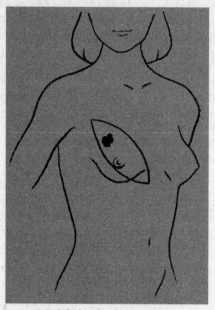

Modified radical mastectomy

breast cancer. In fact, because it has the best long-term results, it is the surgical technique against which the effectiveness of all other treatments for breast cancer are currently measured.

A "modified radical," as it is often referred to, consists of the removal of:

• The entire breast that we can actually see protruding from the chest, including the nipple and the areola

• The nonprotruding breast tissue, which extends toward the breastbone, the collarbone, the lowest ribs, and back toward the muscle at the side of the body (the latissimus dorsi)

• The lymph nodes in the armpit

• The minor pectoral muscle, which is removed only if it interferes with the removal of the lymph nodes. The loss of this muscle is barely perceptible afterward. The major pectoral muscle, which forms the chest wall underneath the breast, is not removed in a modified radical procedure (see "Radical Mastectomy," page 137).

The Incision

The actual surgery should be tailored to the patient's anatomy, taking into consideration the position of the tumor and of any previous biopsy, as well as any plans for reconstruction. The incision extends from the border of the breastbone toward the armpit. It is in the shape of an ellipse; we try to avoid a vertical incision, and we try to keep it slightly away from the breastbone so the scar won't be visible in low-cut clothing. Though we also hope to avoid creating any unsightly folds, unfortunately this often does occur in heavier women.

The Surgical Procedure

The skin and the layer of fat beneath it are cut with a scalpel or an electrocautery instrument. A laser, a surgical instrument that uses a narrow beam of intense energy, is sometimes used for breast surgery. Personally, I don't think it has any advantages; you can achieve the same precision with a scalpel as with a laser, and using a laser prolongs the time the surgery takes.

The breast is then removed from the underlying muscles of the chest wall, along with the covering (fascia) which forms the "sac" that envelops the breast tissue. The major pectoral muscle is not removed.

THE AXILLARY LYMPH NODES

WHY REMOVE THE NODES?

No matter where in the breast a cancer is located, the lymphatic system of the breast drains primarily into the lymph nodes of the axilla, the armpit. For that reason it is crucial that we examine these underarm lymph nodes to see whether cancer is present. Until recently, the only way to accomplish this was to remove all of them for examination. It is now possible to target and sample just a few nodes (the sentinel nodes); if they are free of disease, no additional nodes have to be removed. Only if they show evidence

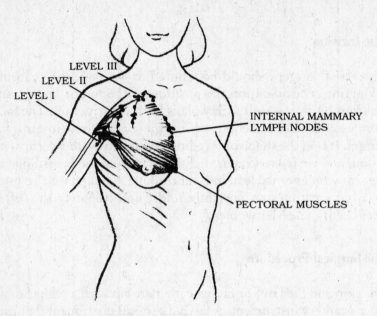

The lymphatic system of the breast

of malignancy do we have to completely remove the lymph nodes in the armpit, as was done in the past.

Lymph node involvement is the single most important factor in planning treatment of breast cancer and in assessing prognosis. As we saw on pages 41–43, it is vital to the process of staging, the essential measuring tool in the treatment of cancer.

WHERE ARE THE LYMPH NODES THAT DRAIN THE BREAST?

The lymph nodes of the breast start in what is sometimes called the tail, the breast tissue that extends up toward the axilla. The nodes in this area are called **Level I** nodes. **Level II** nodes are located just beneath the pectoralis minor muscle. **Level III** nodes are at the apex of the armpit, beyond the pectoralis minor.

The nodes are not arranged in a neat trail, like pearls on a string, but are instead embedded in fat pads. And in this fact lies the answer to many of the questions women have about lymph node excision. Because the nodes are arranged in complex networks and are not all apparent at the time of surgery:

• We cannot predict in advance exactly how many nodes we will get.

• We cannot take the same number from all patients.

• We cannot tell accurately the total number of nodes any individual has or therefore the percentage that have been removed or that are cancerous.

Axillary Dissection

Complete Axillary Dissection

Removing lymph nodes at all levels, I, II, and III, is an operation known as a complete axillary dissection. This provides a full picture of nodes involved by breast cancer. Unfortunately, such surgery is also associated with a risk of subsequent swelling of the arm, called lymphedema.

Sentinel Lymph Node Biopsy

During the last decade an effort has been made to reduce the number of lymph nodes that have to be removed. The concept that underlies the sentinel node approach is based on the fact that the lymphatics of the breast drain first to particular lymph nodes (one or more) in the adjacent armpit. These are referred to as sentinel nodes. To find these nodes, a blue dye that diffuses quickly into lymphatic channels is injected into the affected breast a few minutes before surgery starts. Alternatively, a fluid containing a low level of radioactive material (an isotope) is injected into the breast a few hours to a day prior to the surgery. When an incision is made under the arm, the surgeon can usually see the first nodes that pick up dye, or, with a detector, can find those that have picked up the isotope. The same sentinel nodes are usually detected by both the dye and the isotope. These nodes are removed and may be immediately examined by the pathologist with a frozen section. Only if cancer is found is complete axillary dissection done. To increase the reliability of the sentinel node procedure, the nodes are not only tested by the pathologist using standard tissue-staining techniques but are also examined using a more sensitive cytokeratin test, in an effort to detect even a minute number of cells that may have escaped from the tumor to one of these nodes.

Just as important as the skill of the surgeon in finding and removing nodes is the expertise of the pathologist who does an intensive examination of the lymph nodes once they reach the laboratory, and of the physician in the nuclear medicine department who injects the breast with the isotope.

The sentinel node technique has revolutionized the treatment of breast cancer. It has the potential to:

• Decrease the need for axillary node dissection by 75 percent.

• Make it possible for most breast cancer operations to be done on an outpatient basis.

• Reduce the occurrence of swelling of the arm.

It has not replaced complete axillary dissection, because:

• It is relatively new and not all surgeons have sufficient experience with it.

• The significance of finding minute numbers of cells in lymph nodes stained by the cytokeratin technique is still being studied to determine whether an axillary node dissection is always necessary.

This technique is not used if, prior to surgery, the lymph nodes are enlarged and known or suspected to contain tumor cells, in which case a complete axillary dissection is needed. Furthermore, it may not always be feasible in cases where surgical biopsies have been performed that have left large cavities or hematomas (masses of blood) in the breast.

Nevertheless, this approach offers new hope of reducing the side effects of lymph node surgery, in particular lymphedema (see page 146). You should discuss it with your surgeon and find out if this is right for you, as well as whether he has had enough experience to feel comfortable in performing the procedure. In fact, you should be operated on only by a surgeon who is experienced in performing sentinel lymph node biopsies.

Specific information about the nodes is usually not available immediately after the surgery. It is only after the pathology report that we can tell how many nodes were analyzed and how many were cancerous. In fact, this is all we need to know: The most accurate prediction of the outcome arises out of the *number* of nodes involved, and to a much lesser extent, the proportion of involved nodes to the total removed.

HOW ARE THE AXILLARY NODES REMOVED?

In the standard modified radical mastectomy, these procedures are followed:

1. As the breast is being separated from the muscle, the axilla is approached through the same incision.

2. Fat pads, usually from levels I and II, are removed by separating them from the adjacent structures: the vein that lies in the axilla, the nerves, and the chest wall.

3. Unlike the procedure in a radical mastectomy, in a modified radical, the nodes on level III are rarely removed. If there is reason to believe they are diseased, however, the pectoralis minor muscle can be removed so that we can more easily reach these level III nodes.

4. The pads of fat, along with the breast tissue that was removed, are sent to the pathologist for analysis.

5. When a sentinel node biopsy is performed, the modified radical mastectomy starts with the armpit part of the incision and the removal of the sentinel nodes. Only after this is completed does surgery to remove the breast begin.

HOW IS THE SURGERY COMPLETED?

1. After the breast and nodes have been removed, plastic tubes, called drains, are placed beneath the skin of the breast and the pectoral muscle. These tubes drain the fluid that will collect in the spaces created by the surgery. At the places where the tubes emerge, they are sutured to the skin and attached to a small bulblike device in which there is a vacuum that fills with this fluid.

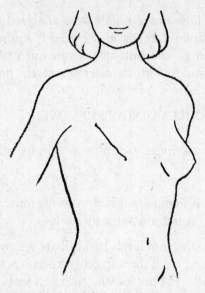

Completed modified radical mastectomy

2. The incision is closed with absorbable sutures or with metal staples. Though there are varying degrees of skill among surgeons, the aim is to close an incision so that when it heals, the scar will be thin and flat on the chest wall. The incision for a modified radical may be fairly long, depending on breast size, and it may be under tension, depending on its placement on the chest. Therefore, the wound may not heal absolutely uniformly. Still, it is important to remember that there are surgeons whose results, from an aesthetic point of view, are regularly quite good.

All mastectomies should be planned with breast reconstruction in mind, whether or not specific plans have been made for it at this point. It is not necessary for a plastic surgeon to be present merely for the closing of the incision. If, however, you and your surgeon have decided that you will have breast reconstruction at the same time as your mastectomy, then of course the plastic surgeon will be standing by. For further information on how such a decision is made and on the details of breast reconstruction, see Chapter 12.

3. The wound is dressed with protective bandages. I prefer to use a light dressing. I don't think you need a lot of pressure from a bulky dressing to "bind" the wound, because the use of suction drains makes it possible for the skin to "stick down" to the chest wall.

TOTAL (SIMPLE) MASTECTOMY

Total (or simple) mastectomy is a procedure that is the same as the first part of a modified radical mastectomy. However, only the breast is removed—*not* the axillary lymph nodes. Total mastectomy is used as the curative procedure for ductal carcinoma in situ. It is also used when prophylactic surgery is performed (see page 140).

RADICAL MASTECTOMY

Radical mastectomy involves the removal of the breast, the muscles of the chest wall, and sometimes so much skin that skin grafting may be necessary. This deforming breast surgery, which women feared for so many years, is rarely performed today, because most breast cancers are found early, before they have invaded the muscle. The physical and psychological results of this operation were traumatic, and very different from what we commonly achieve today.

This procedure was developed in the late nineteenth century by William S. Halstead, and his name is still used to describe a radical mastectomy. It was the only breast surgery available until the development and use of the "modified radical" in 1948 in England, and in the 1970s in America.

Because the major pectoral muscle is removed, the natural contour of the chest wall is lost, arm mobility may be affected for a time, and breast reconstruction (see Chapter 12) is more difficult.

An even more extreme version of this procedure removed the lymph nodes behind the breastbone as well as a segment of the ribs. Called an extended radical mastectomy, or a super-radical, it is no longer in use.

PARTIAL MASTECTOMY

A partial mastectomy is the removal of part of the breast. Depending on the extent of the procedure, this may also be called wide excision or quadrantectomy. The more general and more commonly used term for preserving the breast, treating it without removing it, is *lumpectomy*. In this procedure, the cancerous tissue plus a margin of healthy tissue is removed, as are some axillary lymph nodes. The surgery is always followed by radiation treatment of the breast; and as with a mastectomy, adjuvant hormone therapy or chemotherapy is usually used (see page 186).

Breast conservation is the newest of procedures, and the surgical techniques are still developing. There may be differences in the way equally competent surgeons approach these operations. The material that follows in this chapter is, of course, a description of the techniques and practices that I use. If it differs from what your surgeon plans for you, discuss that with him. His ideas may be absolutely right for you, your cancer, and your anatomy.

LUMPECTOMY/WIDE EXCISION

If the tumor is small in relation to the whole breast, its removal, plus the removal of about 2 centimeters (¾ inch) of healthy tissue all around if possible, is called a lumpectomy, or a wide excision. Sometimes enough tissue is taken at the time of the excisional biopsy that a separate procedure is not necessary.

Quadrantectomy

If 20 to 25 percent of the breast (a quarter, or quadrant) is removed, along with the overlying skin, the procedure is called a quadrantectomy. Obviously, the breast will be smaller after this procedure.

WHEN DO PARTIAL MASTECTOMIES YIELD GOOD COSMETIC RESULTS?

The purpose of partial mastectomy is to cure the disease and preserve the breast. While it is safe, in many cases, to use this procedure with tumors up to 4 centimeters (1½ inches) in size, other factors must also be considered:

• Removing a large tumor from a large breast may result in a nearly normal-looking breast. Taking the same size tumor out of a small breast would not yield an attractive result.

• Because we must always have a clear margin of healthy tissue, wide excisions of tumors in the center of the breast or in the areola may not yield good aesthetic results. Such tumors are better treated with mastectomy. It is sometimes possible to achieve safe and clear margins by removing the nipple and areola—a central quadrantectomy. Some women may prefer this to losing a breast.

• While it is desirable to have generous margins, this is frequently not feasible or necessary at the anterior aspect of the specimen (near the skin) or at the posterior aspect (near the muscle of the chest wall). Therefore, findings with regard to margin need to be interpreted by your surgeon as well as by the pathologist.

• If more than one tumor is present, several wide excisions may also preclude a satisfactory appearance.

Surgical Procedure for Partial Mastectomy

1. The incision for partial mastectomy must be carefully individualized to the woman's anatomy and to the size and location of the tumor. An experienced surgeon can in most instances perform a very safe operation whose results look good afterward.

   • If the tumor is in the upper part of the breast, we try to make the incision in a curved line, as close to the areola as possible, within the boundaries of where clothing would normally fall.

   • In what is called the upper outer quadrant—the upper quarter near the armpit—we may be able to remove the nodes and the tumor through the same incision. For other sections of the breast, a separate incision is required for the armpit. Some surgeons believe you should always use two separate incisions, but this is a matter of personal preference.

- Tumors in the lower part of the breast usually require an incision that extends from the center of the breast to the perimeter. Called a radial incision, it does not need to be big or unsightly in order to be adequate (in most situations).

2. After the incision is made, the tumor is removed, along with a margin of healthy tissue that is as wide as possible without causing deformity.

3. The tissue is sent immediately to the pathologist.

4. If an axillary dissection is needed, the nodes are then removed, either through the primary incision or through an incision in the armpit itself, and sent to the pathologist.

HOW IS THE SURGERY COMPLETED?

The surgery is completed by closing and dressing the wound as described on pages 136–37. In a lumpectomy, the incision is closed with great attention to cosmetic results, since that is a major objective of this procedure. A plastic drain may be placed in the wound in the axilla if a complete node dissection has been done, but it is rarely placed in the breast itself or in the axilla after a sentinel node biopsy.

PROPHYLACTIC MASTECTOMY

This term refers to mastectomies that are done before any breast cancer has appeared. It is discussed later, in Chapter 15, Prevention (page 316), and is primarily considered for women with an established high genetic risk of developing breast cancer. In such cases, total mastectomy is the operation carried out.

ONCOPLASTIC SURGERY

When they remove tumors, excellent surgeons always place incisions carefully so that they are as inconspicuous as possible and

Wide excision

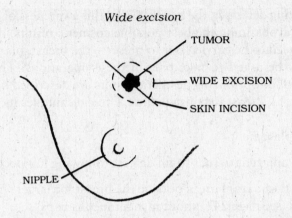

TUMOR

WIDE EXCISION

SKIN INCISION

NIPPLE

Quadrantectomy

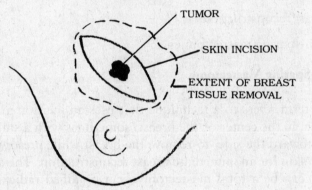

TUMOR

SKIN INCISION

EXTENT OF BREAST
TISSUE REMOVAL

Incisions that are used

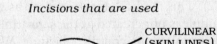
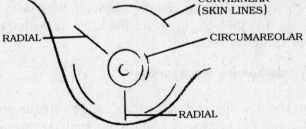

CURVILINEAR
(SKIN LINES)

RADIAL

CIRCUMAREOLAR

RADIAL

avoid creating defects in the breast. Given this awareness of the importance of obtaining the best possible cosmetic results, if larger incisions need to be carried out to preserve the breast, plastic surgeons may be asked to take part in these operations. The techniques used for optimizing aesthetic results are described here and in Chapter 12, Breast Reconstruction. These techniques include:

- Incision placement

- Rotating adjacent tissues to fill defects following lumpectomy

- Bringing tissue from areas outside the breast for larger excisions (see page 242, about myocutaneous flaps)

- Reducing the opposite breast to provide symmetry after a single mastectomy or a lumpectomy

- Breast reconstructions

- Skin-sparing mastectomies

Skin-Sparing Mastectomy

This term refers to a technique that uses an incision around the areola, in the center of the breast, sometimes with a small extension toward the side, to remove the breast while preserving most of its skin for an immediate breast reconstruction. The operation itself can be a total mastectomy or a modified radical mastectomy, and a sentinel node biopsy can be performed. The volume of the reconstructed breast has to be sufficient to fill the skin envelope that has been saved. A TRAM flap is best if it can be done (see Chapter 12). This method does not work as well with an implant. A new nipple is not created at the same time; it is done in a second procedure, following complete healing. With skin-sparing mastectomy, it is possible to create the most normal-appearing breast, with minimal scars.

Nipple-Areola–Sparing Mastectomy

Similar to the skin-sparing mastectomy, this technique preserves the nipple and the areola. It is not commonly performed surgery and should be carried out only by a breast surgeon who has experience with this technique. There are special conditions when it is considered safe; among them are when the mastectomy is a prophylactic mastectomy, when it is for in situ and small invasive breast cancers, and when the cancer is located at a distance from the center of the breast.

After the Surgery

THE RECOVERY ROOM

When you wake up after the surgery, you will find yourself in the recovery room with other postoperative patients.

Your condition will be carefully observed by the specialized nurses who staff these rooms. Your heart rate, blood pressure, and respiration will be monitored, and you will be kept in this room until you are fully awake and your condition has stabilized.

If you feel any pain, tell the recovery room nurse. Orders for pain medication will have been written by the surgeon or the anesthesiologist, and the nurse will be ready to give you the drug if you need it.

You may feel cold after you awaken from the surgery. Shivering is part of the recovery process after anesthesia. Ask for more blankets if you need them. You may want to bring a warm blanket with you to the hospital in case there is not an ample supply. I advise my patients to do this, though you will not be permitted to use it in the recovery room itself.

HOW LONG IS THE HOSPITAL STAY?

Because of government and hospital reimbursement regulations, the current trend is to keep patients in the hospital for as short a time as is feasible. In fact, many patients welcome the opportunity to go home earlier, thanks to improvements in anesthesia and pain medications. Nowadays that means the following:

• For a mastectomy, usually one to two days

• For a mastectomy with reconstruction, one to six days, depending on the method used

- For a quadrantectomy or partial mastectomy with axillary dissection, usually overnight

- For a lumpectomy with sentinel node biopsy, a same-day ambulatory procedure

REMOVING DRAINS, SUTURES, AND STAPLES

- After a mastectomy, if two drains are used, we usually remove one of them on the second or third day after surgery and leave the other drain in place until after the patient goes home from the hospital. It is removed during a subsequent office visit, when the wound is no longer draining. A drain may be needed for one to two weeks. Do not worry if it needs to remain longer; this does not mean that anything is wrong. After the drains are removed, if fluid collects at the site of surgery, it can be easily removed in the doctor's office, with minimal discomfort, using a syringe and needle.

- When the breast has been conserved, a drain may be used only if an axillary dissection was done; it is removed on a subsequent office visit.

- Because we ordinarily use sutures that are absorbed into the body, there is no need to remove them.

- Staples are removed at the time of an office visit.

PAIN

Aside from some pain that may occur from an incision in the armpit, neither partial nor modified radical mastectomies cause much discomfort. Because this is a major concern, I have talked about it with literally thousands of women and have asked them to describe to me what these procedures feel like. Almost every woman reports "an uncomfortable day of surgery and first night, but no real pain," and my patients seem to use very little medication after that first night.

Though it is not pain, many women feel a sensation of tightness at the site of the surgery after a modified radical mastectomy.

This feeling markedly improves after the first few weeks, though some feeling of tightness may linger for several months.

NUMBNESS

During the removal of the lymph nodes, we come in contact with the nerves that control sensation at the back of the underarm area. You may therefore experience temporary or permanent numbness at this site.

With a modified radical mastectomy, there is a general numbness of the chest wall within the area of incision. Most women say that the numbness improves in a few months and eventually disappears. For some, however, it may take several years to improve and, while much better, may never feel completely normal.

INFECTION

Since women know that the lymph nodes are part of the immune system, they quite understandably worry that the removal of underarm nodes will increase their risk of infection. The truth of the matter is that there are many groups of lymph nodes throughout the body and, proportionately, the number that is removed during an axillary dissection is insignificant.

Though there is no general impairment of the immunological system, complete axillary node removal does interfere with the lymphatic drainage of the arm. Because of the altered lymphatic drainage, the arm will be less able to handle infection. To prevent infection:

• Avoid going to manicurists.

• Don't cut or push at the cuticles of your fingernails. This is the place where most arm infections start.

• If blood samples need to be taken in future examinations, ask that the doctor or technician use the arm with intact lymph nodes. Though it is unlikely that this procedure will cause an infection, there is no inconvenience in using the other arm for this purpose.

Many physicians say you should avoid allowing your blood pressure to be measured on the affected arm, but there is no evidence that this causes any trouble.

The fact is that infections develop only rarely, though any needle puncture or breaking of the skin can cause problems. In addition to manicure incidents, the most common offenders are burns, thorns, embedded particles of steel wool, and insect bites.

If by any chance you notice any of the following symptoms, call the surgeon. He will prescribe antibiotics that will usually clear up any infection quickly and safely.

• Splotchy redness on the arm or chest

• Pain or tenderness, often starting along the inner side of the elbow but at times severe throughout the arm

• Pain at the front of the chest wall

LYMPHEDEMA

Swelling, or edema, of the arm used to be more common when radical mastectomy was followed by radiation therapy. This combination often interfered with lymph drainage in the arm. With the modified radical mastectomy, however, more lymphatic channels are left intact. Nevertheless, the removal of lymph nodes, particularly if followed by cycles of low-grade infections in the arm, may lead to swelling of the arm in some women. About 10 to 20 percent of women who have had this surgery may develop noticeable lymphedema after a few years. With lumpectomies such edema is less frequent, and though it is often mild, in some women it is more significant and may cause troublesome problems. You should call your surgeon if you have pain or swelling in your arm. Early intervention with antibiotics may be helpful. If the edema persists, treatment by physical therapists who are trained in special massage techniques may be required. The National Lymphedema Network can provide advice and referrals to qualified therapists (see resources in Book IV).

Given the minimal number of lymph nodes removed by the sentinel node procedure, the risk of swelling or infection of the arm is lessened, but it still makes sense to be careful.

PHLEBITIS

After an incision is made in the axilla, even that of a breast biopsy, a very superficial vein of the affected arm may develop a clot. Called phlebothrombosis, this condition is not serious, because the clot is not in a vital part of the vascular system. On occasion, this may actually be a dilated lymphatic channel, not a vein.

When this condition is present, you may find that after you have already recovered the full range of motion of your arm (see below), you are suddenly able to do less. You may feel as if there were a wire in your arm that keeps you from fully extending it. Though these symptoms may seem alarming, treatment is usually not required. The condition can be uncomfortable, however, and may take four to six weeks to disappear.

ACTIVITY

It seems to me that women recover most quickly and best if they return to normal activities as soon as possible after the surgery. Patients sometimes worry that the stitches won't hold or that the wound will open, or that some other mishap will occur.

As a rule, mastectomy incisions on the chest do not pull apart. You have to be more selective in the kinds of exercises you do if there was an axillary incision; no one ought to lift weights or serve overhand in tennis, for example, with an unhealed wound under the arm. If you have any questions about a particular activity, discuss it with your surgeon.

What follows is not an inflexible schedule, but one that reflects the pace and level of activity under which patients seem to do best. It may be slightly altered if there is breast reconstruction at the same time as the surgery.

• Get out of bed within a few hours after the surgery.

• Begin arm exercises (see below) the morning after surgery.

• Resume a normal schedule of activity a few days after lumpectomy.

• Resume a normal schedule of activity two to three weeks after mastectomy.

ARM EXERCISES

Nowadays most women do not find that the range of motion of their arm is limited after breast surgery. Therefore, exercises specifically for arm strengthening are not necessary.

All we do in my practice is ask women to do simple stretches, while seated, starting the morning after surgery. You should be able to do these fairly easily within a few days. In the first exercise, grasp both hands together in your lap, lift your arms—elbows out—over your head, and finally rest your clasped hands at the back of your neck. In the next exercise, as in calisthenics or aerobics, bring the arms up, out, forward, and down. First raise them straight up, then extend them horizontally, bring them forward and together directly in front of you, and finally lower them onto your lap.

WHEN CAN I BATHE?

You can take a shower when the drains and the staples or any sutures have been removed. You can take a bath when the wound has healed, or earlier if a waterproof dressing is used.

REACH TO RECOVERY

The American Cancer Society trains women who have had breast cancer to act as volunteers in helping current patients. It can be very reassuring to talk to someone who has "been there" and also to receive printed information on matters like the use of a prosthesis (see pages 237–39) and other postoperative questions you may have. Someone in your surgeon's office can usually put you in touch with the Reach to Recovery organization if you think it would be helpful or you can call the American Cancer Society directly at 1-800-ACS-2345.

How Do I Know Which Type of Surgery Is Right for Me?

Our basic job is to get rid of the cancer and prevent its spread and recurrence, if possible, while preserving the breast. In order to accomplish that task, we have to understand the nature or pathology of the malignancy; its stage, including its size and how much it has spread; its location in the breast; and the size of the breast itself. We also have to give serious consideration to what you yourself prefer.

The following sections describe the general circumstances under which each type of surgery is appropriate.

STAGE 0 CANCER

Stage 0 cancers are noninfiltrating cancers confined to the lobules and ducts.

Lobular carcinoma in situ (LCIS), generally speaking, requires no surgery after the biopsy. It should, however, be very carefully watched. Mammography and a physical examination by a doctor should be regularly scheduled, because this in situ cancer is what we call a marker of risk. Twenty percent of women with this symptom develop infiltrating cancers over a twenty-year period, and there is a likelihood that both breasts are at risk. Recent evidence suggests that the risk of developing infiltrating cancer can be significantly reduced with hormone therapy (see page 187). Bilateral prophylactic mastectomies are rarely advised but may be appropriate under special circumstances:

• If there have been recurrent lumps that required biopsy.

• If mammograms show calcifications that are difficult to interpret.

• If there is an extremely strong family history of breast cancer or the presence of an abnormal breast cancer–causing gene: BRCA1 or BRCA2 (see page 114).

In the past, duct cell carcinoma in situ (DCIS) was usually discovered after a biopsy for a nipple discharge or ulceration. With the recent improvements in mammography, we are now able to pick up very early abnormalities, and over 20 percent of the women we treat for breast cancer have DCIS.

To treat DCIS, we usually do a lumpectomy or wide excision (often there is no lump). This is frequently followed by radiation therapy. Alternatively a total mastectomy may be done, usually accompanied by a sentinel node biopsy or the removal of a few lymph nodes near the tail of the breast.

Which procedure to choose poses a dilemma. We know that if we preserve the breast with excision and radiotherapy, there is a 1 percent a year recurrence rate. With a mastectomy the lifetime risk is well under 1 percent, but the patient is left without a breast. Of those who have a recurrence, half will again have in situ cancer and can be successfully treated with a total mastectomy. The other half will have infiltrating disease. Some of them will be cured, but some lives will be lost. Typically, the lifetime risk of dying of breast cancer after wide excision for DCIS is probably under 3 to 4 percent if radiation therapy is added to surgery, while after mastectomy that risk is well below 1 percent. In Chapter 11 we will discuss the role of preventive drug therapy with tamoxifen in lowering the risk of recurrence after lumpectomy for DCIS.

Many women and their doctors say, "If there is any risk of recurrence at all, do a mastectomy." Others decide that 1 percent a year is an acceptable risk, opting for as wide an excision as can be done to avoid deformity, along with radiation therapy.

As we will see below, invasive cancers are treated with lumpectomy, node removal, and radiation. It may seem paradoxical that in some cases of DCIS—that is, of noninvasive cancer—we do a mastectomy because of its near-100 percent cure rate. As one of my patients said, "Is the loss of my breast the reward I get for finding cancer before it has spread?"

There are studies now underway to try to resolve this dichotomy, and to find out whether wide excision alone is adequate treatment in some cases of DCIS. In the meantime, over the past ten years, for many surgeons wide excision followed by radiation therapy has become the treatment of choice for small areas of DCIS. Mastectomy is reserved for those who have the following:

- A large area of DCIS, where wide excision will produce deformity.

- Diffuse DCIS, so that clear margins cannot be obtained.

- Multiple areas of DCIS scattered in more than one quadrant.

- DCIS involving the central ducts near the nipple or Paget's disease of the nipple.

- Diffuse residual calcifications on mammography, which make follow-up observation for recurrence difficult.

When mastectomy is not done, radiation therapy is effective in reducing the risk of recurrence. Efforts to identify characteristics of tumors that make the addition of radiation therapy *unnec*essary continue. Among the criteria being considered are:

- Tumor size

- The width of the tumor-free margin of normal tissue surrounding the DCIS area that is removed

- The type of DCIS—comedo, cribriform, or other (see pages 96–97)

- The presence or absence of necrosis (destruction) of cancer cells within the duct (see page 96)

- Nuclear grade (see page 94)

In the optimal case of DCIS—that is, with the lowest risk of recurrence—the tumor is small; 1 centimeter of normal tissue surrounds the tumor when the material removed at surgery is examined; the type of DCIS seen by the pathologist is noncomedo in nature; no necrosis of cancer cells is present; and the cells themselves are well-differentiated and are of low nuclear grade (see Chapter 5).

If you have an in situ ductal cancer, you and your doctor will have to carefully discuss and weigh your treatment options. While a 1-centimeter margin is a desirable goal, the position of the DCIS near the edge of the breast or the size of the breast itself frequently does not permit that actual measurement. What is important is that your surgeon and the pathologist have carefully evaluated the margins of the specimen to make certain they are clear. In most cases the breast can be saved, and in at least a few cases, radiation therapy can be avoided. The addition of hormone therapy (tamoxifen) may also reduce the risk of recurrence. Because the risks of the breast-conserving approach still need to be fully defined, treatment for intraductal carcinomas in situ can and should be individualized and the options carefully weighed as to their physical and emotional consequences.

STAGE I AND STAGE II CANCERS

The discussion of treatment for these cancers is best begun with a quote from "the horse's mouth," a conference convened by the National Institutes of Health (NIH) to evaluate available scientific information and to "resolve safety and efficacy issues related to biomedical technology." According to the findings of this June 1990 NIH Consensus Conference on early, invasive breast cancer, "Breast conservation treatment is an appropriate method of primary therapy for the majority of women with Stages I and II breast cancer and is preferable because it provides survival rates equivalent to those of total mastectomy and axillary dissection [modfied radical] while preserving the breast."

To clarify, lumpectomy with axillary dissection and radiation therapy is the preferable treatment for small, infiltrating cancers of either the lobules or the ducts.

There are, however, circumstances where mastectomy is the treatment advised for Stage I and Stage II cancers:

• More than one cancerous tumor in the breast.

• Multiple areas of microcalcification (see page 86) in the breast.

• A relatively large tumor in a small breast or a tumor in or near the center of the breast.

• Considerable axillary lymph node involvement.

STAGE III CANCERS

We have up until now been discussing early, relatively small cancers. As we saw in Chapter 3, some women come for treatment with more advanced disease. In such cases the cancer may be in the skin of the breast, it may be of the inflammatory type, it may be accompanied by extensive lymph node involvement, or it may be over 5 centimeters (about 2 inches) in size.

For Stage III cancers, chemotherapy is the first treatment (see "Neo-adjuvant Chemotherapy," page 232). It is used to treat inflammatory cancer and to shrink a large tumor to operable size. Surgery, usually a modified radical mastectomy, is performed after the tumor has shrunk. Sometimes it may even be possible to have a lumpectomy.

STAGE IV CANCERS

Stage IV cancers have spread beyond the breast and the axillary lymph nodes to other places in the body. They are treated primarily with chemotherapy. Surgery—lumpectomy or modified radical mastectomy—or radiation therapy may sometimes be used to assist in local tumor control.

It is important to say here that I have patients in my practice who came to me with a large tumor and who have done well, usually with chemotherapy followed by surgery. In instances where the tumor was inoperable, some women have survived for many years on long-term chemotherapy.

CANCER IN PREGNANCY

As we saw in Chapter 3, breast cancer in pregnant women tends to be discovered at a later stage than cancer in other women. Our general approach is to "abort the cancer, not the baby." However, when cancer is discovered during the first trimester, women usually choose to terminate the pregnancy and then to promptly seek the most appropriate treatment for the disease.

During the second trimester or later, a mastectomy can be

safely performed. We do not use radiation with pregnant women, to avoid risking the well-being of the fetus. Chemotherapy may be started in the latter half of pregnancy.

CANCER IN THE YOUNG

Women in their thirties or younger have a higher rate of recurrence of cancer after breast conservation than do older women. It is not fully understood why this should be. It may be that being young and having a long life ahead means that there are many more years during which additional cancers may arise. Possibly it may be some intrinsic property of these malignancies. It has also been observed that tumors tend to grow more rapidly in young women. As a result of both these observations, mastectomy is often recommended.

Women who develop breast cancer before age forty have a relatively high risk of carrying a mutated BRCA gene (see Chapter 7). If a mutation is found, bilateral mastectomy is advised.

CANCER IN THE ELDERLY

It is important to adjust treatment to the physiologic age of the patient, not only the chronological age. Some women may be older but in excellent health, while others may be affected by a variety of illnesses. Of course, as always, the nature of the tumor is most important. But, there is good evidence that in women over seventy, breast cancers grow more slowly and can be treated less aggressively. If the tumor is under 2 centimeters and the sentinel node biopsy shows no tumor in the axilla, it appears to be safe to omit radiation therapy. If the tumor has estrogen receptors, adjuvant hormone therapy should be used. Survival is correlated with the size of the tumor. For this reason the American Cancer Society guidelines recommend that annual screening mammography be continued unless a woman's general medical condition suggests treatment is not advisable.

Treatment Options

To summarize the treatments that may be recommended for all stages of breast cancer:

STAGE 0

Lobular Carcinoma In Situ

1. Biopsy
2. Observation
3. Possible hormone therapy (see Chapter 11)

or

1. Bilateral mastectomy
2. Breast reconstruction

Ductal Carcinoma In Situ

1. Biopsy
2. Wide excision with observation only
3. Wide excision with radiation therapy
4. Possible sentinel node biopsy
5. Possible hormone therapy

or

1. Unilateral mastectomy
2. Possible sentinel node biopsy
3. Breast reconstruction

STAGE I

1. Biopsy

2. Partial (lumpectomy) or total mastectomy

3. Sentinel node biopsy

4. Possible axillary dissection

5. If mastectomy, possible breast reconstruction

6. If lumpectomy, radiation therapy

7. Hormone therapy, chemotherapy, and/or targeted therapy

STAGE II

1. Biopsy

2. Lumpectomy or total mastectomy

3. Sentinel node biopsy

4. Axillary dissection

5. If mastectomy, possible breast reconstruction

6. If lumpectomy, radiation therapy

7. Hormone therapy, chemotherapy, and/or targeted therapy

STAGE III

1. Biopsy

2. Possible sentinel node biopsy

3. Course of chemotherapy, targeted therapy, and/or hormone therapy

4. Total mastectomy or lumpectomy

5. Axillary dissection

6. Possible breast reconstruction

7. Additional chemotherapy and/or hormone therapy

8. Possible radiation therapy

STAGE IV

1. Biopsy

2. Course of chemotherapy and/or hormone therapy

3. If appropriate, lumpectomy or modified radical mastectomy

4. Continued chemotherapy, targeted therapy, and/or hormone therapy

CHAPTER

9

RADIATION THERAPY

To destroy cancer cells, radiation therapy most commonly uses electromagnetic radiation, consisting of X-rays and gamma rays. It also uses what is called particulate radiation, waves of electronic particles such as electrons, neutrons, and protons.

What is electromagnetic radiation? Waves of energy from various sources, electromagnetic rays include ordinary light, X-rays, and gamma rays. The rays used in therapy have special properties. Though sunlight can shine through a fairly sheer window curtain, X-rays and gamma rays actually have the ability to penetrate solids. It is this property that allows us to use them to treat tissue within the body and to "see through" the skin to what is inside. The dentist, for example, uses minute levels of radiation to examine our teeth. In fact, he uses a lot less than one centi Gray (cGy), the unit of measure of radiation absorbed by the body. About the same or lower levels are used in other diagnostic X-rays.

When radiation is used at high energy levels, it has the ability to destroy what is in its path, both normal and abnormal tissues. Why, then, do we use it to treat people who have had cancer?

Because we have learned how to harness its enormous power in the battle against cancer. Think of a radiation device as a high-tech, superbly focused searchlight that can be accurately aimed at cancer cells so that its rays may destroy them. While the doses used in radiation therapy may damage normal cells in their path, they *destroy* rapidly multiplying malignant cells. Normal cells have the ability to repair themselves. Furthermore, in the treatment of breast cancer, the side effects are local—limited to the specific area of the radiation and not involving the rest of the body.

THE COURSE OF RADIATION THERAPY

AFTER LUMPECTOMY

Almost without exception, women who have had lumpectomies for infiltrating cancers are now treated with radiation therapy, as are most women with ductal carcinoma in situ. That statement inevitably raises three good questions:

1. IF THE CANCER WAS REMOVED, WHY DO I NEED FURTHER TREATMENT?

The decision to use radiation is based on overwhelming evidence that there is an unacceptably high rate of recurrence in the affected breast when the cancer is treated by lumpectomy alone. This rate can be reduced three- to fourfold when we add radiation therapy. In fact, by combining lumpectomy and radiation to the whole breast, we can get results that are comparable to those from mastectomy—while still preserving the breast.

2. IF RADIATION THERAPY IS SO EFFECTIVE, WHY DID I NEED THE SURGERY IN THE FIRST PLACE?

The smaller the malignancy, the better radiation works. When we surgically remove all the cancer we can detect, the radiation is left to deal primarily with undetected microscopic disease. That is why, in doing lumpectomies, we perform the widest excisions possible, with clear margins all around.

In addition, by surgically removing all the cancer we can find, we make it possible to use doses of radiation that are small enough to do only minimal damage to normal tissue.

3. WHY DOES THE WHOLE BREAST NEED TO BE RADIATED? WHY NOT JUST TREAT THE AREA IN WHICH THE TUMOR WAS FOUND, THE LUMPECTOMY SITE?

Some radiation oncologists have suggested that treating only the area of the lumpectomy, partial breast radiation, may suffice. Several studies using different techniques are under way to compare the benefits of partial and whole breast radiation, and the early results with partial breast radiation are promising. We do not yet know whether in the long term there will be more recurrences in those parts of the breast that were not irradiated. If less of the breast can be safely treated, it would be more convenient, because treatment could then be completed over one to two weeks, instead of the present five to six weeks (see pages 174–75).

4. WHEN DOES RADIATION THERAPY START?

Radiation therapy is started after systemic therapy is completed if chemotherapy is planned. If hormonal therapy is to be used, radiation can be administered after the wound has healed.

AFTER MASTECTOMY

Though radiation is not routinely used with mastectomy, sometimes when a tumor is large or when the cancer has spread to many lymph nodes, radiation will be used to make sure all the disease is eradicated.

LYMPH NODE TREATMENT

Radiation may be used to treat the lymph nodes behind the breastbone or above the collarbone if those nodes are at high risk of containing cancer cells. For example, we would suspect this to be the case if a great deal of cancer is found at the inner side of the breast or in the axilla.

EXTREMELY LARGE TUMORS

When the tumor is too large to be operated on, chemotherapy is commonly used to shrink it to operable size. Then after surgery, because of the relatively high risk of recurrence at this stage of the disease, radiation may be employed to attack any microscopic malignancy that may have escaped surgical removal. If a large tumor does not shrink to operable size after chemotherapy, radiation may be used before or instead of surgery.

LOCAL RECURRENCE

Occasionally after a mastectomy, a small malignancy may appear at the site of the original disease or in the skin or on the underlying muscle of the chest wall. Because there is no apparent spread to other parts of the body, this is called a local recurrence. The tumor is removed, and radiation is used to sterilize a wider area of the chest wall. Chemotherapy and/or hormone therapy may be given before or after the radiation.

METASTASIS

When breast cancer has spread to other parts of the body, chemotherapy is both the first line of defense against further progression and the frontline attack against the existing disease (see Chapter 11). Sometimes, however, cancer that has spread to the bones may cause pain and bone destruction. If cancer affects the brain or presses on a nerve, function may be lost. Radiation therapy is very successful in relieving these conditions.

WHO IS THE RIGHT PHYSICIAN?

You must go to a *radiation oncologist,* a physician trained in the planning and administration of radiation for medical treatment. There are radiation oncologists whose particular area of interest and expertise is the treatment of breast cancer. This is the kind of person you should look for.

She should have training and experience in radiation therapy and be either board-certified or board-eligible. Board-certified physicians have passed an examination in radiation therapy. Board-eligible physicians have had the training and experience but have not taken the examination.

Finding a qualified radiation oncologist, however, is only part of the job. The treatment facility must have available to it the services of a qualified *radiation physicist* who has a Ph.D. or an M.S. degree. Such a person is key to the precise planning of the radiation therapy.

There must also be licensed *radiation technologists* at the facility who are qualified to operate the radiation therapy equipment.

There should also be trained *radiation therapy nurses,* who work closely with the physicians and the technologists and who are knowledgeable about the treatment and are able to answer many of your questions. Since you will be seeing the technologist and the nurse every day for a considerable period of time, you should feel comfortable with their manner and behavior as well as with their competence.

How do you know the radiation facility is staffed with competent personnel? All states require that radiation departments or facilities have qualified physicians and other technical personnel. The credentials of these individuals are routinely reviewed at regular intervals by local and state agencies. The certificates of education and certification of each staff member should be conspicuously posted in the office. If you do not see every certification you're looking for, ask. It's worth any momentary embarrassment to make sure you are at the right place for your treatment.

WHERE DO YOU FIND A RADIATION ONCOLOGIST?

Radiation oncologists and other radiation specialists are found in hospital or cancer center radiation oncology departments and also in private practice. Because extremely fine skills are required to destroy the cancer yet avoid damaging the body, finding a good radiation oncologist takes very careful consideration. It is so important that it may be worth making arrangements to receive the treatments in another community if there is not an excellent facility near where you live.

As you will see, treatment lasts for several weeks, so this may not be a suggestion that is easy to follow; but the effort may be worth it in terms of the quality of treatment, the results, and the follow-up. In fact, when we first started doing lumpectomies, relatively few physicians were experienced with this new way of treating breast cancer, so it was quite common for women to go to another city for the weeks of their treatment. Even today, when there is no excellent local facility, some women spend Monday through Friday in the city where the radiation oncology facility is located and then go home for the weekend.

Your surgeon will usually refer you to a radiation oncologist to whom he has already sent patients and whose work he respects. Even so, carefully consider whether this is the right doctor and the right facility for you. Refer to Chapter 2 and review the material on finding and evaluating a doctor. If you have any questions about the radiation oncologist, by all means discuss them with your surgeon before you go for treatment.

INFORMED CONSENT

At the beginning of your first visit, you will be asked to sign an informed consent form, which specifies the type of treatment you will be receiving and the possible risks and side effects. It asks you to certify that the procedure and its risks have been explained to you and that you agree to the treatment.

Read the form carefully. If there is any discrepancy between what you have been told your treatment will be and what is stated on the form, ask that the language be explained to you clearly enough so that you understand it or, if necessary, ask that it be changed. You should feel comfortable with the form and not have to worry about any fine print.

However, as we saw when we looked at informed consent in the chapter on surgery, though the form plays some role in protecting the physician from later charges of malpractice and though it spells out for the patient the precise nature of the treatment, in the end—regardless of what the form says—doctors, like other professionals, are responsible for their work.

EQUIPMENT

A machine called a linear accelerator, which employs electrical current to generate low-energy photons and electrons, is now commonly used to deliver radiation therapy.

Also in use is a cobalt machine, which emits gamma rays from a radioactive source of the element cobalt.

Generally speaking, either device may be used to treat breast cancer. The linear accelerator is particularly versatile. It can provide photons to treat the whole breast and electrons for the "boost" treatment, at the site of the tumor, that is discussed on page 168.

THE TREATMENT

PLANNING

Though the radiation oncologist may be consulted before the tumor is even removed, you are more likely to see her after your surgery. Your surgeon should have thoroughly discussed your case with the radiation oncologist by the time of your first visit. He will have sent her a report of your preoperative mammogram, the results of any biopsies you may have had, and the pathology report. (In addition, some radiation oncologists prefer to review the pathology slides themselves.) The surgeon should have told the radiation oncologist any pertinent details of your medical history or of the operation. Your medical oncologist should also have discussed any treatment plans, their nature, and schedule.

How do you know that this exchange of information has taken place before you get to the radiation facility? *Ask.* If the surgeon has already done this groundwork, if the radiation oncologist is well-prepared to receive you, nothing has been lost by your question. If not, you will perhaps have nudged the process along.

Should other treatments be planned in addition to radiotherapy (see Chapter 11), at her first meeting with you the radiation oncologist must integrate her plans with those of other specialists.

PINPOINTING THE AREA

Your second visit to the radiation oncologist will take about an hour and will be devoted to accurately determining the area to be treated. This planning, which is called simulation, requires the use of specially designed equipment, as well as computer technology, to precisely locate and mark the parts of the body that are to receive radiation—the fields—and to determine the angles at which the radiation will be delivered.

A wire model of the breast contour is constructed and then transferred to graph paper to outline the volume to be treated.

This region on your chest is marked with water-soluble ink, and a treatment simulator is then used as a stand-in for the actual treatment machine.

Again, think of a searchlight and the circle of light it casts. The radiation source also emits its rays in a particular shape and depth—*in its own geometry* is the term often used. A simulator, also referred to as a localizer simulator, is used to duplicate precisely where the radiation will go in your body. How will the machine be angled for treatment? What will be the port of entry of the radiation? The size of the port? In relation to the radiation's range, where are the vital organs? The lungs? The heart? Using a simulator before taking X-ray pictures is like a dress rehearsal before the actual performance.

In addition to the simulator, a CAT scan (see page 264) may be employed if the size of the breast or the position of the tumor makes it difficult to get the necessary detailed information.

The simulation is not painful. However, it requires patience to be able to hold still for a period of time.

The radiation physicist then feeds the information into a computer that has been programmed to calculate the distribution of the radiation in the volume to be treated. This helps determine the proper field size and the angles at which the radiation should be delivered to achieve the most exposure to the breast and the least exposure to other tissue. This process of localizing the radiation area is carried out meticulously, to assure that we destroy any cancer cells without exposing the heart, lungs, or ribs to unnecessary radiation.

MARKING

Once this work has been accomplished, the radiation oncologist will mark the area of treatment on your skin with lines of indelible ink or, more commonly, with tiny tattoo marks no bigger than the head of a pin. These marks make it possible to reproduce the

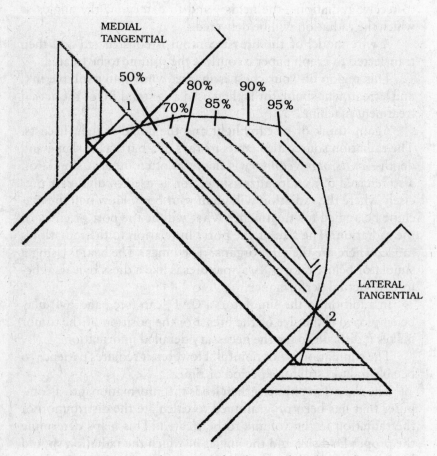

Computer-generated treatment plan showing the radiation dose distribution (in percentages) within the breast. This will be used for prescribing the amount of radiation to be given.

daily treatment in precisely the same area. They also assure that this area not be treated again in the future.

The tattooing may prick a bit, but it does not really cause much discomfort. Usually, the dots are minute, and because tattooing cannot wash off, you don't have to worry about bathing.

Some women do seem to hate the idea that the site of their cancer will be forever marked on their skin, although lasers can now be used to remove the tattoos. If you feel that way, ask that ink be used. However, "indelible" ink does eventually wash away. You need to avoid washing the area too vigorously, and you have to make sure that when the marking is done initially or freshened up later, it doesn't get on your clothes.

SCHEDULE

For the first weeks of your treatment, phase one, the entire breast is treated, the whole area that would ordinarily be encompassed by a mastectomy. Generally speaking, the underarm area does not have to be treated.

In a second phase, most women will get a supplemental treat-

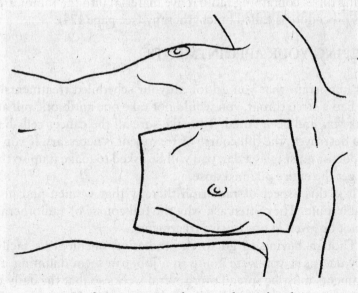

Marking or tattooing the area to be irradiated

ment, called a boost, that concentrates the radiation in the area where the tumor was located.

Phase One

Treatments are given five days a week, Monday through Friday, for about five to six weeks. The weekend pause is not only for convenience but because normal cells need a little time to recover between treatments.

Phase Two

This first course of treatment is called external radiotherapy. Immediately following it, the patient will usually receive additional radiation treatment, which is given only in the area of the breast that contained the tumor. This is called a "boost." Depending on the planned dose, treatment will be given every weekday for one to two weeks. The boost dose is also commonly administered by external radiation, by X-rays, gamma rays, or electron beam.

It can also be given in the form of internal radiation, by inserting tubes containing radioactive material into the tumor area. This procedure is called brachytherapy (see page 174).

KEEPING YOUR APPOINTMENTS

It is important that you go for all your scheduled treatments. If you had a strep throat, you would not take one antibiotic pill and think you had been cured. To make sure all the cancer cells have been destroyed, the full course of treatment is necessary. If you or the doctor must miss a day, you will be asked to make it up so that you get the entire planned dose.

It is this aspect of radiation therapy that women find most troublesome. They often ask why the full course of radiotherapy cannot be given in one or two treatments.

Though having to go to the radiation oncologist's facility every day, as if you were going to a job, can seem daunting, the treatments must be spread over several weeks so that the daily radiation dose is relatively small. In this way, the total dose can be achieved with less damage to the skin and other tissues than a single high dose might produce.

HOW MUCH RADIATION WILL I RECEIVE?

The total dose will be calculated at the time of your first planning visit. Questions like these will be considered by the radiation oncologist and the radiation physicist:

- What is the total dose the entire breast should receive?
- What dose should be given in the boost?
- For how many weeks is it estimated treatment will continue?
- For how many minutes will each treatment be administered?

Also taken into consideration are the size of the breast, the location and size of the tumor, the involvement of the lymph nodes, and the stage of the disease. In general, during the first phase of treatment, a total of 4,600 to 5,000 cGy is given to the whole breast over a period of five to six weeks. The boost dose is usually 1,000 to 1,600 cGy, given over about one to two weeks.

A COMPANION

Take someone, preferably your personal advocate, with you to the first, planning visit, as well as to your first treatment. As with other aspects of your treatment, such a person can give you moral support, can help you ask questions, and may also help you remember the information you receive. These treatments are painless and are not associated with uncomfortable side effects, so you will probably find that you won't need anyone with you after the first couple of times.

WHAT IS THE DAILY ROUTINE?

1. You will be given a clean paper or cloth gown and asked to remove all clothing and jewelry from the upper part of your body.

2. You will be taken to the treatment room and asked to lie down on the table beneath the machine with your arm raised and supported with an armrest away from your breast in a position determined at simulation. Usually you will be flat on your back, though sometimes you may be asked to lie on your side or stomach.

3. Once the technologist and radiation oncologist have positioned you for the first field to be treated and adjusted the angle of the machine, they will leave the room, closing the door behind them. The machine will be turned on, and you will be asked to lie completely still, though, unlike the routine during X-ray pictures, you can breathe normally during your treatment, which can take a minute or two.

   Do not worry about being left alone. You are being monitored by closed-circuit television, and there is a microphone in the room so that you can be heard outside if you have something to say.

4. After the first radiation has been administered, the technologist will return and position you for the next field of treatment. Usually one or two fields are irradiated each day.

5. The whole process takes about twenty minutes, though the radiation treatment itself takes only a fraction of that time.

6. At the time of the first treatment, and then at intervals during the course of your treatment, a blood test will be taken to make sure that the radiation is not affecting your blood count—something that rarely happens with breast radiation.

7. You will be asked to avoid using deodorants, powder, or perfumes, because some of their ingredients may cause skin irritation during treatment. If you have not had a tattoo, you will also be cautioned to only lightly wash the area where your body has been marked, to avoid rubbing off the ink. You may resume normal activities after treatment is completed.

SKIN CARE

1. It is best to wear loose cotton shirts during the weeks you are receiving radiation. If possible, limit the use of a bra, especially an underwire bra.

2. Ask your radiation oncologist to recommend a moisturizing cream to use on the skin of your treated breast. The most commonly suggested creams are pure aloe gel (those prepared directly from the plant are best), or vitamin A and D ointment.

3. No creams should be applied to the breast immediately before your daily radiation treatment. Creams can sometimes act as irritants if present during radiation. It is therefore best to apply the moisturizing cream after the treatment or at bedtime.

4. Once all radiation therapy has been completed, you can usually return to the moisturizer of your choice. It may need to be applied more frequently than usual for the first several weeks after radiation.

WILL IT HURT?

Radiation treatment does not seem to cause anyone any pain. A few women say that they feel some tingling or warmth in the area being treated, but even that sensation seems to be rare.

WILL I BE SICK DURING THE COURSE OF TREATMENT?

You can carry on your normal life to a great extent while you are receiving radiation therapy. There are rarely any really trouble-some problems, and only a few discomforts:

• Think of radiation as giving you a sunburn, not just of the skin but of the entire area the treatment encompasses. As the tissues absorb the radiation, they tend to retain water, so, as with a sunburn, there may be some swelling. For that reason, you may want to wear a cotton T-shirt rather than a bra, or under a bra, during the weeks you are being treated.

• In addition to the swelling, your skin may get a little red— again, as if you had a sunburn. This is particularly likely to happen after the fourth or fifth week of treatment.

• There is some pattern of increasing fatigue as the treatments continue. Part of this may be due to the strain of getting to the radiation facility every day, but it is so prevalent that there is reason to believe it is also related to the generalized effect of the treatment, particularly if more areas than the breast alone are being irradiated. Try to go with what your body is telling you. Don't radically change your life, but, especially toward the end of your treatment, program yourself to allow time to rest when you need to.

You will be seeing the technologist daily. But it is also important that the radiation oncologist examine you each week during treatment to make certain that your general reaction to the therapy, and in particular its local effects on the skin, are proceeding as expected.

WHAT ARE THE LONG-TERM SIDE EFFECTS?

The question that causes the most concern is, Will the radiation treatment itself cause a later cancer? There is no evidence that it does so, either in the treated breast or in the other breast.

In the past, when low-energy X-rays were used, there was some increased incidence of a disease called sarcoma, a malignancy of blood vessels, bones, or connective tissues. With modern radiation equipment that produces high-energy X-rays, these cancers are extremely rare, but they can occur at the site of treatment. This is a serious malignancy, called hemangiosarcoma, and requires a mastectomy.

Younger women in particular worry about the effects of this therapy on their reproductive system. It has been estimated that during the course of treatment, the ovaries do receive from 30 to 40 rads of radiation, depending on the patient's size and the site of the treatment. This is due to scattered radiation within the body, and it cannot be decreased by adding lead protection. Thirty to 40 rads are not considered biologically significant. Neither menstrual periods nor fertility is affected.

You will probably not be able to nurse a baby with a breast that has received radiation. The other breast will be able to lactate, and some women who have had this treatment have nursed their babies.

Very occasionally, radiation can cause a hairline fracture of a rib. This doesn't usually cause problems, and there may be no evidence of its presence until it shows up on an X-ray. Similarly, radiation can sometimes injure the lungs. Properly planned and administered radiation therapy rarely causes these problems.

Though there has also been concern about possible effects on the heart, particularly when the left breast is radiated, long-term studies show no additional risk of heart attacks with modern radiation therapy.

Most swelling of the breast usually disappears after a few weeks, but if the boost radiation was near the nipple and areola, the swelling may take longer to subside. (Also, if a tumor near the center of the breast was removed, there is a greater likelihood of long-term edema from damaged lymphatics.)

Some women report a feeling of warmth in the treated breast that continues for several months after the treatment.

You may find some changes in sensation, but there is no uniformity to this reaction. Some women say their breast is much more sensitive; others say it is less so. The sensitivity of the breast to touch or pressure may persist for many years. Episodes of discomfort, aching, and even sharp pain are not unusual. It is important to know that these are not signs of a recurrence of breast cancer.

There are some cosmetic side effects, but these are usually quite minor: The superficial layers of skin will die, and this will leave a slight discoloration; the skin may darken and thicken slightly. Use a vitamin A and D cream or other nonirritating preparation to moisturize the skin. Don't expose the treated area to the sun during the period of your treatment and for a few weeks thereafter. Use a sunblock of medium strength (SPF 15 to 30) on the treated area after this time.

A treated breast is usually somewhat firmer than normal. In most patients the breast remains the same size, but in some instances it may shrink or become larger. This is another reaction that varies from woman to woman.

Many women ask about the effect of radiation on their immune system. It has been found that immunological changes as a result of local radiation therapy have no bearing on the course of cancer, nor have we found changes in immunity to other diseases.

PARTIAL BREAST RADIATION

The following are methods currently being used to treat only the area of the breast where the lumpectomy was done. Usually such treatment is performed as part of a study comparing partial and complete breast radiation.

- Mammosite—A catheter with a balloon at its end is placed into the cavity of the lumpectomy at the time of surgery. Radioactive seeds are inserted into the balloon through the catheter twice a day for five days; the catheter is then removed.

- Brachytherapy—A series of fine tubes are inserted at the time of surgery into the area of the breast to be treated. Radioactive seeds are later placed into these tubes, and the patient is admitted to the hospital, usually for one night. The tubes are removed before discharge.

- Intraoperative radiotherapy (IORT)—After surgery, while the patient is still in the operating room, specialized equipment delivers radiation directly into the lumpectomy cavity before the wound is closed.

- External beam—Radiation is given to the lumpectomy site by standard technique or by intensity-modulated radiation therapy (IMRT). IMRT divides the radiation beam into many smaller beams, with the intensity of each beam individually controlled. This permits more accurate delivery of radiation therapy to the tumor site while sparing surrounding normal tissues.

Another term you may hear is *accelerated therapy,* which means that a higher daily dose of radiation is used. All the methods described here share a common goal: to reduce the duration of treatment from the usual five to seven weeks to as little as twenty minutes in the operating room.

DOES RADIATION EXPOSURE EVER CAUSE CANCER?

Under certain conditions there have been radiation-induced cancers. The connection seems to have to do with the radiation dose and the age of the person who is exposed. People nineteen and younger are at the highest risk for radiation-induced cancer. After thirty-five, the risk is negligible.

The incidence of radiation-induced malignancies increases with an increase in dose up to a range of 300 to 1,000 rads. Thereafter, the incidence decreases as the dose goes up.

At the lower doses, more normal cells are transformed into malignant cells. At the higher doses, cells that show malignant transformations are destroyed and the number of transformed cells actually goes down. In fact, when the radiation dose reaches therapeutic range—more than 4,500 rads—the risk is negligible.

Women in Hiroshima, particularly young women, who had been exposed to radiation from the atomic bomb had an increased incidence of breast cancer. The level of radiation they received was 300 to 400 rads, and about 60 to 70 women per 100,000 developed breast cancer. In the unirradiated population the rate was about 25 per 100,000.

In the past, women who had many fluoroscopic examinations for tuberculosis had a higher incidence of breast cancer. Each examination delivered 4 to 20 rads, and many women received more than one hundred fluoroscopies. Such women had an 80 percent higher incidence of breast cancer than the general population.

There is a similar situation among women who were treated for postpartum mastitis in the early part of the twentieth century with radiation doses of 100 to 600 rads.

Radiation therapy continues to be used successfully for the treatment of Hodgkin's disease. When radiation therapy is given to the lymph nodes of the neck, armpit, and center of the chest, it is referred to as mantle therapy. Women who received this treatment in their teens and early twenties have a higher incidence of breast cancer, which is felt to be related to their radiation treatment.

What is the connection between these statistics and the treatment of breast cancer? Radiation therapy after lumpectomy uses at least 4,500 rads. There has been no increased breast cancer observed either in the treated or in the opposite breast of women who received this treatment. The incidence of new cancers in the opposite breast is the same for women who received radiotherapy as for those treated with mastectomy alone.

An extremely rare cancer, hemangiosarcoma (mentioned on page 172), can occur at the site of radiation treatment to the breast after a lumpectomy. Its presence is suspected when a bruise-like discolorization appears on the breast.

RECURRENCE AFTER RADIATION THERAPY

Once we have treated a breast with radiation, we can seldom use this treatment again. If there is a local recurrence (that is, at the site of the original cancer), further surgery—usually a mastectomy—needs to be done. A repeat sentinel node biopsy should be considered. Occasionally, if the recurrence is an in situ cancer, lumpectomy alone may be adequate, or, if a new cancer has developed in another quadrant of the breast, it may be possible to use direct localized radiation treatment. Systemic hormone therapy and/or chemotherapy are often indicated. If a new cancer develops in the opposite breast, radiation can safely be used to treat that breast.

Surgery and radiation therapy are the essential partners in breast conservation. The track record of this two-pronged attack on cancer is remarkably good.

CHAPTER
10

PROGNOSIS

❦

Whether you had a lumpectomy followed by a course of radiation, or a mastectomy without radiation, you have now reached the point at which you and your doctors must plan the next strategy.

Cancer—an enemy if ever there was one—has been beaten back, but we want to make certain it stays that way. The first step to achieving that goal is to ask a simple question: Should we now use further therapy to prevent the recurrence or spread of the cancer?

For most physicians, the answer depends on the patient's prognosis and her prospect of recovery and continued good health. Decisions about using chemotherapy and hormone therapy are often made on the basis of prognosis.

To use a military analogy, the more powerful the enemy and

the further our intelligence service tells us he has advanced against us, the more powerful must be the force we use against him. Moreover, since we are fighting in our own home territory, we have to eliminate him without destroying ourselves.

DETERMINING THE RISK OF RECURRENCE

How do we look into the future and arrive at a prognosis? On the basis of risk factors, we examine individual criteria in each patient to determine the likelihood that she will remain disease-free. Each of these factors gives us some information about the future, and taken together, they can provide some guidance to the physician about what treatment is most apt to be helpful.

No one knows for sure the risk of recurrence of any particular cancer for any particular person. We only know statistically that given such and such circumstance, in a group of patients, such and such is likely to happen if the disease is untreated.

But even after the most exhaustive analysis of risk factors, scientists have had to concede that there are more individual questions than there are general conclusions. When we say, "Here is the prognosis for someone with three cancerous lymph nodes and a 2-centimeter invasive breast tumor," we're really saying, "Here is the pattern of consequences that we've observed in a lot of people who were in that situation." We cannot say to any particular person, "This is what's going to happen to you."

Why, then, do we want to assess any one person's risk factors? Because many people believe that these may provide guidance as to what treatment should be used next. But the fact is that even when we consider risk factors in the light of making treatment decisions, the impact of factors other than tumor size and the number of involved nodes is fairly limited. We've seen that surgery is the primary treatment for almost all breast cancer, and when the surgical choice is lumpectomy, radiation therapy usually accompanies it. When we get into the heart of the next chapter, on chemotherapy and hormone and targeted therapy, you will also see that there is fairly consistent agreement that some form of systemic therapy is usually indicated to further reduce the risk of recurrence.

However, some important gray areas remain: for instance, what the specific regimens should be for each patient and the circumstances in which chemotherapy, hormone therapy, or targeted therapy can be avoided. It is in these situations that determining prognosis becomes especially important.

We evaluate prognosis primarily by the stage of the cancer (see Chapter 3), the combination of factors by which the extent of the illness is defined. Those primary factors are:

• Infiltration

• Size of tumor

• Lymph node involvement

Let's now propose an unthinkable scenario: Suppose we did the surgery and perhaps the radiation, but we chose to do no chemotherapy or hormone therapy, whatever the patient's condition might be. What would the recurrence and survival statistics be, given a particular tumor size, a particular degree of infiltration, a particular number of involved lymph nodes? What risk factors would point to a favorable or unfavorable outcome?

INFILTRATION

As we saw in Chapter 3, cancers can be in situ—that is, confined to their site of origin. When they have broken through the wall of the duct or lobule, they are said to have infiltrated—that is, they have spread to the adjacent local tissues.

The risk of recurrence of an in situ cancer after mastectomy is almost zero. With infiltrating cancers, the size of the tumor is important, but risk is also related to the pattern of infiltration. For example, cancer in the lymphatics of the breast itself is not as significant as the involvement of the lymphatics of the skin or, as very rarely happens, involvement of the chest muscle. The latter cancers are more likely to spread to other parts of the body, no matter what the size of the primary tumor.

As we will see in the chapter on systemic therapy (Chapter 11), infiltration is often the risk factor that determines whether or not we will recommend further treatment.

TUMOR SIZE

The larger the tumor, the higher the risk of recurrence of cancer, either within the breast, in the local area, or at a distant site. If there were no further treatment and if the nodes were negative, here are the statistical chances—according to tumor size—that five years after diagnosis the patient would be cancer-free:

• Less than 1 centimeter (about ⅜ inch): more than 90 percent cancer-free

• Up to 2 centimeters (about ¾ inch): 75 percent cancer-free

• 2 to 5 centimeters (about ¾ inch to about 2 inches): 30 to 40 percent cancer-free

• 5 centimeters (about 2 inches) or larger: 25 percent cancer-free

LYMPH NODE INVOLVEMENT

There is some correlation between tumor size and the likelihood of lymph node involvement. In a group of patients with tumors smaller than 1 centimeter, a little over 20 percent had some cancerous lymph nodes. Among patients whose tumors were larger than 5 centimeters, 60 percent had lymph node involvement.

We get our first decisive information about the lymph nodes in the armpit after breast surgery when, as we saw on page 131, they are removed and examined. These nodes provide us with information vital to evaluating the disease.

As to the influence of node involvement on the recurrence of cancer, in general:

• The more nodes involved, the greater the risk, with the highest risk among patients who have ten or more cancerous nodes.

• The larger any tumor in the nodes, the greater the risk.

• If the tumor breaks through the capsule of the node and they adhere to each other, the risk of recurrence increases.

As we have seen, the lymph nodes are grouped in three levels, from those that extend from the top of the breast to those high up in the armpit. Five-year survival, in one study (in which treatment was limited to surgery), was 65 percent when level I nodes were involved, 45 percent when level II nodes were involved, and only 20 percent for women whose disease had spread high in the armpit to the level III nodes. While a tumor spreading to the nodes is usually detected by routine pathology staining methods, isolated cancer cells can sometimes only be seen in lymph nodes with a special cytokeratin-staining technique at the time a sentinel node biopsy is done. In cases of in situ breast cancer, the finding of isolated tumor cells in a sentinel node does not change the excellent prognosis. With an infiltrating cancer, however, it indicates that more lymph nodes may be involved.

OTHER RISK FACTORS

PATHOLOGIC GRADE

A few types of ductal cancers have more a favorable prognosis (see page 96), but for most cancers it is the differentiation of the cell nucleus that reflects its biologic activity. Grading systems such as that of Bloom and Richardson (see page 94) try to describe a tumor's characteristics more completely by adding other aspects of tumor appearance to that of the nucleus. Grade is seldom a major consideration in determining preventive treatment.

HORMONE RECEPTOR LEVELS

We discussed the question of whether tumors are hormone receptor-positive or -negative on page 98. These findings affect the prognosis.

Cells can be classified by whether they are mature (differentiated) or immature (undifferentiated). In general, mature cells are not very good at dividing and multiplying, but they do specialized work very efficiently, and they produce estrogen and progesterone receptors.

The less mature a cell, the less likely it is to have hormone receptors on its surface and the greater its ability to divide and multiply. If immature cells are normal, they will develop into mature cells and take on their characteristics. But when cancer is present, it arrests these cells in the course of their maturation process, sometimes before they have developed the ability to produce hormone receptors.

There is a modest improvement in outlook if both estrogen and progesterone receptors can be detected in the tumor. Women with one or the other of the receptors have an intermediate advantage. Women with tumors that have no receptors are at a somewhat higher risk of recurrence. As an indicator of prognosis, the presence or absence of hormone receptors is less significant than the size of the tumor or the number of nodes involved. Recent studies suggest that while women whose tumors are without receptors are at a higher risk for recurrence during the first three years after surgery, their risk decreases after that. Women whose tumors have receptors have their highest recurrence rates in the first five years after surgery, but their risk of recurrence may remain significant for a much longer period of time. New treatment strategies are being developed that take this extended period of risk into consideration.

THE GENETIC MATERIAL OF THE CELLS

In the past few years, we have learned that the increased presence and heightened activity of certain genes, called *oncogenes,* are associated with the capacity for more vigorous cell growth. The presence of one of these genes is now considered an important risk factor for the recurrence of breast cancer. This gene goes by several names, any of which you may hear from your team of doctors: HER-2, HER-2/neu, or erbB-2. Whatever the gene is called, scientists have discovered that an increased number of copies of it are produced in about 25 percent of breast cancers. This is referred to as overexpression. The more copies, the more serious the prognosis. However, since such cells differ from normal cells by producing an excess of the protein whose production is controlled by HER-2/neu, they are uniquely sensitive to attack by drugs directed against this protein (see page 197). Preliminary studies suggest that certain chemotherapy drugs are more effective than others against tumors that overexpress HER-2/neu. Further studies are needed, however, to confirm these results. Herceptin (see page 202) is a targeted therapy that has been specifically developed to treat women with HER-2 overexpression.

Another gene that may limit growth in normal cells is the suppressor gene p53 (see page 328). Overproduction of abnormal, improperly functioning protein by this gene is associated with a less favorable prognosis.

GENE EXPRESSION PANELS

The nucleus of a human cell has programming information that dictates everything the cell can accomplish. This programming is written in DNA using a triplet code, which has four letters (nucleotides), combined in sets of three, known as codons. The particular sequence of the letters in a set determines its message. Sets of codons used for a particular purpose are called genes. Cancer cells have changes in this programming that permit them to grow in an uncontrolled fashion and to invade tissues that normally exclude them. Using new technology developed in the last ten years, scientists have begun to determine which genes are abnormally expressed in breast cancer. Sets of such genes have recently been identified that give information about the prognosis for patients once their tumors have been studied for the expression of these genes. This pattern is sometimes referred to as a "molecular signature."

While there are several reported grouped gene tests, only two are available commercially. These are the Onco*type* DX and MammaPrint tests. The Onco*type* DX test consists of twenty-one genes. It can be performed on tissues that are formalin-fixed and have been fully processed for pathologic testing. Results are classified as low, intermediate, or high risk. The MammaPrint test requires that a fresh, unfixed tissue specimen be sent to Holland for testing. It relies on a panel of seventy genes, and is said to identify patients with very good or very poor prognoses. This test is generally not available in the United States. The American Society of Clinical Oncology (ASCO), the professional organization for oncologists, in a technology assessment completed in late 2007 considered the Onco*type* DX test to be the more established of these two. The current use of these tests is primarily for patients with very small tumors that contain positive hormone receptors and no involved nodes, patients who might otherwise be considered to be at too low a risk to warrant getting preventive chemotherapy or targeted therapy and can be treated with hormone therapy alone.

OLDER TESTS

There are tests that measure actual cell proliferation. This is referred to as the "proliferation index." Though the terms and methods of measurement differ from test to test, in general the fewer cells proliferating, the smaller the risk. In one test, when 18 percent or more of the cell population is proliferating, that is considered high risk.

The validity of other prognostic tests has also been questioned. These include the presence of small numbers of tumor cells in the bone marrow or within the circulatory system.

What can we make of all this arcane information? How can we use such data for any particular patient to decide whether the risk of a recurrence of cancer warrants the use of chemotherapy and hormone therapy?

Well, from my point of view, you can't hang your hat on any one of these factors. First of all, there are a lot of complexities. For example:

• Small tumors are better than large tumors, aren't they? Not if there's lymph node involvement. That might indicate that even though the tumor is still small, it's vigorous enough to have already spread to the nodes.

• Patients with no hormone receptors have a higher risk of recurrence in the first three years, but the risk may decline more sharply after that than for those whose tumors do have these receptors.

The fact is that most women who have had breast cancer now receive chemotherapy, or hormone or targeted therapy. The question of whether or not to give further treatment remains open only for women with small invasive tumors.

Still, the improvement in breast cancer detection methods is increasing the number of patients diagnosed with early tumors. How does the oncologist balance the increasing number of favorable and unfavorable characteristics that can be described for such smaller tumors to determine whom to treat? The matter is, of course, simpler if there are many more favorable than unfavorable aspects to a particular tumor, or, unfortunately, the reverse. However, in many cases the situation is less clear and you may get different opinions if you see more than one oncologist.

One tool that is somewhat helpful to oncologists in this setting is the Adjuvant! model, a probability-generating program that is available to oncologists on the Internet (adjuvantonline.com). Since the results often require considerable interpretation, it is not available at this time to patients. Adjuvant! comes in several versions that try to integrate most, but so far not all, available prognostic information for a patient. It then predicts risk with or without chemotherapy or hormone therapy.

Occasionally you may see laboratory reports referring to findings as "favorable" or "unfavorable." Given the uncertainty of how to sum up the significance of the lesser prognostic tests, whose results are often contradictory, such simplified interpretations are misleading. For instance, in situ cancers (see pages 35–36), if tested, frequently are associated with poor risk factors, yet the cure rate for this form of breast cancer is close to 100 percent.

So, though we are getting a lot more sophisticated information now than we have ever had before, we do not yet have absolute correlations between prognostic test results and outcomes in a specific patient. For that reason, it is my view that we should collect as much evidence as we can and continue to do thorough research to measure the impact of what we are learning on patient outcome. But in the meantime, when there is any doubt about where the prognosis is pointing, we should use some kind of systemic therapy. As the next chapter indicates, it is far better to err on the side of safety than to later regret not having used all the weapons at our command.

CHAPTER
11

HORMONE THERAPY AND CHEMOTHERAPY

You have come through breast surgery and perhaps a course of radiation therapy, and now your surgeon may be telling you that the next step to be considered is chemotherapy, targeted therapy, or hormone therapy. No wonder many women throw up their hands and say, "Enough! The cancer's gone. I don't want any more treatment, and I certainly don't want anything done to me that's going to make my hair fall out."

This chapter will explain the lifesaving usefulness of systemic preventive therapy, the treatment processes, the details of the drug regimens that may be suggested for you, their side effects and benefits, and how you can evaluate whether these therapies are right for you.

WHY CHEMOTHERAPY, TARGETED THERAPY, AND/OR HORMONE THERAPY?

Why should you even consider systemic treatment, treatment with drugs that circulate throughout your body? After all, your surgeon has probably assured you that he has removed all the cancer.

Systemic therapy is being considered because there is a possibility that the cancer has traveled to other parts of the body, even though there may be no discernible evidence of this. Surgery has greatly reduced the risk that the cancer will spread, but some risk does remain, as we discussed in the previous chapter. Systemic therapy is used to bring us as close as we can now get to eliminating that risk.

Removing the breast, as we have seen, cures in situ cancer. In the case of infiltrating cancer—breast cancer that has moved outside the duct or lobule in which it originated—even though it may still appear to be confined to the breast, we cannot be certain that it has not spread to other parts of the body.

Systemic therapy interferes with the growth and spread of cancer. It is often referred to as adjuvant therapy, because it is used to supplement the effectiveness of surgery. Unlike surgery or radiation, which acts locally on the breast and nearby lymph nodes in the armpit, systemic treatment, because it travels through the bloodstream, also acts against cancer in distant sites and significantly reduces the risk of recurrence. In fact, it can reduce that risk by fifty percent or more, and can markedly increase the life span of a woman who has had breast cancer.

But to get that result, treatment must begin fairly soon after surgery, with what I describe to my patients as "due, deliberate speed." Despite the natural reluctance of most people to undertake still another course of therapy after surgery and possibly radiation, adjuvant therapy isn't something you can postpone. You can't say, "Okay. You've convinced me. The next time I get sick, I'll do it."

To put it plainly, waiting until there is a problem reduces the effectiveness of systemic treatment; it is much more powerful an adversary against cancer when it is brought to bear against what is called subclinical disease, disease that is so limited that we cannot find it through the usual tests available to us.

This may sound like medical voodoo, and it is logical to ask, "If you can't find it, how do you know you've cured it? Maybe it wasn't there in the first place."

We know it was there from statistical evidence that has accumulated since 1975 in studies of large numbers of women in various regions of the United States as well as abroad. These data show that the recurrence of cancer for patients at relatively high risk, as well as for those at a much lower risk, can be significantly reduced by early intervention with adjuvant therapy.

Recent studies suggest that systemic treatment may also benefit those who have had in situ cancers. This has been found both for patients with lobular carcinoma in situ (LCIS) and ductal carcinoma in situ (DCIS). In both conditions the concern is not the prevention of distant spread of the disease that was originally removed, but local recurrence or, more important, the later development of new, more dangerous, invasive tumors in the same or opposite breast.

WHO SHOULD GET SYSTEMIC THERAPY?

For women with breast cancer, it is in the use of chemotherapy that most of the complex questions and choices among options arise. There is considerable controversy about which patients should receive chemotherapy, whether it should be with or without targeted therapy, and what mix of drugs should be used, whether hormones should be administered, and whether such treatment should be routine for all women who have had breast cancer. Much of this difference of opinion has to do with:

• The size of the tumor

• Whether the tumor is in situ or invasive

• Whether the tumor has receptors for estrogen and/or progesterone (see page 98)

• Whether the tumor overexpresses HER-2

- Whether the disease has spread to the lymph nodes
- Whether you were pre- or postmenopausal at the time the tumor appeared

   In general:

- Chemotherapy works best in premenopausal women.
- Hormone therapy works best for postmenopausal women whose tumors were estrogen or progesterone receptor-positive.

BUT

- We have learned that chemotherapy, often combined with or followed by hormone therapy, does have a place in the treatment of postmenopausal women.
- Similarly, hormone therapy can add to the benefits of chemotherapy for premenopausal women, specifically those whose tumors were estrogen and progesterone receptor-positive.
- For both pre- and postmenopausal women, hormone therapy may be helpful in treating in situ cancers.
- Targeted therapy has a major role to play in the treatment of HER-2–positive tumors.

   Though we will come back to these questions at the end of this chapter, it may be simpler to begin by looking at the issue this way: If you had an infiltrating cancer, most physicians at this time would recommend chemotherapy with or without targeted therapy and/or hormone therapy, unless the tumor was very small. If your tumor was in situ, then physicians may recommend only hormone therapy.
   You should follow the recommendations for adjuvant therapy for the following reasons:

- No one dies of cancer in the breast, only of cancer that has spread outside the breast.

- Systemic chemotherapy, targeted therapy, and hormone therapy can prevent the spread of cancer.

- Such treatment, particularly hormone therapy, will help to reduce the risk of a local recurrence or the development of a new tumor.

- Chemotherapy, targeted therapy, and hormone therapy are saving tens of thousands of lives, particularly of women with an average risk of recurrence.

- Women who would have had no chance of even surviving in the past now have the possibility of cure.

Why, if these things are true, aren't women rushing enthusiastically to systemic therapy? We all know the answer. People are terrified of the side effects. They do not want to be nauseated, lose their hair, or gain weight. For women who have just had breast surgery, the threat of further cosmetic assault and physical discomfort is almost unbearable. Many women are as terrified of chemotherapy as they are of the potential consequences of not taking the treatment.

We will discuss side effects in greater detail as this chapter proceeds, but there are a few reassuring amulets you can carry with you through these pages:

- The drugs used in systemic therapy are not poison. In general, when used prudently, they will destroy bad cells, and spare good cells.

- Most side effects will pass relatively quickly. They are not permanent.

- A good physician can ameliorate the most feared side effects.

WHO IS THE RIGHT PHYSICIAN?

The first task, as in every phase of illness, is to find a good physician to administer systemic therapy. Luckily, you are not starting from scratch. In most instances, your surgeon regularly refers patients to one or two physicians with whom he has worked and whom he trusts.

Even so, cautions are necessary. Here are the qualifications you should look for:

- The medical oncologist who administers the chemotherapy should be board-certified or board-eligible in medical oncology, the medical treatment of tumors, particularly malignant tumors. That is, she should have completed a fellowship in this specialty and then passed an exhaustive examination. (Board-eligible or, as it is sometimes called, board-qualified specialists have taken their training, but not the examination.)

- She should have extensive experience and skill in the treatment of breast cancer.

- She should be someone to whom you can comfortably relate.

Chemotherapy can be dangerous. Do not accept treatment from a surgeon or local physician just because he says he can do it. Expertise in the use of these techniques is essential.

A COMPANION

You will find it especially helpful to have with you during at least your first visits to the chemotherapist someone who knows you well and with whom you feel comfortable. Though you will probably find that the treatment is less traumatic than what you may have been dreading, for the first few times take your personal advocate, a friend, or a family member with you to help you raise questions with the doctor, to remember what she said, or simply to provide a supportive presence.

The Physician's Office

Though this is not something that came up when we were discussing the qualifications of other doctors, the physical arrangement of the oncologist's office is particularly important. This is not a matter of interior design; it is the reality that it is hard to treat patients with dignity unless there is room to treat them separately.

You should be given some privacy during your chemotherapy, and this may not be possible in a room where several people are receiving treatment at the same time. On the other hand, you may at times wish to be with others. The choice should be yours.

The Pretreatment Examination

During the initial visit, the physician will take a complete medical history and do a thorough physical examination. Make sure to take with you to that first appointment a list detailing your medical history, as well as a list of *all* medications you are now taking, including vitamins and any other supplements. Make sure to note the dosages. You will also need the operative report, the pathology report, and the pathology slides. The operative report is often not available in the first few weeks after surgery, but a summary from your surgeon will still be very useful. (See pages 271–73 for information on how to get these.) Before the visit, write down any questions you may have about why chemotherapy, targeted therapy, or hormone therapy is being recommended, and during the visit raise any concerns you have about the effectiveness and side effects of the particular plan the doctor is proposing. You and she should discuss these matters thoroughly.

Optimally, you should be seen by the physician every time you go for a treatment. Her first questions will give her an overview of your general condition: How have you been feeling? What is your general condition like?

After that broad view, the doctor will explore with you the subtleties of your condition since your previous treatment:

- Appetite—Are you eating normally? Are there any foods you especially like or dislike?

- Energy level—Are you living your normal life? Do you go out? Go shopping? Go to work?

- Sleep—Are there changes in your normal sleep pattern? Do you fall asleep easily? Wake up at your normal time?

- Pain—Do you have any pain? Where exactly is it? How severe? Do you take any medication for it?

- How are your other body systems working? Do you have headaches, sore throat, runny nose, earache, cough, sputum production, nausea, vomiting, diarrhea, constipation, or a burning sensation when you urinate?

By no means will you have all—or even any—of these symptoms, nor will your treatment be the cause of everything you may feel, but this is a time when you and the doctor want to know as precisely as possible what is going on in your body.

Each time you arrive for a treatment at the oncologist's office, a nurse or technician will prick your finger in order to take a blood count.

A brief physical examination is often done at every visit. It includes:

- A breast examination for any gross changes

- A general examination that concentrates on nearby lymph nodes and the chest

At intervals, the doctor may order scans of your body, X-rays, or other tests to monitor your condition, including any effects of the therapy. A more thorough general physical examination will also be conducted from time to time, as well as a very thorough palpation of the breasts.

At each visit you should review with the doctor any questions you may have; as always, write these down beforehand so that you don't forget to ask them. This question period helps crystallize information about your general condition; it can also be a chance for you and the doctor to pick up on anything that may have been missed during the last visit.

As with the description of other procedures, all this may sound formidable. The truth is, it takes almost as long to describe as to do. In fact, the entire examination and discussions during your treatment visits should take only fifteen to twenty minutes. They are, however, a vital aspect of the treatment itself and an important reassurance to you that you are getting careful and concerned attention.

THE TREATMENT

We will begin this section with certain general information on the use of adjuvant chemotherapy for patients who have had breast cancer. Much of this applies to targeted therapy as well. The mechanics of treatment may differ from doctor to doctor. As noted above, make sure that you discuss in detail the treatment your oncologist plans for you and that you understand and feel comfortable with it. Raise any questions you now have, and continue to do this if other concerns arise later.

HOW ARE THE DRUGS ADMINISTERED?

While some chemotherapy drugs are taken by mouth, most are given intravenously—that is, directly into a vein. This is usually done by starting an intravenous infusion (IV) of dextrose and water or saline and then administering the drug by adding it to the IV.

It can also be done by an injection of the undiluted medication directly into a vein—usually at the top of the hand. This is called a direct push, and it is a very simple way to administer the drugs. It spares the patient from waiting the thirty minutes or so that it takes for an infusion to be completed.

WHO ADMINISTERS THE DRUGS?

It takes a very skilled, experienced person to administer either an infusion or a direct push injection. Women often worry about whether chemotherapy causes a "breakdown" of the veins. That is not a common occurrence if those administering the drugs are good at what they do. The proper needle must be used, and the patient should press on the spot where the needle was placed for a few minutes after the treatment is completed.

Usually the person who gives the treatment is specially trained and is often a certified oncology nurse. She knows how to insert the needle in the vein without damaging it. She also knows how to test that it is actually in the vein before administering the injection itself. This is important if we are to prevent leakage under the skin, which can cause problems with certain chemotherapy drugs.

WILL THEY HAVE TO POKE AROUND TO FIND A VEIN?

In most cases there is no problem in locating a good site for the injection. In instances when women have more body fat or very tiny veins, however, it can be more difficult to "find" the vein. In such cases, it may be necessary to tap the skin to bring the vein up toward the surface. If you think that you require special attention and that the person who is treating you does not have that level of expertise, speak up. Your physician has probably done many thousands of such injections over the years, and when it is necessary, you should have the most experienced hands available to you. It is reassuring to know, however, that in some patients who have required long-term therapy, drugs have been administered for years without discomfort.

ARE THERE OTHER WAYS TO ADMINISTER CHEMOTHERAPY?

In some situations, plastic tubing is inserted under the skin and connected to one of the larger veins leading to the heart. This is a surgical procedure that is performed in the hospital, and the device remains in place until it is no longer needed and is removed.

In the Hickman or the Broviac device of this type, the tubing comes out through the skin and ends in a cylinder with a rubber diaphragm, into which medication can be directly injected. These are used only when frequent treatments over a short period of time are planned.

For drugs given weekly or less often, over longer periods of time, an Infus-a-Port and other, similar devices are placed. The entry to the tubing is via a flat, buttonlike port, the size of a nickel or smaller, that is implanted under the skin. The needle must go through the skin into this port each time an injection is given. Such devices can remain in place for long periods of time.

Generally speaking, this type of apparatus is not necessary in order to avoid vein "breakdown." Ordinarily, with care, the vein will not be damaged. And though they may seem a convenient way to administer intravenous medication, these devices can cause problems:

- They have to be surgically implanted.

- They can be a source of infection.

- They may cause clots to form in the vein into which they have been inserted.

- They must be flushed regularly with an anticoagulant to prevent them from becoming clogged.

Very occasionally, there are compelling reasons for the use of these tubing devices. A woman may not tolerate repeated injections into a small vein. Sometimes there may be swelling in the arm that makes access to the vein difficult. And some people prefer the ready access to their veins that such devices provide.

On balance, of course, this choice is an individual matter, but something else does need to be considered: The patient should feel that when she leaves the office, she is fine. In the office, she is, unavoidably, a patient, but when she leaves, she is a normal person, and should be able to go about her business normally. It is hard for many people to see themselves in this way with plastic tubing embedded in their chest.

Targeted therapy is currently given by vein. Though a new pill form has become available, its use for prevention depends on further testing.

THE DRUGS

The hormones used in hormone therapy for breast cancer normally play a role in regulating breast cell growth and survival. When they are given therapeutically, they cause dramatic shrinking of breast tumors without damaging cells in the rest of the body. Drugs used for chemotherapy are called *cytotoxic,* which means that they act largely by destroying cells. The question that is inevitably raised is this: Won't cytotoxic drugs destroy normal cells, too?

The answer is that when properly administered, cytotoxic drugs will kill some normal cells, but not many. The drugs used in chemotherapy are useful because cancer cells are much more sensitive to their effects than are normal cells. This difference in sensitivity is the edge we utilize to treat the cancer without injuring the patient.

Targeted adjuvant therapy at this time refers to drugs that act against HER-2, a switch on the cell's surface that stimulates cell growth. These drugs kill tumor cells that overexpress HER-2. Clinical trials are testing new agents targeting HER-2, as well as newer drugs that target the formation of the new blood vessels that tumors require to grow.

DOSAGE

In the systemic treatment of breast cancer, most women are given the same dose of hormones by mouth. Tamoxifen (Nolvadex), which is still the hormone most commonly used in premenopausal women and is also employed in the treatment of some postmenopausal women, is given in a daily dose of 20 milligrams. Other hormone-related drugs such as aromatase inhibitors (see pages 280–82), are also given in a single, standard dose for all women.

In chemotherapy, on the other hand, dosage is individually tailored according to height and weight, in order to give the highest dose possible that will kill the cancer cells without harming the patient. If the dose is too low, the cancer cells will not be destroyed. If it is too high, the side effects will be unacceptable.

Though there may seem to be high-dose and low-dose advocates among oncologists, there is in fact a fairly narrow range of doses that is effective and well tolerated. Both the schedule and the dosage are, however, important factors in administering these drugs. Cancer cells can be sensitive to chemotherapy in some stages of their growth and resistant to it in others. What is *not* possible is to give a single dose so high that it kills all the cancer cells at one time. That level of dosage cannot be tolerated. The higher the dose, the less frequently it can be given; the lower the dose, the more frequently.

There are various programs of chemotherapy: weekly, biweekly, every three weeks, and others. The frequency varies with the program, the drugs used, and the doses. Despite these variations, there are two very important strategies in using chemotherapy to fight cancer.

Hit hard, and as early in the course of the disease as possible.

That doesn't mean we should load the patient up with a megadose of the most aggressive drugs available. But neither does it make sense to "lead up to" the program that will eventually be used. The physician should make careful plans about the drugs that will be used, how they will be combined, their dosages, and the schedule—and then go to it.

The proper dosage for targeted therapy is currently calculated on the basis of weight.

Use a proven treatment.

Your physician should use a regimen that has been tested and validated. She should not "invent," or tailor, a special treatment for you, and the treatment should be administered using proven doses and schedules.

This approach works best because there is reason to believe that not only does the number of tumor cells increase as the disease progresses, but so does the possibility that cells will develop that are resistant to chemotherapy. For that reason, we should act vigorously from the start and insist on the use of proven standard regimens.

TIMING

Tamoxifen should begin within about four weeks of surgery or after radiation therapy is completed (see pages 203–04). Studies in patients whose tumor was confined to the breast at the time of surgery (Stage I, see page 152) indicate that tamoxifen should be given for a period of five years. At ten years, an analysis of combined data showed reductions in risk for those taking tamoxifen for one, two, and five years to be respectively 21 percent, 29 percent, and 47 percent. Taking tamoxifen beyond five years may not provide additional benefit, but ongoing studies are seeking to determine whether longer periods of tamoxifen are helpful.

Newer hormone-related agents, referred to as aromatase inhibitors, such as anastrozole (Arimidex), letrozole (Femara), and exemestane (Aromasin), have been introduced as a means for preventing recurrence. Extensive studies indicate that these drugs are more effective than tamoxifen in postmenopausal women, whether given immediately after surgery, after two to three years of tamoxifen, or following five years of tamoxifen. However, giving a drug such as Arimidex *together* with tamoxifen eliminates the advantage of the aromatase inhibitor.

Until the last few years, since there was no evidence that more than five years of hormone therapy offered any additional benefit, hormone therapy was routinely stopped after five years. However, starting with research using Femara, we have since discovered that the introduction of an aromatase inhibitor after five years can significantly reduce the recurrence rate. As a result we are now uncertain about the optimal length of time to give adjuvant hormone treatments. Studies are under way to see if ten years or more of an aromatase inhibitor will be more effective in preventing late recurrences of breast cancer than taking the drug for only five years.

Adjuvant chemotherapy should also begin about two to eight weeks after surgery. If you need both radiation (see Chapter 9) and chemotherapy, the sequence of the treatments will vary according to the individual situation. Chemotherapy is usually completed before radiation since, in general, delaying radiation therapy by several months has not been shown to be detrimental.

In the few cases where there is a high risk of local recurrence, radiation therapy may be offered first.

As to the duration of chemotherapy, we know that a single treatment does not destroy every cancer cell. Our goal is to get rid of all cancer cells, because even if 99.9 percent of the billions of cancer cells that were present were to be destroyed, the remaining .1 percent would still leave a significant number capable of multiplying and causing grave harm. We also know that because the drugs only attack the DNA of multiplying cells, any one treatment may "miss" those cells that are not actively preparing to divide at that time. Like hibernating bears, these noncycling cells may awaken later on and become active.

For these and other reasons, repeated treatments of chemotherapy are used over a period of time that may vary from several months to half a year. The stage of the disease, the particular drugs used, and the risks are all taken into account in determining the duration of treatment.

When Adriamycin is used, targeted therapy for patients whose tumors overexpress HER-2 generally does not start for at least two months after chemotherapy begins. This is to prevent the excessive side effects that may occur if Herceptin use overlaps that of Adriamycin. Once started, Herceptin treatment is continued for one year, but ongoing studies are evaluating alternative treatment durations.

COMBINING DRUGS

At present, using only one single drug for preventive therapy against cancer simply isn't effective. Most modern chemotherapy programs for breast cancer combine two or three drugs, and as many as six. We're not sure why this strategy works, but perhaps it is because cells that respond to one drug don't respond to another. By using several substances, we get an overlapping effectiveness. However, some newer drugs may be effective as single agents and are being studied as such.

THE TYPES OF DRUGS

There are five types of drugs currently in use for adjuvant treatment of breast cancer:

- **Alkylating agents,** the first group, damage the genetic programs that control growth in the chromosomes of the tumor cells.

- **Antimetabolites,** the second group, interfere with the manufacture of nucleotides, the simple substances that make up DNA.

- **Natural products,** the third group, interfere with cell structure and cell division.

- **Targeted agents,** the fourth group, are directed against genes and gene products that control growth.

- **Hormones,** the fifth group, affect the growth of breast cancer cells.

ALKYLATING AGENTS

The most widely used alkylating agent is Cytoxan (cyclophosphamide). It can be given by mouth or intravenously, and it is not activated until it is processed in the liver. For the small number of patients who cannot tolerate Cytoxan because of its side effects, Leukeran (chlorambucil) is usually used.

A related but not typical alkylating agent is Adriamycin (doxorubicin). This drug must be given intravenously and must be carefully administered, because it can be extremely damaging to the skin if it leaks out of the vein. Ellence (epirubicin) is a drug very similar to doxorubicin.

Other alkylating agents that are currently not widely used for breast cancer but are being considered in special situations are Platinol (cisplatin) and Paraplatin (carboplatin).

ANTIMETABOLITES

Methotrexate and 5-fluorouracil are the two antimetabolites widely used for the treatment of breast cancer. In adjuvant treatment they are usually given intravenously.

Leucovorin, a vitamin derivative of folic acid, is sometimes used in combination with these drugs to modulate their activity. It may be given by mouth or intravenously.

NATURAL PRODUCTS

Oncovin (vincristine) and Velban (vinblastine) are derived from the periwinkle plant. A chemically altered product of the same plant, Navelbine (vinorelbine), is also available. These work in tiny concentrations.

Recent additions to this drug group are Taxol (paclitaxel) and Taxotere (docetaxel), whose original sources are, respectively, the barks of the Pacific and European yew trees. Taxol is presently produced synthetically. All these drugs, which are given intravenously, can cause damage if they accidentally leak into the skin.

TARGETED AGENTS

Herceptin is a monoclonal antibody (an antibody produced by a clone of cells, that is directed at a single target); it binds to HER-2 receptor sites on the surface of breast cancer cells (see pages 183 and 208). Growth factors that bind to HER-2 trigger cell growth. Herceptin blocks this activity, thus preventing the cells from growing. There are other growth-promoting receptors on cell surfaces. Several new drugs are being prepared to act against them (see Chapter 16).

HORMONE-RELATED SUBSTANCES

Prednisone, a drug related to cortisone, probably works in adjuvant therapy because as a hormone, it enhances the effects of the other, cytotoxic drugs. It may also have other, more direct, antitumor properties.

Tamoxifen, as noted, is the most widely used hormone-related drug. It is an antiestrogen, or hormone antagonist, because though it is itself a weak estrogen, it interferes with the action of estrogen on cancer cells and inhibits tumor growth. It is given by mouth.

Arimidex (anastrozole), Femara (letrozole), and Aromasin (exemestane) all act against the enzyme aromatase, which converts materials circulating in the blood to estrogens. These drugs are called aromatase inhibitors (AIs; see page 199). They are effective only in postmenopausal women. They are also given by mouth.

How Are These Drugs Combined?

The following section is a brief survey of the way these drugs are combined in systemic therapy. You may want to read the material now, or you may want to wait and use it as a reference when you and your physician discuss your planned treatment.

TAMOXIFEN

We begin with this hormone-related substance because it is so frequently used, often alone, sometimes in combination with other drugs.

A study completed in 1990 compared the benefits of tamoxifen alone with those of tamoxifen and chemotherapy after surgery in 1,200 women, age fifty or over, who had hormone receptor-positive tumors (see page 98) as well as lymph node involvement. The study showed that chemotherapy added significantly to the effects of tamoxifen in preventing tumor recurrence. Additional studies have since confirmed this observation.

An analysis of the ten-year results of treating 37,000 women with tamoxifen, using pooled data from fifty-five separate studies, has revealed that the long-term benefits of tamoxifen extended equally to premenopausal and postmenopausal women whose tumors were hormone receptor-positive. These results were found to be "irrespective of ... whether chemotherapy had been given to both groups."

In these studies, tamoxifen and chemotherapy were usually given at the same time. A more recent clinical trial in postmenopausal women explored the effectiveness of giving first chemotherapy, and then tamoxifen. The results showed a significant advantage for the sequential treatment, and that has become the more common practice.

We do not yet know whether aromatase inhibitors, such as Arimidex and Femara, interfere with chemotherapy, but until we do, it is probably also best to start these drugs after adjuvant chemotherapy is completed.

AC

Adriamycin and Cytoxan are given intravenously every two or three weeks, for a total of four times.

AC/TAXOL

Two drug regimens are given in sequence. The treatments are administered either every three weeks in the standard program or every two weeks in the more frequently used "dose dense" protocol. The first four treatments consist of Adriamycin and Cytoxan, given together. Then Taxol is given for four doses. These regimens were initially recommended for higher risk patients, those with positive nodes, but they are increasingly being used for patients whose nodes were negative but whose tumors appeared more aggressive on pathologic examination. There is evidence that an every-two-week schedule is more effective than when drugs are given every three weeks.

AC/TH

AC/TAXOL plus Herceptin for the adjuvant treatment of HER-2 positive breast cancer. Weekly Herceptin is added to the regimen with the start of Taxol treatments and continued for one year.

AC/TAXOTERE

Similar to AC/TAXOL but Taxotere is given instead of Taxol either weekly or every three weeks over a twelve-week period.

TAC

The TAC treatment combines Taxotere Adriamycin, and Cytoxan. It is similar to AC/TAXOL or AC/TAXOTERE (Taxotere and Taxol are both taxanes), but the three drugs are given at the same time. Side effects are somewhat greater than when the taxane is given after the Adriamycin/Cytoxan. It is given every twenty-one days for six cycles.

ACT

Similar to TAC but uses slightly different dose of the same drugs on an every-three-week schedule.

TC

This is a treatment in which Taxotere replaces the Adriamycin of AC. TC is given four times at an every-three-week interval. In a study comparing TC to AC given every three weeks, the TC program was somewhat more effective. TC is usually given four times at twenty-one-day intervals.

TCH

Taxotere, Paraplatin (carboplatin), and Herceptin are combined for the adjuvant treatment of HER-2 positive breast cancer. This is a relatively new program that has been considered as an alternative for AC/TAXOL and Herceptin for the treatment of patients who have had HER-2 positive breast cancer but want to or need to avoid Adriamycin. It is given every twenty-one days, six times. After the chemotherapy is finished, the Herceptin is continued every three weeks to the end of one year.

CMF

CMF—Cytoxan, methotrexate, and 5-fluorouracil—is the pro-totype chemotherapy combination because of its documented record of improving survival rates in several groups of women. In recent years it has been supplanted as the most commonly used adjuvant chemotherapy program by Adriamycin-based regimens.

The most frequently used schedule for the administration of this combination of drugs is giving all three intravenously, once every three weeks for six months.

Others believe that there is an advantage to giving Cytoxan by mouth over a longer period. They use the original schedule of this treatment program. In this variant:

• Cytoxan is taken daily, by mouth, for the first fourteen days of every four-week month (that is, every twenty-eight days, rather than the thirty or thirty-one days of a calendar month).

• The other two drugs, methotrexate and 5-fluorouracil, are given intravenously on the first and eighth days of the four-week month.

CMF is usually administered for six months. Studies that evaluated the use of this treatment program for up to two years showed no additional benefits over the six-month course.

CAF

This program combines Cytoxan, Adriamycin, and 5-fluorouracil. Much like CMF, it is nowadays usually given on an every-three-week basis. In a variant of this schedule, these drugs are adminis-tered on the first and eighth days of each four-week month, with no medication during the remaining two weeks of the month. Treatment continues for four to six months, depending on the dose of each drug used.

FAC

Similar to CAF, and using the same drugs, this program empha-
sizes somewhat higher doses of Adriamycin, generally given with
the other two drugs on the first day of a twenty-eight-day cycle.
Only 5-fluorouracil is given on day eight. Another variant of this
program treats with all three drugs one day every three weeks.

FEC

This is similar to CAF, but in this regimen Adriamycin is replaced
by epirubicin, a related drug, long a mainstay in Europe and
Canada. The treatment is given every three weeks, six times.
Since Ellence (epirubicin) is significantly more expensive in the
United States than Adriamycin, the program is infrequently used
in the U.S.

CMFVP

In this plan, vincristine and prednisone (or prednisolone, a similar drug) are added to CMF. This combination of drugs is used in
my own practice once every week for six months. The program
is administered by some physicians for six to eight weeks on a
weekly basis, and then for two out of four weeks. The duration of
the treatment is usually from six to nine months. Like CMF it is
much less widely used since AC/TAXOL became a de facto standard for adjuvant chemotherapy for most oncologists. However,
this program and others such as TC have a particular role for the
treatment of patients with heart problems who are less able to tolerate Adriamycin.

MF

This program combines methotrexate and 5-fluorouracil with
the folic acid derivative leucovorin, and thus avoids the use of
Cytoxan, which, as we will see, may have troublesome side effects.
It has been effective in treating women with no lymph node

involvement. There is evidence, though it is by no means conclusive, that this regimen is more likely to permit women to retain their fertility, because it does not include an alkylating agent.

HERCEPTIN

Herceptin, a monoclonal antibody directed against HER-2, has proven highly effective against advanced breast cancer. It is the first "targeted drug" to be used against this disease. In 2004, its value as an adjuvant treatment for women whose breast cancers are HER-2–overexpressing was reported. The results of two American studies, when combined, showed that, when used with AC/TAXOL chemotherapy, Herceptin produced an astounding 52 percent decrease in the risk of recurrence.

VERY HIGH DOSE CHEMOTHERAPY IN CONJUNCTION WITH STEM CELL TRANSPLANT

Though not established as a treatment for patients with advanced-stage breast cancer, people who have blood-related cancers, such as leukemia and lymphoma, have been treated successfully for many years with doses of chemotherapy so large that they destroy not only cancer cells but normal bone marrow cells as well. After this treatment, patients have no residual bone marrow to produce the white blood cells that protect against infection, or the platelets that prevent bleeding.

In order to counteract this effect, before such chemotherapy, drugs are used to stimulate the patient's marrow to produce large numbers of immature white blood cells, which are released into the circulating bloodstream. These "stem cells" are also removed and stored. After a very high dose of chemotherapy is completed, the stem cells are given back to the patient.

Such treatments began to be used for breast cancer in the late 1980s and soon became a treatment of choice for patients with a very high risk of breast cancer recurrence, such as those with ten or more lymph nodes involved by metastases. The initial results were promising, but multiple studies comparing the effects of very high dose or bone marrow/stem cell transplant therapy with conventional treatments have shown no overall advantage.

GENERAL SIDE EFFECTS

Hormone therapy may produce increased sweating, chilliness, or typical "hot flashes." Some produce mild arthritis and aggravate the usual loss of bone density with age. In general, however, its side effects are not particularly troublesome.

On the other hand, side effects are the aspect of chemotherapy treatment that concerns patients most. The concern is valid, but:

• Chemotherapy does have side effects, but they are usually transitory.

• Several side effects cause particular difficulty right after treatment, but they soon fade.

• There is no way to avoid side effects completely, but an experienced and careful physician can alleviate many of the adverse symptoms.

PAIN?

There is usually no pain associated with the administration of chemotherapy. Very occasionally, the drug may feel cold as it goes into the vein, but that feeling rarely lasts for more than a few seconds.

NAUSEA

Nausea is for most of us one of the most unpleasant of physical sensations. For that reason, apprehensiveness about nausea is sometimes worse than the actuality.

Most drugs do not cause immediate nausea unless a particularly large dose is being used and it is being pushed into the vein very fast. If you feel queasy during the treatment, mention it at once, and ask that the procedure be done more slowly.

Though this is not always the case, as we will see below, nausea is often a result of excessive acid secretion in the stomach caused by certain of the drugs. This nausea can be controlled with the use of preparations like Maalox, Pepcid, Zantac, Nexium, or Prevacid. Eating a bowl of oatmeal can also help settle your stomach.

Especially with the use of higher doses of chemotherapy, the nausea may be severe enough that the doctor has to prescribe a medication to reduce this symptom before beginning treatment. The introduction in the early 1990s of a new category of antinausea drugs, including Zofran and Kytril, has almost eliminated the immediate nausea associated with many forms of chemotherapy. These are available in both intravenous and oral preparations. They are often given together with Decadron, a cortisone-like drug that further increases their effectiveness. When nausea persists for a day or two after treatment, it is usually less intense and can be treated with an older antinausea drug, such as Compazine. If the delayed nausea is a more significant problem, you may be offered Emend. This drug works by a different mechanism than the drugs already mentioned. Given on the day of treatment and for the following two days, it can prevent or reduce delayed nausea.

HAIR LOSS

This is the side effect that causes women the greatest sadness. At a time when they are extremely vulnerable, their appearance may be radically changed, and their illness given a visible and very upsetting public manifestation.

True. *But every strand of hair will grow back.*

With that fact in mind, let's examine the question of hair loss.

With very high doses of Adriamycin and standard doses of Taxol or Taxotere, temporary hair loss cannot be prevented as of this writing. It occurs over a few days about three weeks after the first dose of chemotherapy is given. You should therefore arrange to buy an attractive hairpiece at the start of your treatment so that it will be on hand for the temporary period when you lose your hair. Try to get one that is close not only to your own color but also to your own hairstyle so that you will not have to cope with a new image of yourself when you look in the mirror.

Depending on the drugs used, hair loss can be total and include eyebrows, underarm, and pubic hair. LOOK GOOD . . . FEEL BETTER, a program of the American Cancer Society, is an incredibly valuable resource for women undergoing chemotherapy, providing classes and personal advice about makeup and hair care.

With vincristine in drug combinations such as CMFVP, we can prevent hair loss in women under sixty—and prevent or reduce it in women over sixty—by the use of a kind of tourniquet around the head during treatment. A narrow blood pressure cuff is particularly effective for this purpose. The headband does not keep all of the drug from the scalp, but it does prevent the highest levels of the drug from reaching it. This precaution preserves the hair, and there has been no indication that it reduces the benefits of adjuvant therapy. Soft rubber tourniquets or headbands are left in place for ten minutes after the patient is given her chemotherapy.

With such treatments hair loss may also be ameliorated by using an ice pack on the head for fifteen minutes before and fifteen to thirty minutes after treatment.

FATIGUE

High doses of chemotherapy can cause a great deal of fatigue, especially on the first day after treatment. You should, however, feel little fatigue after a couple of days, though occasionally you may feel tired late in the day. If you do continue to feel exhausted, or if you have days when you are what some patients call "zonked out," tell the oncologist. Recent studies have shown that prolonged fatigue in this setting may have many causes, such as lack of sleep, skipping meals, or anemia. Your doctor may be able to help with relatively simple suggestions or treatments. Procrit, a red blood cell growth factor, is a drug that can be used to correct anemia caused by chemotherapy and therefore help reduce fatigue.

If you are extremely tired the first day or two after treatment, you should rest, but try to resume your normal level of activity as soon as possible. Many women find they can continue to work, though they may need some flexibility in their schedules. For some women an active exercise program is the best way to overcome fatigue.

OTHER SIDE EFFECTS

Although modern antibiotics have reduced the risk, infection can be a problem with chemotherapy, because most anticancer drugs affect bone marrow and therefore the production of the white blood cells the body uses to fight infection. This is one of the reasons you have a blood count taken every time you go for treatment. If there is a problem with your white blood cell count, your therapy will be adjusted. A colony-stimulating factor (a hormone that stimulates white blood cell growth), such as Neupogen, may be prescribed to help restore white blood cell levels to normal more quickly. *If you develop a fever, report it to your doctor.*

The platelets are the cellular component of the blood that prevents bleeding. Since chemotherapy can affect the number of platelets, we must stop or postpone chemotherapy when blood counts show that platelet counts have fallen below normal levels. For safety, the levels during chemotherapy are usually well above those associated with bleeding. You should also avoid taking aspirin, because it interferes with platelet function. There is one natural product, interleukin 11 (Neumega), available that stimulates platelet production. However, its effects on platelet counts are less dramatic than those of Neupogen on white blood cell counts, so Neumega is not widely used.

The term *phlebitis,* as we saw, describes an inflammation of the vein as well as the formation of a blood clot. It occurs infrequently in the legs as a side effect of hormone therapy or chemotherapy, but it must be promptly treated.

Weight gain is a common and often unavoidable side effect of several of the drug programs. Ironically many women about to undergo a course of chemotherapy are afraid that they are going to grow thin and gaunt; instead, they find that the opposite happens.

The discomfort of the excess acid in the stomach that some of the drugs cause can be mistaken for hunger. Sometimes, also, women eat because they are nauseated; still others seem to gain weight whether they eat more or not. Try to follow a sensible weight-controlling diet, but don't chastise yourself for putting on a few pounds, and don't go on a radical diet while you are on chemotherapy. If necessary, and it often is, your physician may prescribe drugs that reduce acid production. Eat nutritious and attractive food, and remember that "this, too, shall pass." Most women go back to their normal weight six months to one year after chemotherapy.

Some people develop arthritis during hormone treatment or when chemotherapy is discontinued. The former is usually managed by switching to another hormonal drug that has similar benefits but may produce less arthritis for particular patients. Arthritis that first appears after chemotherapy is a condition that will gradually disappear, usually within a year of its onset. Vitamin B6, 200 milligrams a day, has been prescribed for such arthritis and may be helpful.

Sweating and "hot flashes" similar to those some women experience during menopause are among the general side effects of chemotherapy or hormone therapy. These symptoms can be partially relieved by the use of drugs such as Paxil or Effexor.

You may also stop menstruating during systemic therapy, though you should not rely on this occurrence for contraception. Whether your period resumes depends on your age. Younger women are more likely to return to a normal menstrual cycle. Women in their forties and those closer to menopause are less likely to begin menstruating again. The drugs responsible for this are Lupron and Zoladex, which cause the pituitary gland to release a large amount of a hormone that may temporarily suppress ovarian function. These drugs are sometimes used prior to initiating chemotherapy in women who have never had children or those who are in their later thirties or early forties, in the hope of preventing or reducing ovarian damage secondary to chemotherapy.

Fertility, of course, is closely related to this. When your period returns, you have a significant chance of conceiving, although the likelihood may be somewhat lower than if you never had chemotherapy at all. And though couples quite naturally worry about this, there is no evidence that chemotherapy or hormone therapy causes either mutation to the eggs or birth defects. Pregnancy does occur after chemotheraphy, as many delighted former patients have found out (see pages 358–59). If you are concerned, however, some fertility experts suggest that you harvest and store eggs before you start chemotherapy.

Some women report that they have more difficulty remembering recent information, such as people's names or where they left their glasses or keys, while on chemotherapy. Whether this is due to the chemotherapy, antinausea or other drugs, or just stress alone is unclear. Memory in such patients appears to return to normal soon after the chemotherapy program is completed.

SPECIFIC DRUG-RELATED SIDE EFFECTS

In addition to the general symptoms we've been reviewing, the following side effects specific to particular drugs can occur. Though this is by no means a complete list of side effects, I have selected those that in my experience are most significant and most likely to be troubling to patients.

Remember: You may experience only a few—or even none— of these symptoms during the course of your treatment. Side effects can often be controlled by well-regulated dosages and schedules.

PREDNISONE

Like other cortisone products, this drug can cause emotional ups and downs, weight gain, insomnia, hyperacidity, ulcers, and an elevation of blood sugar levels. If given daily, the drug is most commonly used for a course of treatment lasting no more than eight weeks. For longer therapy, it is much better tolerated if it is taken every other day, rather than daily. Prednisolone, a closely related preparation, has similar side effects.

TAMOXIFEN

Tamoxifen has relatively few significant side effects in most patients. Occasionally a woman will have mild nausea or weight gain, and younger women may experience annoying menopausal symptoms while they are taking the drug. Very rarely, a woman may notice some light-colored facial hair growth as a result of using tamoxifen. Phlebitis has been reported in 2 percent of patients and requires prompt treatment. Because the drug is itself a weak estrogen, it does not cause the loss of bone calcium associated with low estrogen levels. In fact, there is reason to believe tamoxifen helps prevent osteoporosis and lowers blood cholesterol levels.

As to gynecological symptoms, a slight vaginal discharge is common. Vaginal dryness may also occur and may have to be treated with moisturizers. While some gynecologists recommend estrogen creams for this purpose, most oncologists prefer to avoid using estrogens after breast surgery. Tamoxifen, like estrogens used for hormone replacement therapy after menopause, modestly increases the risk of developing endometrial cancer. You should therefore see a gynecologist regularly.

ANASTROZOLE, LETROZOLE, AND EXEMESTANE

While these drugs, which are all aromatase inhibitors, are generally well-tolerated, like tamoxifen, they can cause hot flashes, nausea, and fatigue. Compared with tamoxifen, they are less likely to produce phlebitis or to have any effects on the uterus. This group of drugs does not share tamoxifen's protective effects on bone, and may cause osteoporosis and an increase in fracture risk. Fosamax and Actonel are among the drugs that can be added to the treatment to stop bone loss.

LUPRON FOLLOWED BY AROMATASE INHIBITOR

Since aromatase inhibitors reduce the risk of recurrence in postmenopausal women when given after five years of tamoxifen, some oncologists treat premenopausal women who are at higher risk with the drug Lupron at five years. This stops their periods. Then an aromatase inhibitor is added. Studies of the effectiveness of this approach are still under way.

ADRIAMYCIN

Adriamycin can have a toxic effect on the heart, causing potentially significant heart muscle damage. Such damage is rarely seen if the total dose of Adriamycin does not exceed a threshold of between 750 and 1,000 milligrams. This threshold can be calculated depending on the patient's size. For that reason, optimal programs are designed to keep Adriamycin well below that threshold.

The urine may be slightly red immediately after an Adriamycin injection. This is no cause for concern. Hair loss, nausea, vomiting, and inflammation of the mouth lining are also associated with the use of this drug. There can be marked skin damage if the drug infiltrates the skin during injection.

CYTOXAN

The end products of Cytoxan after it has been "used" by the body can irritate the bladder and cause serious damage to the bladder wall. It is very important to increase your normal intake of water while you are using this drug; each doctor will have his own recommendations about how to accomplish this. For instance, you may be told to drink three glasses of water, in addition to your normal intake, within three hours of receiving Cytoxan. Ample water intake is especially important in hot weather. Cytoxan can cause leukemia. This is rarely, if ever, seen in patients who have been on relatively low-dose programs such as CMF or CAF, but it may be a bigger problem for women who receive high-dose intravenous Cytoxan. Currently more attention is being given to limiting the dose of Cytoxan to less than a maximum of 1,200 milligrams a day (the dose varies with a person's height and weight). Two important research studies show no advantage for higher doses.

CMFVP

Patients receiving this drug combination may develop persistent elevated temperature and a mild cough that may indicate a serious infection. Report any fever to your oncologist as soon as possible so that he can prescribe specific antibiotics. *Bactrim,* taken together with *erythromycin,* appears to be the most effective.

5-FLUOROURACIL

This drug can cause irritation of the lining of the mouth and of the intestinal tract.

If mouth irritation occurs, avoid using commercial mouth-washes that contain alcohol or other irritants. Rinse your mouth regularly with a solution containing ⅛ teaspoon of baking soda dissolved in a glass of lukewarm water. Brush your teeth gently, and use a soft brush. This irritation is rarely severe, but numbing agents are available if they are necessary. A popular remedy for this purpose is Magic Mouthwash. It comes in several variations but all contain a numbing agent and several other drugs to soothe the mouth.

If severe diarrhea becomes a problem, the treatment must be stopped, though this usually occurs only at high doses or in the case of somewhat lower doses of 5-fluorouracil when given in combi-nation with leucovorin.

There may be a mild, reversible darkening of the skin after pro-longed use of 5-fluorouracil. Thickening and peeling of the skin of the palms may also be seen.

METHOTREXATE

This drug may cause soreness of the mouth, and diarrhea. In ad-dition, nausea and vomiting may occur. Methotrexate may cause fat accumulation in the liver, but this is usually reversible once the drug is stopped.

TAXOL/TAXOTERE

Taxol may cause an allergic reaction. To prevent this, Decadron, a cortisone-like drug, is taken by mouth twelve and six hours before Taxol is administered. Benadryl and cimetidine (the latter more familiar as the antiulcer drug Tagamet) are also used before Taxol for this purpose. Taxol will cause the white blood cell level to fall, and Neupogen is used to counteract this. After a while Taxol can cause numbness in the hands and feet. Taxotere, while in many ways similar to Taxol, does not cause an allergic reaction. It might, however, produce marked swelling of the legs after several doses. This cannot be corrected by using a diuretic such as Lasix; instead, to prevent such swelling, patients must take Decadron for several days, starting the day before treatment. Nail changes can occur with either drug but are more prominent with Taxotere. If they are troublesome, immersing your fingertips in ice water during the time Taxotere is being given may be helpful.

VINCRISTINE

In large doses, this drug is given only for a short time, six to eight weeks. That is because it can cause nerve damage that is sometimes permanent and that may result in constipation; numbness and tingling in the hands, feet, and fingers; and a loss of reflexes in the legs. These symptoms are not common when, instead of high doses, low doses of vincristine are used over a longer period of time.

HERCEPTIN

The most important side effect of Herceptin is its effect on the heart. Given alone, the number of patients with clinically significant heart symptoms because of Herceptin is low (circa 0.5 percent). It is higher when the drug is combined with Adriamycin. Patients' heart function should be tested before treatment and at regular intervals after treatment. To avoid an allergic reaction to Herceptin, Benadryl (see above) is given before Herceptin.

IS SYSTEMIC THERAPY THE RIGHT STEP?

Let's begin with some general statements.

The purpose of chemotherapy or hormone therapy is to prevent the recurrence of cancer. That no one would choose to go through the experience of breast cancer more than once goes without saying. But there is another reality to be faced: It is extremely difficult to cure a recurrence. For that reason, the current consensus is that most patients with breast cancer should receive adjuvant therapy to prevent recurrence.

This point of view is particularly compelling because the side effects of adjuvant therapy are not life-threatening to the vast majority of patients. The most dangerous effects—heart muscle damage and the risk of infection—may occur in programs using Adriamycin, but only a very small percentage of women are affected. Most side effects of adjuvant therapy are temporary and can be ameliorated by a carefully modulated program.

It is these considerations that have led me to the belief that adjuvant chemotherapy and/or hormone therapy should be used wherever there is an invasive cancer and therefore a risk of the disease's recurring. I think this is the most prudent policy. Moreover, it appears to be prudent even in circumstances where the risk is fairly small, as in the case of an invasive ductal cancer of less than 1 centimeter. Unless there are other prognostic factors suggesting a higher-than-average risk of recurrence, I favor hormone therapy alone for patients in whom hormone receptors are present who have in situ lobular cancers; who have in situ ductal cancers and had breast-conserving surgery; or have tumors that were minimally invasive (that is, an invasion of less than 5 millimeters into the surrounding tissue).

WHAT ADJUVANT THERAPY WILL I RECEIVE?

You will get different answers to that question from different oncologists. That is because, as we have been learning in this chapter, there are many options to be considered, as well as many risks.

When the oncologist proposes a program for you, she has to take into account what might be called the risk/benefit formula. If the disease has progressed far enough to put you at considerable risk, the oncologist will be more likely to recommend "aggressive" treatment, despite the possible toxicity, if she thinks it will lead to long-lasting benefits. In such cases, the risk the cancer poses to survival needs to be weighed against the side effects of the treatment, though successful "aggressive" treatment does not necessarily have to be hard on the patient.

TAILORING ADJUVANT THERAPY TO RISK

How do we tailor the treatment to the specific patient? First we determine her risk. Next we consider whether she is pre- or postmenopausal and does or does not have overexpression of HER-2.

Then we figure out from statistical evidence and from experience what has worked best for other women in each category.

When we are trying to decide what therapy is appropriate for a particular patient, we consider the following factors most important:

• Invasion

• Size of tumor

• Hormone-receptor status of tumor

• HER-2/neu overexpression by tumor

• Lymph node involvement

To review the general guidelines:

• Noninvasive in situ cancers have such a low risk of metastasizing that no chemotherapy is used. However, tamoxifen or an aromatase inhibitor should be considered.

• If the tumor was restricted primarily to the inside of ducts or lobules (in situ cancer) but shows early signs of invasion, that is 1 millimeter or less in depth (microinvasion), then tamoxifen or an aromatase inhibitor is more likely to be used.

• If the tumor was invasive but was restricted to the breast and less than 1 centimeter in size, many oncologists give adjuvant therapy. Others feel that the risk for these women is too small to warrant using systemic therapy.

• If the tumor was invasive and one centimeter (about ⅜ inch) or more in diameter, systemic hormone therapy or chemotherapy is generally advised, whether or not the lymph nodes were involved.

• If the lymph nodes were involved, chemotherapy or hormone therapy should always be used, even if the tumor was less than 1 centimeter in diameter. There are differences of opinion only about how vigorous the treatment should be in correlation with the number of nodes involved.

THE RANGE OF TREATMENT

It would be wonderful if we had a simple, logical gauge for who should get what treatment. Women would be faced with far fewer difficult choices if we could finely calibrate the risks and the treatments and come up each time with a precise plan of what to do. You would then get pretty much the same advice from every doctor you spoke to.

Unfortunately, the treatments now available to us do not permit such fine-tuning. What is considered "aggressive treatment" very much depends on whom you are talking to. The routine approach of one doctor may be considered aggressive by another.

There are, however, a few criteria by which such judgments are commonly made:

• If the oncologist were to propose using only MF, that would be considered a less aggressive treatment.

• If she used a combination like AC followed by Taxol, or CAF, certain other physicians might consider that more aggressive.

• The intervals between treatments, the intensity of dosage, and alternating drug combinations are other variables used to differentiate how vigorous the treatment is.

What is the advice you are likely to get, given your particular circumstances? The following chart may help explain what treatment an oncologist may recommend for you. (Refer to earlier sections of this chapter for explanations of the drug combinations that follow, as well as the various rationales for their use.)

```
                        − Nodes +
Group   0 1 2   3   4       5           6
Lower risk├──┼──┼──┼──┼──────────┼──────────┤ Higher risk
```

Group 0 = In situ carcinoma
Group 1 = Microinvasion, no involved nodes
Group 2 = Tumor less than 1 cm, no involved nodes
Group 3 = Tumor more than 1 cm, no involved nodes

Group 4 = 1–3 involved nodes
Group 5 = 4–9 nodes
Group 6 = 10 or more nodes

PREMENOPAUSAL WOMEN

If you are in Group 0:

- No treatment is needed after mastectomy for in situ ductal carcinoma.

- No treatment if after lumpectomy the tumor proves to be small, low grade, and removed with a large margin of normal tissue surrounding it

- Radiation only following lumpectomy, without systemic therapy

- Tamoxifen for five years after lumpectomy with or without breast radiation

If you are in Groups One and Two:

- No treatment may be recommended because of your relatively low risk.

- Tamoxifen for five years if the tumor was receptor-positive

- A "less aggressive" treatment, like MF with leucovorin, may be suggested.

- CMF or less toxic variations of CMFVP may be used by some oncologists.

- TC

- Adriamycin/Cytoxan (AC)

- Adriamycin/Cytoxan followed by Taxol (AC/T)

- Adriamycin/Cytoxan followed by Taxol and Herceptin if tumor was HER-2 positive

- In all cases where chemotherapy is given, it is followed by tamoxifen for five years if tumor was hormone receptor-positive.

If you are in Group Three, chemotherapy is desirable, and one of the following drug combinations may be suggested:

- AC

- TC

- CMF

- AC +/– Taxol

- AC +/– Taxotere

- AC/Taxol, plus Herceptin if tumor was HER-2 positive

- TCH, plus Herceptin if tumor was HER-2 positive

- CMFVP

- CAF

- FEC

- Herceptin may be added to other drug combinations that do not contain Adriamycin or epirubicin, a drug related to Adriamycin.

- Tamoxifen is added for five years after chemotherapy if tumor was receptor-positive.

If you are in Group Four, one of the following treatments will be proposed:

- AC followed by Taxol

- AC followed by Taxotere

- AC followed by Taxol or Taxotere, plus Herceptin if tumor was HER-2 positive

- TC

- TCH, plus Herceptin if tumor was HER-2 positive

- CAF and its variants

- FEC

- CMF

- CMFVP

- Herceptin may be added to other drug combinations that do not contain Adriamycin or epirubicin (a drug related to Adriamycin).

- Tamoxifen is added for five years if tumor was receptor-positive. If you are near menopause and then have no periods for two years after the initiation of chemotherapy, then the tamoxifen may be replaced with Arimidex or another aromatase inhibitor.

If you are in Group Five, one of the following treatments will be proposed:

- AC followed by Taxol

- AC followed by Taxotere

- AC followed by Taxol or Taxotere, and Herceptin if tumor was HER-2 positive

- TCH, plus Herceptin if tumor was HER-2 positive

- TAC/ACT

- FEC

- CAF and its variants

- FAC

- Herceptin may be added to other drug combinations that do not contain Adriamycin or epirubicin (a drug related to Adriamycin).

- Tamoxifen for five years may be added if tumor was receptor-positive, followed by an aromatase inhibitor for patients who by then are two years postmenopausal. If you are still having your periods, a combination of Lupron and Arimidex, or other aromatase inhibitor, may be suggested.

If you are in Group Six:

Group 6 patients will be presented with the greatest range of options. CMF alone is not effective, but each of the following programs offers some promise of helping. Most oncologists have developed regimens for this group that they feel provide optimal responses:

- AC followed by Taxol

- AC followed by Taxotere

- AC followed by Taxol or Taxotere plus Herceptin if tumor was HER-2 positive

- TAC/ACT

- TCH, plus Herceptin if tumor was HER-2 positive

- FEC

- CAF

- FAC

- Tamoxifen for five years may be added if tumor was receptor-positive, followed by an aromatase inhibitor for patients who by then are two years postmenopausal. If you are still having your periods, a combination of Lupron and Arimidex, or other aromatase inhibitor, may be suggested.

POSTMENOPAUSAL WOMEN WITH HORMONE RECEPTOR-POSITIVE TUMORS

As noted earlier, aromatase inhibitors, such as Arimidex, Femara, and Aromasin, have largely replaced tamoxifen as adjuvant hormone therapy for postmenopausal women who have breast cancer. These drugs cannot be used alone in premenopausal women because they cause more rather than less estrogen to be produced in women with normally functioning ovaries. It is still unclear how long women who are postmenopausal should take an aromatase inhibitor after chemotherapy.

The exception is for in situ ductal carcinoma, where tamoxifen is still often used for prevention.

If your tumor was hormone receptor-positive, the following treatments may be suggested:

If you are in Group 0:

- No treatment after mastectomy for in situ ductal carcinoma

- No treatment after lumpectomy if tumor is small, low grade, and removed with a large margin of normal tissue

- Radiation therapy only after lumpectomy

- Tamoxifen for five years after lumpectomy and breast radiation

If you are in Group One or Two, one of the following may be suggested:

- No treatment because of the relatively low risk

- Arimidex or other aromatase inhibitor

- A "less aggressive" treatment, such as MF with leucovorin

- CMF or less toxic variations of CMFVP

- TC

- AC

- AC followed by Taxol

- AC followed by Taxotere

- AC followed by Taxol or Taxotere and Herceptin if tumor was HER-2 positive

- Herceptin may be added to other drug combinations that do not contain Adriamycin.

If you are in Group Three, with negative nodes and a tumor that was larger than 1 centimeter, you may be offered one of the following:

- Arimidex or equivalent drug

- AC

- TC

- AC/Taxol

- AC/Taxotere

- AC/Taxol or Taxotere, plus Herceptin if tumor was HER-2 positive

- TCH plus Herceptin if tumor was HER-2 positive

- CMF

- CMFVP

- CAF and its variants

- FEC

- Herceptin may be added to other drug combinations that do not contain Adriamycin or epirubicin (a drug related to Adriamycin).

- In all cases, if tumor has hormone receptors, when chemotherapy is given it is followed by Arimidex, or other aromatase inhibitor, which is given for a minimum of five years.

If you are in Group Four with three or fewer positive nodes, you may be offered one of the following:

- Aromatase inhibitor or tamoxifen followed by an aromatase inhibitor

- AC

- TC

- AC/Taxol

- AC/Taxotere

- AC followed by Taxol or Taxotere, plus Herceptin if tumor was HER-2 positive

- TCH followed by Herceptin if tumor was HER-2 positive

- FEC

- CAF or its variants

- CMFVP

    If you are in Group Five, with four to nine involved nodes, you may be offered one of the following:

- AC/Taxol

- AC/Taxotere

- AC followed by Taxol or Taxotere, plus Herceptin if tumor was HER-2 positive

- TCH, plus Herceptin if tumor was HER-2 positive

- TAC/ACT

- FEC

- CAF

- FAC

- Herceptin may be added to other drug combinations that do not contain Adriamycin or epirubicin (a drug related to Adriamycin).

- In all cases where chemotherapy is given it is followed by an aromatase inhibitor which is given for a minimum of five years, if tumor was hormone receptor-positive.

    If you are in Group Six, with ten or more involved nodes, you may be offered one of the following:

- AC/Taxol

- AC/Taxotere

- AC followed by Taxol or Taxotere, plus Herceptin if tumor was HER-2 positive

- TAC/ACT
- TCH plus Herceptin if tumor was HER-2 positive
- FEC
- CAF
- FAC
- Herceptin may be added to other drug combinations that do not contain Adriamycin or epirubicin (a drug related to Adriamycin).
- In all cases where chemotherapy is given, it is followed by an aromatase inhibitor which is given for a minimum of five years, if tumor was hormone receptor-positive.

POSTMENOPAUSAL WOMEN WITH HORMONE RECEPTOR-NEGATIVE TUMORS

For women who are postmenopausal and hormone receptor-negative, chemotherapy can also be of value. Some oncologists may use Arimidex or another aromatase inhibitor in addition to chemotherapy if either estrogen or progesterone receptor levels are measurable, even if they do not reach the threshold level considered "positive." However, using the most recent information available, tamoxifen is no longer likely to be given to women whose tumors have no detectable levels of receptor to either hormone.

Group 0

If you are in Group 0, the following options may be suggested:

- No treatment after mastectomy
- Radiation therapy following lumpectomy
- Tamoxifen, since subsequent new tumors, whose prevention is intended, may be hormone receptor-positive

For Group One, no treatment may be used, because of the relatively low risk.

For Groups Two and Three on the chart—women with no node involvement—one of the following may be used:

- AC

- TC

- AC/Taxol

- AC/Taxotere

- AC plus Taxol or Taxotere, plus Herceptin if tumor was HER-2 positive

- TCH plus Herceptin if tumor was HER-2 positive

- A "less aggressive" treatment such as MF with leucovorin

- FEC

- CMF

- CMFVP

- CAF and its variants

- Herceptin may be added to other drug combinations that do not contain Adriamycin or epirubicin, a drug related to Adriamycin.

For Group Four the following options may be suggested:

- AC

- TC

- AC/Taxol

- AC/Taxotere

- AC followed by Taxol or Taxotere plus Herceptin if tumor was HER-2 positive

- TCH plus Herceptin if tumor was HER-2 positive

• FEC

• CAF and its variants

• CMF

• CMFVP

• Herceptin may be added to other drug combinations that do not contain Adriamycin or epirubicin, a drug related to Adriamycin.

If you are in Group Five, the following options may be suggested:

• AC/Taxol

• AC/Taxotere

• AC followed by Taxol or Taxotere, plus Herceptin if tumor was HER-2 positive

• TCH plus Herceptin if tumor was HER-2 positive

• TAC/ACT

• FEC

• CAF

• FAC

• Herceptin may be added to other drug combinations that do not contain Adriamycin or epirubicin (a drug related to Adriamycin).

For Group Six, suggested treatments may include the following:

• AC/Taxol

• AC/Taxotere

• AC followed by Taxol or Taxotere, plus Herceptin if tumor was HER-2 positive

- TCH plus Herceptin if tumor was HER-2 positive

- TAC/ACT

- FEC

- CAF and its variants

- Herceptin may be added to other drug combinations that do not contain Adriamycin or epirubicin (a drug related to Adriamycin).

TRIPLE NEGATIVE BREAST CANCER

Triple negative breast cancers are those which are both estrogen and progesterone receptor-negative as well as HER-2 negative. They are found more frequently in African-American women and in women with a BRCA1 mutation. Recent studies suggest they have a more serious prognosis. However, such tumors do react well to chemotherapy, which should be used for adjuvant treatment. Studies are under way to determine whether specific preventive approaches are more effective in this group of patients.

NEO-ADJUVANT THERAPY: CHEMOTHERAPY TO REDUCE TUMOR SIZE BEFORE SURGERY

Chemotherapy (or neo-adjuvant chemotherapy, as it is called in this context) is sometimes used to treat tumors too large to remove safely, so as to permit later surgery, or to downsize (downstage) tumors so that the breast can be saved. The programs commonly used for this purpose include Adriamycin-based programs such as AC, AC followed by Taxol or Taxotere, and TAC. Taxol or Taxotere together with Herceptin are increasingly being used in patients whose tumors are HER-2 positive. TCH is another alternative. Sometimes hormones alone are used for this purpose, mainly aromatase inhibitors, although their full value remains to be established.

IN SUMMARY

I recommend hormone therapy to most patients with in situ cancers, and hormone therapy and/or chemotherapy with or without Herceptin to all patients with invasive cancers, because it seems to me that even a small risk of a life-threatening recurrence of breast cancer is unacceptable if there is a chance that risk can be reduced. There are situations, as with very small in situ and invasive tumors, where it is very hard to ask a woman to go through a course of treatment that she probably dreads and that may have some temporary side effects. But even in these instances, it seems clearly better to do everything we can to prevent a recurrence of cancer.

The development of preventive therapy has changed the prospects of tens of thousands of women. It has also given us hope that someday, with improved therapy, all women will be cured of breast cancer.

SEQUENCING RADIATION, HORMONE THERAPY, AND CHEMOTHERAPY

Radiation therapy alone is used mainly for in situ breast cancer. There is some recent evidence that tamoxifen may increase the sensitivity of breast tissues to radiation. Therefore, when hormone therapy is the only additional treatment, it may be recommended that radiation be given first. When chemotherapy is used, it is usually administered before any radiation. Giving radiation therapy after chemotherapy does not significantly decrease its effectiveness, although it may require a delay of up to six months from the time of surgery until the completion of chemotherapy. The alternatives include:

• Radiation therapy only

• Radiation therapy concurrent with or followed by hormone therapy

• Radiation therapy followed by chemotherapy

• Chemotherapy followed by radiation therapy

• Sandwich therapy, with radiation therapy given between two periods of chemotherapy

• Concurrent radiation therapy and chemotherapy

The optimal schedule for integrating Herceptin (a targeted therapy) with radiation has not been determined. Currently Herceptin is often continued while radiation therapy is being given.

Which sequence your doctor chooses will depend on the risks she perceives to be most important in your case. If the risk of recurrences elsewhere in the body is high, chemotherapy is usually used first. Radiation is more likely to be used early if there is a danger of recurrence within a breast because of the size of the tumor removed or because the tumor is found to be near a surgical margin.

12

BREAST RECONSTRUCTION

❧❦

Replacing the breast after mastectomy by means of breast reconstruction is elective surgery. That means there is no compelling medical reason for the operation. Whether or not you choose to have this procedure is entirely your call. The choice became more complicated in 1992, however, when the Food and Drug Administration ordered that the use of silicone gel implants for cosmetic purposes be discontinued, because certain manufacturers might not have been forthcoming about the potential risks of using these implants. Several scientific studies have subsequently proven the safety of silicone implants. Nevertheless, as a result of major lawsuits alleging damage, several manufacturers went out of business. Silicone-filled implants are primarily used for breast reconstruction after mastectomy, and then under "limited supervisory" conditions. Effectively, they have been replaced by saline-filled implants. This matter is discussed more fully later in the chapter.

We know that women have very different reactions to the removal of their breasts. There are also a variety of reasons that some do not want breast reconstruction:

- They want to treat the cancer only and do not want to have more general anesthesia or to undergo further surgery.

- They seem relatively undisturbed about having lost a breast, glad to be alive without worrying too much about the cosmetic effects of mastectomy.

- Especially if they were small-breasted to begin with, there may not be enough real difference in their appearance when they are dressed to bother them.

- They are satisfied with their appearance when they are dressed and wearing a prosthesis (see pages 237–39) inside their bra.

- They feel that it is a betrayal of what they have lived through to hide the fact that they had breast surgery in order to conform to society's definition of what a woman's body should look like.

- They are concerned about the questions that have been raised about the safety of silicone gel implants.

On the other hand, there are many, many women who, after mastectomy, feel that having both breasts is vital to their physical and emotional health. For them, what is at stake is their own self-image and their sense of the wholeness of their body.

It is this feeling, of course (and its effectiveness), that has made the lumpectomy procedure as common as it is today. But the truth is that the choice between mastectomy and lumpectomy no longer needs to make such a radical difference cosmetically. The techniques of breast reconstruction have become so refined that though women might still prefer to have been able to preserve their breasts, those who have had mastectomies and reconstruction also feel good about their appearance. And because reconstruction is usually done at the time of the mastectomy, even the trauma of waking up after surgery with one side of the body totally different from the other can be avoided.

The Choices

DO NOTHING

You can choose to do nothing cosmetically after mastectomy, as women regularly did in the past and many continue to do now. What are the consequences? They vary.

I asked one of my patients who had been quite vehement about not having reconstruction what she thought about her decision six months after her surgery. She said hastily, "I'm fine, I'm fine. I'm just careful when I get dressed in the morning not to look in the mirror. I never look in the mirror when I'm undressed."

It seems to me this woman is not as "fine" as she said she was. On the other hand, another patient—a particularly chic professional woman—seems genuinely accepting of a double mastectomy. She now wears clothes that are cut differently from those she wore before the surgery, but finds that no great hardship. She has been married for a long time and says that her husband has grown more appreciative of her since the cancer than he was before.

The conclusion about doing nothing? Many women seem to fare well, others less well.

WEAR A PROSTHESIS

You can decline to have reconstruction and instead consider wearing a prosthesis, an artificial breast form.

1. CAN I TRY A PROSTHESIS BEFORE ACTUALLY BUYING ONE?

There is an easy way to accomplish this. Usually, after you have had a mastectomy, a volunteer from the American Cancer Society's Reach to Recovery program (see page 148) or someone from the hospital breast service will visit you in the hospital. This person will provide you with a bra that contains a temporary cloth prosthesis and will encourage you to wear it home from the hospital and during the following weeks. It won't fit as well as a permanent prosthesis, but it will give you the idea of how your clothes will look with the prosthesis in place.

2. WHAT IS A PERMANENT PROSTHESIS LIKE?

The prosthesis is often a plastic form that contains silicone gel and is therefore fairly resilient and soft to the touch. Another type is made from nylon and cotton and is cushioned with a fiber mixed with tiny glass beads that are said to give the form weight and balance. The results, when you are dressed or wearing a bra, are so good that you will look the same as you always have.

3. WHEN WILL I BE READY TO USE ONE?

You can be fitted for a permanent prosthesis within two to three weeks after your surgery, when there is no longer any swelling and your surgeon says the wound no longer needs care.

4. WHERE DO I GET A GOOD PROSTHESIS?

The local unit of the American Cancer Society, a Reach to Recovery volunteer, or the nurse in your surgeon's office will be able to give you a list of vendors.

Corset shops and the lingerie departments of many large stores employ salespeople with special experience in working with women who have had mastectomies. There are also shops that specialize in postmastectomy fittings. They usually stock a variety of forms and will also sew pockets in your own bras to accommodate the prosthesis. These shops tend to be less impersonal and more sensitive to the needs of women after breast surgery.

Try to find out whether other people have been satisfied with the work of the store you're considering. A good fitter is important. If you are small-breasted, it may only be necessary to use some light padding. If you are fairly heavy-breasted, the weight will have to be evenly balanced so that your bra does not ride up on one side and so that you avoid back and shoulder strain.

5. COST

Medicare and private insurance plans pay for prostheses. Women who do not have this coverage and cannot afford a prosthesis may contact the American Cancer Society Reach to Recovery program at (800) ACS-2345 or Breast Cancer Network of Strength at (800) 221-2141. Free wigs may also be available to women nationwide who are in financial need.

RECONSTRUCTION

Though many women are satisfied to wear a prosthesis, others are not:

- "Every time I put it into my bra, I remember that I had breast cancer."

- "Even with the form, I feel unbalanced."

- "When I'd go out for my run in the morning, especially in the summer, I'd always be worrying that the prosthesis was going to pop out."

- "A prosthesis isn't the point. I'm not worried about what other people think about the way I look; I'm the one I care about. I don't like the feeling that I'm missing a vital part, especially one that's been so important to my life. I don't only mean my sex life—I mean things like nursing my babies, and looking in the mirror and admiring my great shape."

More and more women are choosing breast reconstruction after mastectomy. According to the American Society of Plastic Surgeons, in 2007, about 57,102 women had breast reconstruction. More frequently, the reconstruction was performed at the same time as the mastectomy. Implants and expanders of artificial origin are used more frequently than TRAM flap surgery using the patient's own tissues.

For about 43,090 of those women an implant or expander was used; for about 14,012 it was their own body tissue that was employed to reconstruct the breast. Though the latter procedure continues to be less common, there is reason to believe that in coming years surgical advances will encourage more women to choose to be reconstructed with their own tissues.

WHO DOES BREAST RECONSTRUCTION?

You should go to a reconstructive surgeon, a plastic surgeon who regularly does breast reconstruction. A plastic surgeon who sees mostly post-accident patients or primarily does cosmetic procedures probably does not have sufficient current experience in breast reconstruction. As with the search for other specialists, the governing philosophy is that the more of this procedure the surgeon does, the better.

He should be board-certified, with special training and experience in plastic surgery and breast reconstruction, having passed an examination in the specialty.

Almost certainly, the best referral you can get is from your breast surgeon. For one thing, it's important to him that you be satisfied with the combined results of mastectomy and reconstruction. There will be at least one or two people with whom he has worked and whose results he respects.

In addition, discuss with other women who have had reconstruction which plastic surgeons they used and whether they were satisfied with the results. For specific advice on finding a doctor, refer to Chapter 2.

You may want to talk to more than one plastic surgeon before making your final decision, to make sure that your goals for the procedure and those of the person you choose coincide. For example, if you are quite small-breasted, some plastic surgeons may recommend that for aesthetic reasons the second breast also be augmented. Don't have surgery merely to conform to someone else's idea of what is cosmetically pleasing. If you've always wanted larger breasts, this may be the time to achieve that goal, but that should be exclusively your own judgment. On the other hand, if you are especially full-breasted, it may not be possible to make your reconstructed breast as large as the remaining one, and the second breast is frequently reduced. This may be welcomed by women who have been bothered by having large and heavy breasts all their lives.

THE COST OF RECONSTRUCTION

The cost varies according to the type of procedure and where in the country you're having it. For reasons that will become clear as we discuss each procedure, the simple insertion of an implant costs less than a free flap reconstruction. The creation of a nipple raises the cost of all reconstruction.

As one example of what these procedures cost, in New York City reconstruction with an expander costs $3,500 to $7,000 and flap surgery can add $10,000 to $24,000 to the cost of a mastectomy.

Reconstruction after mastectomy is not considered "cosmetic" surgery, as many people believe. Federal law requires health insurance plans to pay for reconstruction after mastectomy. This includes the cost of any implants, as well as augmentation or reduction surgery on the opposite breast when this is needed to restore symmetry. Check with your benefits representative or with the insurer.

WHEN IS RECONSTRUCTION DONE?

Because it used to be thought that breast implants at the site of mastectomies might mask the recurrence of cancer or even cause it, reconstruction was delayed until it was considered "safe," usually at least five years after mastectomy. Years of experience have shown that breast reconstruction after mastectomy does not appear to interfere with any postsurgical follow-up you may need. It does not mask or interfere with the detection of cancer by physical examination or increase its risk *after a mastectomy has been performed*. Most of the time the procedure is now done at the time of the mastectomy, as soon as the breast surgeon has finished his work. That means that the plastic surgeon must practice at the same hospital as the breast surgeon and must be available at the

time of the operation. This can limit the choice of plastic surgeons, though the scheduling conflicts can usually be overcome.

Mammography is not performed on a reconstructed breast
unless there is particular concern about a skin recurrence of cancer. The remaining breast needs to be screened according to mammography guidelines (see page 60), keeping the patient's increased
risk in mind.

Now that lumpectomy is so prevalent a form of treatment,
women who had counted on preserving their breast are sometimes very disheartened if they are advised that this procedure is
not appropriate for their particular condition. When immediate
breast reconstruction is an option, it can make the prospect of
mastectomy seem much less traumatic.

Other women prefer to wait until they've recovered from their
surgery and had a chance to catch their breath, think about it at
leisure, and discuss it with family and friends. There are a great
many important decisions to make and much to absorb emotionally and physically in the weeks after breast cancer is diagnosed,
so it is not at all uncommon to feel you need time before making
another decision.

In such instances, where the reconstruction is not done at the
time of the mastectomy, most surgeons recommend that you allow a three-month period for the mastectomy site to heal. Breast
reconstruction is feasible any time after that—even years later. It
is really never too late.

TYPES OF RECONSTRUCTION

To replace the breast that has been removed, a shape (mound) has to
be created and covered with your skin so that it is similar in appearance to your other breast. There are two types of reconstruction:

- When a prosthesis is used, it is called an *implant-expander
reconstruction.*

- When your own tissues are used, it is known as a *myocutaneous
flap.* This is because muscle *(myo),* fat, and skin *(cutaneous)*
are transferred from elsewhere in the body and used to create
the new breast.

If your own tissues are used, they must have a blood supply. If they are moved together with their arteries and veins, this is referred to as a *pedicle flap*. If the arteries and veins are detached at their original site, the tissues must be reattached to a blood supply in the breast area. This is referred to as a *free flap*.

THE IMPLANT

An implant is really an internal prosthesis, a plastic envelope filled with a saline solution or with silicone gel or with a combination of these.

Implants are inserted in a surgical procedure, usually under general anesthesia.

The implant is not placed, as many people think, directly under the skin. Instead, it is inserted under the chest muscle, in a pocket created by the surgeon. The muscle lies over the implant, girdling it.

Most frequently, reconstruction is done by the plastic surgeon

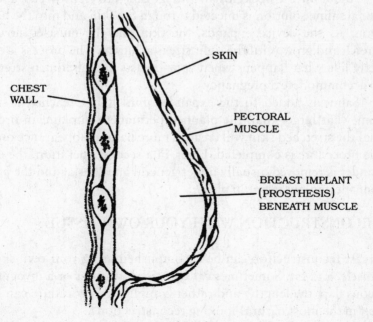

Breast implant placement

immediately after the mastectomy has been completed by the breast surgeon.

A drain is inserted to remove any fluids that accumulate in the days after surgery. This is later removed.

The incision is closed with sutures, as with any surgery.

Implant surgery takes from forty-five minutes to one and a half hours.

In addition to these standard elements of all breast implants, there are variations in the procedures.

In a simple implant, the full-size implant can be put in place in one operation, especially if the skin is sturdy and can be stretched, the chest muscle is healthy, and the woman is small- or average-breasted.

The permanent implant is rarely placed in a single operation. To permit the muscle and skin at the mastectomy site to accommodate a full-size implant, reconstructions usually start with a procedure called tissue expansion. A small balloonlike device, an expander, is placed under the chest muscle. It contains a valve into which saline solution can be injected.

About once a week, for an average of six to eight weeks, additional saline solution is injected through the skin and into the balloon. As the device expands, the skin and the muscles slowly stretch and grow until the right size is achieved. The process is exactly like what happens when your breasts and abdomen stretch to accommodate a pregnancy.

Saline is added to the expander until it has reached a size somewhat larger than the planned permanent implant, in order that the stretched skin will create a more natural appearance once the procedure is completed. Later, in a second operation, the expander is removed, usually under general anesthesia, and the permanent implant is put in place.

RECONSTRUCTION WITH YOUR OWN TISSUE

Breast reconstruction can be accomplished using your own skin, muscle, and fat. Sometimes called a tissue transfer or a myocutaneous flap, the lengthy and rather complicated procedure can result in the most natural-looking reconstructions.

There are several types of flaps. Among them are the latissimus

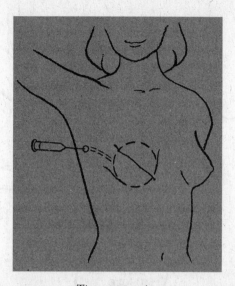

Tissue expansion

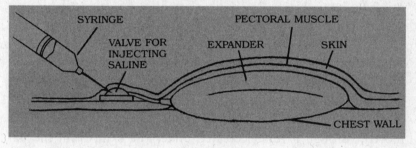

SYRINGE   PECTORAL MUSCLE

VALVE FOR   EXPANDER   SKIN
INJECTING
SALINE

CHEST WALL

Tissue expander

dorsi reconstruction; the TRAM flap (for *transverse rectus abdominal muscle*) as a pedicle or free flap reconstruction; the DIEP (for *deep inferior epigastric*) flap reconstruction; and the gluteal (buttock) reconstruction, which is always a free flap.

LATISSIMUS DORSI

This procedure takes about four to six hours and is done under general anesthesia. It is used primarily after a radical mastectomy to replace the pectoral muscle, but it may also be used to reconstruct a small breast in its entirety without the addition of an implant. During the procedure, the surgeon makes an incision

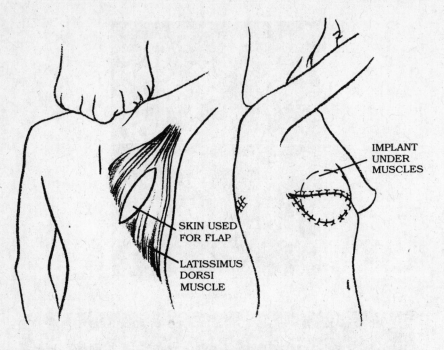

Latissimus dorsi flap reconstruction

beneath the shoulder blade in the back to expose the large, flat muscle called the latissimus dorsi.

The muscle and a portion of the skin that covers it are then moved, through a tunnel created under the skin, from the patient's back to the site of the mastectomy. An implant is usually needed, and it is placed under the latissimus dorsi muscle now relocated at the mastectomy site. Drains are inserted to remove any fluid that may accumulate over the following few days, and sutures are used to close the incision. (See Chapter 8 if you wish to review general procedures for breast surgery.)

Obviously, because the skin just under the shoulder blade is being cut, there will be a scar on the back as well as on the chest.

TRAM FLAP

This procedure can take four to six hours, is done under general anesthesia, and can result in a quite natural reconstruction. The

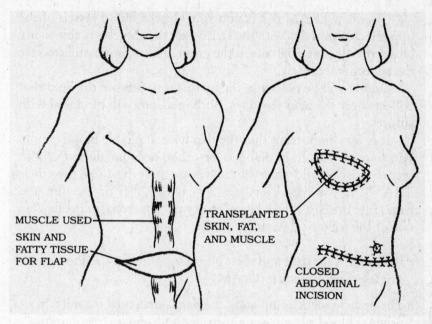

MUSCLE USED

SKIN AND
FATTY TISSUE
FOR FLAP

TRANSPLANTED
SKIN, FAT,
AND MUSCLE

CLOSED
ABDOMINAL
INCISION

TRAM flap reconstruction

newly constructed breast will respond to changes in weight just as the rest of the body does. The TRAM flap is not suitable for women who are very thin or extremely obese, who have abdominal scars from previous surgery, or who are heavy smokers.

During the TRAM flap procedure, your own tissue is moved from one part of your body to another. If the blood vessels are retained, it is called a pedicle flap; if they are cut, it is called a free flap. The surgeon makes an elliptical incision in the lower abdomen. He then moves the skin, the fat, the blood vessels (pedicle), and one or both of the abdominal muscles, through a tunnel he creates under the skin, from the abdomen to the mastectomy site.

This flap of muscle, skin, and fat is contoured into the shape of your breast and because the abdomen is wider than the breast, the excess skin is discarded. The procedure does, of course, leave a large scar across the abdomen. The results of the abdominal surgery are very much like those of a cosmetic procedure called an abdominoplasty, or "tummy tuck."

Usually a TRAM flap is nourished by the blood vessels of the upper rectus muscle. With the DIEP flap, the surgeon is able to use blood vessels that originate in the groin, making it possible to save the abdominal muscle.

Drains will be placed in the incisions to remove the fluid that collects over the next few days. Both incisions will be closed with sutures.

It is very important that the flap have a reliable blood supply. For women who have diabetes or other vascular diseases, both rectus muscles and their blood vessels may be used (bipedicle TRAM). If you have ever been a heavy smoker or are thin and have large breasts, it may be necessary to "supercharge the flap" in one of the following ways:

• Both rectus muscles and their blood supplies are used to build a single breast (bipedicle TRAM).

• The pedicle is cut completely, the flap is detached from its original blood supply, and the artery and vein are reconnected (free flap). This permits a more direct blood flow through larger vessels.

• A preliminary procedure is performed before the actual reconstruction, called a delay, in which a blood vessel to the flap is tied off before it is transferred and time is given to permit the remaining vessels to enlarge and improve the circulation in the flap.

Because a free flap spares more muscle, with this procedure the wall of the abdomen will remain stronger than with a pedicle flap.

BILATERAL TRAM FLAP

It is possible to reconstruct both breasts at the same time if there is enough abdominal wall tissue. A very natural appearance can be expected. If a prophylactic mastectomy is considered because the second breast is at high risk for also developing cancer (for instance, because of genetic reasons), the decision regarding the timing of a second mastectomy should take this issue into consideration, because a TRAM flap can be created only once.

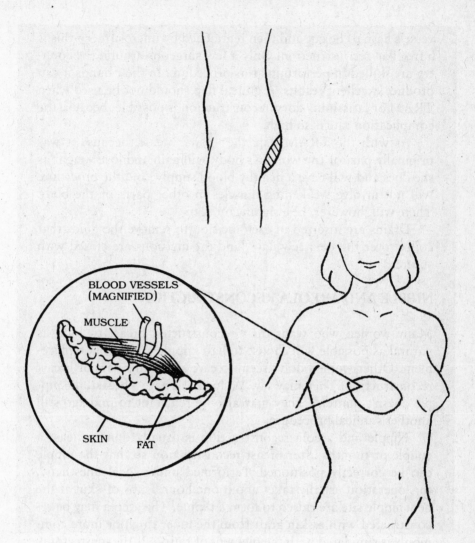

Gluteal (buttock) free flap reconstruction

GLUTEAL (BUTTOCK) FREE FLAP RECONSTRUCTION

This procedure takes about eight hours and is done under general anesthesia.

For a gluteal flap, the skin and muscles of the buttock are removed as a wedge and used to replace the breast. Since the blood vessels have to be cut and then reattached by microsurgery, this is a free flap reconstruction. Only a few surgeons around the country are skilled in performing this procedure. In their hands it can produce excellent results. A gluteal flap should not be used when TRAM or latissimus dorsi reconstruction is possible, because the complication rate is so high.

As with the TRAM flap, the "new" breast, because it was originally part of the woman's body, will gain and lose weight as she does and will have a healthy blood supply; and the procedure will not involve weakening muscles in other parts of the body. There will, however, be a significant scar.

Drains are inserted in each incision to remove the fluids that collect over the next few days, and the incisions are closed with sutures.

NIPPLE AND AREOLA RECONSTRUCTION

Many women who want their reconstructed breast to look as natural as possible will choose to have nipple and areola replacement. Other women don't seem to care about this part of breast reconstruction. They may say, "As long as I have a breast, the nipple doesn't matter." They may also be reluctant to undergo still another surgical procedure.

Nipple and areola reconstruction is usually done at least a couple of months after breast reconstruction so that the nipple can be correctly positioned. Performed under local anesthetic, this operation usually takes about one hour. Flaps of skin at the new nipple site are raised to form a nipple. The areola may be reconstructed with a skin graft from the inner thigh or more commonly is simulated with the pigment of tattoo. If the mastectomy performed spared the nipple or areola (see page 142) this may not be necessary.

To achieve a good color match, the proper pigments are carefully selected. Occasionally the nipple is also tattooed. This tattooing is done in the doctor's office, under local anesthetic.

SIDE EFFECTS OF BREAST RECONSTRUCTION

PAIN?

There is, of course, some pain associated with all surgery, since it involves the cutting and manipulation of tissue. There is relatively little pain as a result of mastectomy. Breast implants, however, do cause more temporary discomfort because of the pressure of the prosthesis against the chest wall as well as the stretching of the muscle.

When tissue is moved from one part of the body to another, there will be two wounds that may cause you discomfort, and with the TRAM flap you will have the greater discomfort that is associated with abdominal surgery. Women are pleased with the flat abdomen, but there may be persistent numbness in the lower central abdomen and some widening of the waist.

During a TRAM flap, a hernia, or hole, may develop in the fascia, the fibrous tissue that gives the abdominal wall its strength. This is a rare occurrence, but these hernias eventually have to be repaired.

Since tissue transfers may involve considerable blood loss, you may need a transfusion. Prepare for this in advance of the surgery by donating your own blood or having friends and family do so. This blood will be stored specifically for your use, in case you need it.

HARDENING OF THE BREAST

When there has been an implant, it is expected that scar tissue will form around it as the body works to encapsulate this "foreign" insertion. The extent of the scarring depends on the woman's own physiology. Sometimes this capsular contracture, as it is called, may become quite hard, and it can sometimes be painful. After flap reconstruction, masses may form, which are due to fat necrosis (see page 47). Because these feel like lumps, they sometimes need to be biopsied to be certain of the diagnosis.

RIPPLING OF THE IMPLANT SURFACE

Saline implants may have a "wavy" appearance, depending on the position of the prosthesis and the thickness of the fatty tissues beneath the skin that covers them.

WEAKENING OF THE ABDOMINAL MUSCLES

Because the TRAM flap (see pages 246–48) involves an incision and the transfer of muscle from the abdominal region, stomach tone may be lost. (On the other hand, since fat is removed, it may also make your stomach look better, because, as we have noted, the procedure actually does result in a tummy tuck.)

TISSUE FAILURE

The major complication of flap reconstruction is the occasional failure of the transferred tissue to survive. If this happens, part or all of the tissue will have to be removed, and the wound may require an extended period of treatment and revision by the surgeon before it heals. Free flaps have a higher complication rate, and 5 percent of patients may need a second operation a few days after reconstruction to reestablish blood flow in the connected vessels.

INFECTION

Infections may develop at the site of any surgery in the period just after the procedure. They are treated with antibiotics and generally respond well. During an infection, an implant may have to be temporarily removed. Most often it can be reinserted several months after the infection is gone.

LEAKAGE

When a saline solution is used, there may be some leakage from the prosthesis. Leakage of this type poses no danger, since the "saltwater" is simply absorbed into the body tissues. The implant, however, will deflate and have to be replaced.

It is leakage from silicone gel–filled implants that was the cause of concern and actions by the Food and Drug Administration. There have been reports that silicone gel leakage may be associated with serious autoimmune diseases, such as scleroderma and arthritis. The American College of Rheumatology stated in late 1995 that there is no evidence of a causal relationship between silicone gel exposure and any of the rheumatoid diseases.

Furthermore, as we have noted, a number of scientific studies have confirmed the safety of these implants. These studies were reported *after* the FDA banned the use of these implants for cosmetic purposes and imposed "supervisory" conditions over their use for breast reconstruction after mastectomy. However, much damage has been done by the class action lawsuits against the manufacturers. In 2006, the Food and Drug Administration approved silicone-containing breast implants, but required studies in 40,000 women over the following ten years to assure they are safe. Also, women in the study group will be asked to have an MRI of the reconstructed breast every two years to ensure that the implants are not leaking. An MRI is the best radiologic procedure for demonstrating a leak.

Implants have been used for over forty years, primarily—over 80 percent—for cosmetic, not reconstruction, purposes. None of the recent data have made the distinction between the two uses, so we don't know precisely what percentage of postmastectomy patients have had difficulty with silicone gel implants.

Silicone Implants

As of this writing, silicone gel–filled implants are again becoming available for breast reconstruction. The Food and Drug Administration is also allowing physicians to insert them for cosmetic purposes except in women younger than twenty-two years of age. Women who already have such implants and are not experiencing problems do not need to have them removed. All women with implants should be regularly examined by their surgeons.

Most medical procedures have side effects. As we saw when we talked about mastectomy and lumpectomy, there are factors to be weighed, risks and benefits to be balanced.

On the whole, breast implants provide the simplest solution to breast reconstruction. The expander can be placed at the time of mastectomy and involves a procedure that adds little time to the surgery and hospitalization. But saline injections into the expander must be given over a period of weeks, and at least one additional operation is needed to remove the expander and insert a permanent implant in exchange. Moreover, implants sometimes do not age well. Over a period of years they may require additional surgery if the capsule around them hardens or their position changes, or (in the case of silicone implants) if they leak.

The TRAM-type operation generally provides a reconstructed breast whose appearance and texture are much better than those produced with an implant. It may be close in appearance to a normal breast, and because it was originally a part of the woman's body, it will gain and lose weight as she does. This is a bigger operation, with a longer period of recovery, but with the exception of the nipple-areolar reconstruction, it can be accomplished in a single procedure that immediately follows the mastectomy.

You do not have to have reconstructive surgery at the time of mastectomy, but many women who need to have a mastectomy do opt for immediate breast reconstruction. While the appearance of the reconstructed breast is not identical to the original breast, most women find this outcome satisfactory. When a skin-sparing or nipple-areola–sparing mastectomy has been performed, the results can be remarkable.

There is little doubt that reconstruction procedures have made an enormous difference in the overall well-being of most patients who have used them. Breast reconstruction after mastectomy has enhanced the lives of many women by enabling them to live with a feeling of wholeness and with no apparent sacrifice of their physical well-being.

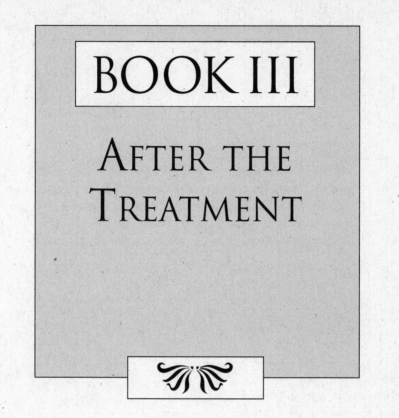

BOOK III

AFTER THE TREATMENT

FOLLOW-UP

N ear the beginning of the book, to show how complex the experience of breast cancer can be, we used as a contrast the example of appendicitis, which has a straightforward protocol of treatment. Dealing with breast cancer is complicated not only because of all the treatment options but also because of what is required after the disease has been treated.

When the stitches have been removed after an appendectomy, and you have regained your strength, you can say good-bye to your surgeon and not concern yourself with the illness anymore. It's over.

After breast cancer, taking care of yourself properly involves a lifetime of surveillance. That doesn't mean you're going to be in a state of high anxiety all the time, or that you will have to go for frequent and expensive tests and examinations for the rest of your life. But it does mean that you require careful follow-up and monitoring of your condition, by an experienced physician, especially for the first four or five years after your surgery.

WHY THE FOLLOW-UP?

Follow-up is essential because breast cancer has a tendency to recur locally and to spread to other parts of the body. That is why you are likely to have received preventive radiation and perhaps hormone therapy and/or chemotherapy in addition to your surgery.

The purpose of careful follow-up is to detect any recurrence, either local or systemic, at the earliest possible time so it can be treated most effectively. (Recurrence will be discussed in Chapter 14.)

AFTER MASTECTOMY

Even if you had a mastectomy, there is the possibility that you may have a local recurrence of breast cancer in the area where the breast used to be, most commonly at the site of the mastectomy incision on the chest wall, in the areola if it has been retained, or in the skin covering the reconstructed breast. Microscopic cancer cells may have been lurking in adjacent tissue. Such cells can remain undetected for an indeterminate time—perhaps a few months, perhaps many years, and then grow into a small lump.

Cancer may also recur in the lymph nodes in the axilla and the neck. This is called a regional recurrence. Distant recurrence is used to describe the finding of cancer that has spread to other parts of the body.

AFTER LUMPECTOMY

Even following radiation therapy after a lumpectomy, there is a certain risk that microscopic cancer remains in the tissue adjacent to the site of the original cancer. Therefore, in the first few years after lumpectomy, the most common place for the cancer to recur is in fact in the area of the original tumor site.

A recurrence in the breast is less worrisome than recurrences that appear in other parts of the body, because it does not indicate that the original cancer has metastasized. There is an excellent chance that with further surgery and adjuvant therapy, we can eliminate the problem.

A new cancer can also develop elsewhere in the breast, just as a new cancer can develop in the opposite breast. Such new and separate breast cancers—as well as regional and systemic cancers—do remain a risk over a woman's lifetime, in the sense that the risk factors that played a part in the first cancer may still be present.

WHO'S IN CHARGE OF THE FOLLOW-UP?

As we have emphasized throughout the book, in an important sense you are the one in charge. In this instance, it is up to you to make sure that no one says to you after surgery and any adjuvant treatment, "Okay, you're fine. Case dismissed." It is also important that you yourself don't say, "Okay, it's over. Good-bye. Leave me alone."

Neither you nor your doctors can resign. Stay alert yourself and put into place a team that will take the "necessary precautions":

1. Make sure there is a follow-up plan in place. (See below.)

2. Decide which doctor is going to be in charge. This question was important during the treatment of your breast cancer and is important now. You are not in any way obligated to remain with the last person to treat your breast cancer for the follow-up. You can give the matter some thought, and if you decide to make a change, choose who, among the specialists who have been treating you, would do the best job.

3. The surgeon was the leader of the team before, during, and after the operation, and he may be the best person to act as coordinator in the years that follow, to help evaluate or interpret the various options that may arise. This is especially true if further surgery is indicated. A surgeon, whether the original one or someone you now choose, should also do

ongoing examinations of your breasts after lumpectomy, or of the remaining breast after mastectomy.

4. If you need long-term hormone therapy or chemotherapy, or if further surgery is not planned, it may be that you select your oncologist to stay in charge of your case.

5. Some women want their follow-up to be supervised by their own family physician, usually an internist, especially if they have had a good long-term relationship with her. That doctor should certainly be kept informed, and she can help you judge how your treatment is progressing, but it is almost certain that you will be better off being monitored by a cancer specialist. In this regard, the specialist will serve as a consultant to the doctor who is responsible for other aspects of your health.

6. Though who becomes the head of your team may come about naturally and satisfactorily, you may want to speak directly to the physician you consider the most caring, meticulous, and alert, and specifically ask her to stay on top of your case.

7. In addition to treating you, the person you choose as the "main woman" or "main man" must maintain careful records of all the tests and treatments you will receive, of the state of your health in terms of cancer as well as of your general medical condition, and—it seems to me—of how your whole life is going.

THE FOLLOW-UP SCHEDULE

There is no standard "calendar of events" that plots how often you should see each physician in the years ahead. The frequency depends to a large degree on the extent of the illness at the time of diagnosis and also on how much time has passed since your treatment.

Unless you had a mastectomy without any other therapy or reconstruction, it's likely that you'll be seeing some combination of surgeon, chemotherapist, radiation oncologist, or plastic surgeon on and off for at least six months, and probably for the first year, after your surgery.

After this period of intensive treatment, for the first four or five years you should see the surgeon every six months.

If you had a lumpectomy followed by radiation therapy, ideally you would alternate visits to the surgeon with visits to the radiation therapist every six months.

If you are receiving long-term chemotherapy, the medical oncologist, as you have seen, will also be examining you on a regular basis and conducting tests.

It is because you will be visiting several different specialists that you need someone at the center of your care to keep track of what each physician is doing and finding.

WHAT DOES FOLLOW-UP INVOLVE?

HISTORY

At the time of your visit to the physician he should review with you any health-related matters that have occurred in the interval since your last visit. It is during this period of "history-taking" that you should report any health concerns that you wish to call to his attention. Let your doctor know if any relatives have developed breast or ovarian cancer and if any genetic testing has been done.

PHYSICAL EXAMINATION

Every six months you should have a complete physical examination, from head to toe. If you are seeing a medical oncologist, it is usually she who will perform this examination. Otherwise an internist familiar with your case should examine you. Whoever the physician is, he should be experienced in the surveillance of cancer and in breast examinations.

If a mastectomy was performed, the doctor will physically examine the chest wall as well as the lymph nodes in the region of the armpit and neck. He will also carefully examine the remaining breast.

If there was a lumpectomy, the treated breast will be carefully palpated to see whether there is any suspicion of a new lump, and the other breast will also be examined.

TESTS

In order for us to achieve fairly uniform reporting of results, many of the same tests are used for all patients. In addition, specific tests are tailored to each patient's circumstances. (The most common exceptions arise when a patient is enrolled in a clinical study. In that case, her follow-up is governed by the rules of the study. Such studies are discussed in Chapter 16.) It is important to say from the start, though, that no single test can ever be relied upon for a definitive diagnosis of breast cancer.

The American Society of Clinical Oncology, a professional group for oncologists, considers history-taking, physical examination, and mammography to be "the cornerstone of breast cancer follow-up." Other tests are advised only if the patient has symptoms. Whether more testing is needed depends on the benefit to the patient of getting early indications of recurrence. Some of us believe that early intervention may permit better outcomes but this remains to be proven in clinical studies.

BLOOD TESTS

A complete blood count should be done every six months. It tells us a number of things: the total number and size of red blood cells; the total volume of the red cells in proportion to the total volume of blood (called the hematocrit); and the hemoglobin content—that is, the quantity in the blood of the protein that carries oxygen.

The blood count also measures the number of circulating white blood cells and of platelets, the cell particles in the blood involved in forming clots.

A mildly reduced hematocrit or hemoglobin may be a sign of chronic illness or of diabetes, arthritis, or heavy menstrual bleeding. If the hematocrit or hemoglobin is very low, anemia is present, and we have to be concerned about the possibility that this is due to tumor recurrence. The same is true if there is a very low white cell or platelet count.

Blood chemistries, another type of blood test, measure various chemicals in the bloodstream. One enzyme that is of special interest in breast cancer is alkaline phosphatase. When it is present in elevated amounts, we are concerned about recurrence in either bone or the liver, though there are other possible causes of this elevation. Other chemistries raise concern about liver involvement specifically.

Blood tests called tumor marker tests usually show abnormal results only when a tumor is large enough to release detectable quantities of certain substances. As such, their role in routine surveillance has been questioned, but your physician may still request them since these tests alert us to the presence of tumors of significant size that may otherwise be missed.

CEA (carcinoembryonic antigen), one such marker, is released in normal amounts by glandular tissue but in increased amounts by tumor cells. Increased production of a milk-fat globule protein, CA 15-3, another marker, is a more sensitive test for breast cancer. A test similar to CA 15-3 is BR 27.29.

Blood cholesterol and lipid metabolism measurements are also useful in monitoring general health.

MAMMOGRAPHY

Every woman who has had breast cancer should have a mammogram once a year. If she had a single mastectomy, the remaining breast should be X-rayed. If she had a lumpectomy, both breasts should be X-rayed. A reconstructed breast generally is not X-rayed. Sonography (see pages 71–72) may be advised to supplement the X-ray study. As MRI technology is rapidly improving, you may be asked to have an MRI to supplement the results of a negative mammogram.

CHEST X-RAYS

A chest X-ray will tell us whether a cancer has spread to the lung, a common site of metastasis. A chest X-ray may be recommended yearly, particularly for the first five years after surgery. It certainly should be done if you have a cough or shortness of breath.

BONE SCANS

Since, if there is a recurrence of cancer, the skeletal system is frequently one of the sites it first spreads to, we order bone scans when there is cause for particular concern. For example, there is no question that a bone scan is necessary if there are symptoms such as persistent back, joint, or other bone pain. These symptoms are worrisome and a negative bone scan can provide peace of mind.

In preparation for a bone scan, a radioactive liquid is injected into the bloodstream and allowed to circulate throughout the body. The liquid will travel to the bones and reveal the skeletal system. It will concentrate in areas of increased blood circulation, which are referred to as hot spots. These include areas of arthritis or bone fractures, as well as those where cancer is present.

For that reason, though a bone scan is a very sensitive tool for finding bone metastases, its results have to be confirmed with X-rays to identify more precisely the reason that it shows increased blood circulation in any particular bone.

OTHER TESTS

The tests we have discussed are the ones routinely used in follow-up care to guard against a recurrence of breast cancer. If blood tests suggest that there may be an abnormality of the liver, the most practical tool to investigate this is a CAT scan. Computerized axial tomography (CAT or CT scan) uses X-rays to create cross-sectional pictures that are combined by a computer to produce extremely detailed images. They are valuable for distinguishing the density of tissue in many parts of the body and are therefore used extensively for medical diagnoses. Usually the chest, abdomen, and pelvis are scanned at the same time. MRI (see pages 73–74) may also be used for further study.

Should both CAT and MRI scans be negative, a PET scan may be helpful. For this test, radioactively labeled glucose (a form of sugar) is injected and concentrates wherever cell metabolism is very active. Tumors consist of such active cells, and PET scans can often locate cancers that are too small to see or that for technical reasons are difficult to distinguish from their normal surrounding tissues. However, PET scans only indicate where to look. They show a spot, not a structure. For more information, PET scans and CAT scans are taken at the same time and the pictures "fused" to reveal more precisely where in the body the increased PET-scan activity is located.

Patients at high risk for familial breast cancer syndromes should be referred for genetic counseling. They will need more careful follow-up of a remaining breast, including the use of MRIs. Carriers of BRCA1 and BRCA2 will also need to be watched carefully for the development of ovarian cancer if a bilateral salpingo-oophorectomy has not been carried out. These patients should usually have their ovaries removed after they have completed their childbearing years.

FOR HOW LONG WILL I NEED THESE TESTS?

Earlier in the book we discussed five-year survival rates. While there's nothing magical about that five-year anniversary, the fact is that most local recurrences, as well as metastases, occur in the first two or three years after surgery. However, when the breast was treated with lumpectomy and radiation, there can be later local recurrences. There are also metastases that occur after five years. We are beginning to understand why some women may remain at risk for such a long time. As noted in Chapter 11, Hormone Therapy and Chemotherapy, newer treatments are being developed to deal with this problem. The method that is most common at the present is to treat postmenopausal woman whose tumors had hormone receptors with an aromatase inhibitor after five years.

If you reach the five-year mark without recurrence, then you will probably no longer get tests like chest X-rays and scans. You will, however, continue to need your breasts examined twice a year, as well as your annual physical examination, blood tests, and mammogram. Make certain that these breast examinations are part of your physician visits.

WATCHING OUT FOR YOURSELF

In addition to the professional tests and examinations, you should continue breast self-examination. Some women say that they're reluctant to start examining themselves again after breast surgery, either because they dread finding another cancer or because they're a little squeamish about touching their treated breast or the chest wall after a mastectomy. This reluctance seems to pass after a few months.

Even if you share these reactions, do not neglect your self-examination:

• Examine your breasts and the operative area carefully every month.

• If you had a breast reconstruction, ask the plastic surgeon to show you how to examine your treated breast. He should point out to you the location of any valve or other protuberance in an implant so that you don't mistake it for a lump.

• Whether you had a lumpectomy or a mastectomy, ask the surgeon to show you how to examine the scar. First, notice whether there is a rash over the incision. Then carefully move the pads of your fingers up and then down the skin over the scar, palpating in the same way discussed on pages 54–56.

• If you had a mastectomy, you are watching for a lump on the chest wall, beneath the skin, frequently beneath the scar.

• If you had a lumpectomy, you are watching for a lump or change in breast consistency in the treated breast.

• A lump in the neck or under the arm may indicate an enlarged lymph node and should be reported.

• You should also report any persistent symptom to the supervising physician, especially bone pain, cough, shortness of breath, or persistent abdominal pain.

• If any additional women or men in your family have developed cancers, tell your physician.

• If you are on tamoxifen, you should be seen by your gynecologist each year. He may request a pelvic sonogram to monitor the endometrium, the lining of the uterus, since there is a higher incidence of uterine cancer in women taking tamoxifen. A change in the appearance of the endometrium may necessitate a biopsy even though this usually is an effect of the therapy and not of tumor recurrence. If you are taking an aromatase inhibitor such as Arimidex, you will need to check your bone health at intervals by having a bone-density measurement.

The reason for this intensive attention to detail is not to turn you into someone preoccupied with illness. In fact, all the procedures of good follow-up care after breast surgery can be taken care of in a relatively short time. The point is simple: The investment can be really important to your well-being.

CHAPTER
14

RECURRENCE

L ife is often not fair, and the recurrence of a cancer you thought had been safely beaten back and destroyed is particularly hard to take. Who could keep from worrying about survival and dreading the prospect of a new round of treatment?

These emotions are completely understandable, and there is no easy way to explain why any particular person becomes ill again. The risks of recurrence of breast cancer have gone way down in recent years. As we have seen in Chapter 11 on adjuvant therapy, and with new research, there is reason to hope that those risks can be even further reduced. Unfortunately, however, as of this moment, even with the best treatment and the most meticulous follow-up care, cancer may recur.

What to do now? Haven't you already used all available re-sources?

By no means. Fortunately, of all carcinomas, breast cancer is one of the most sensitive to treatment. There is a large array of treatments that can be called upon to bring the illness under control and to permit women to live normal lives, often for many years, even after recurrence. What is required—from both the patient and the physician—is a determined effort, a forceful attack. And that brings us to the crucial first step in treating a recurrence of breast cancer.

FINDING THE RIGHT DOCTOR

Many times before in this book, in Chapter 2 and elsewhere, we've discussed the crucial importance of the right physician at every step along the way. But it is at this juncture, when there has been a recurrence, that the task of choosing someone to manage your case is especially subtle and especially important.

Why is this choice an issue yet again? Why shouldn't you just continue with the physician who has been handling your case up to now, the one who has been acting—with your agreement—as the leader or coordinator of the team of doctors you've been seeing?

Despite the recurrence, there is a good chance that going back to one of the doctors who originally treated you is an excellent thing to do. Nevertheless, even if all you want is the reassurance of a fresh evaluation, you should certainly get more than one opinion. It makes sense to review all your previous treatment and to consider alternatives. You may eventually decide to find a new "leader" to work with, or you may decide to remain with one or more of the doctors on the original team. But because a recurrence poses special risks, you will need a doctor who is thoroughly familiar with what has been called the natural history of cancer.

She should have treated many patients with recurring breast cancer so that she understands the hazards that may lie ahead and the steps that must be taken to avoid them.

Her approach should be vigorous. That does not mean she

should rush into therapies that are unnecessarily harsh or risky. It does involve a quality we referred to in Chapter 2: Particularly at this stage of the illness, you want someone who will approach the disease as an impassioned advocate determined to secure the best possible outcome for you. The art of diagnosis is especially important in dealing with a recurrence. Look for a doctor who is meticulous and who will have the time and the patience both to analyze what is wrong with you and to seek out the latest information on the treatment that is most appropriate for your condition.

New techniques are constantly being developed. The physician you choose should present you with a state-of-the-art treatment plan tailored specifically to your needs. In order to do this, she should be up-to-the-minute on the latest research so that she can incorporate proven new approaches into your treatment. But she should use such treatment not because it is "the latest thing" but because there is strong reason to believe that it will benefit you.

Though a recurrence should be fought aggressively, the doctor must bear in mind that you are not only a patient but also a person with a life to live, with your own interests and responsibilities. The treatment plan must take that into account. The aim should be to provide the most effective care possible; to try to limit side effects; and to give treatment that is consistent with your express wishes so that you can continue as much as possible to lead the kind of life you prefer.

Recurrences are potentially life-threatening events. This is a particularly good time to have your entire case reviewed by an expert in breast cancer with considerable experience in the field and whose practice is focused on this disorder. Such experts are usually associated with major hospitals, academic centers, or cancer centers. They may discuss your case with their colleagues at Tumor Board meetings, where your case is presented to a variety of experts including surgeons, radiotherapists, and medical oncologists. Treatment recommendations are then shared with your physician. Obtaining an opinion does not mean you will transfer your care but it will certainly help to reassure you that your care is consistent with the very best medicine available at this point in time.

While opinions are important, I strongly feel that the best outcomes are achieved when a person not only has a very well-informed physician, but also one who is committed to guide the patient directly through the thicket of choices that have to be made and sees herself not as an impartial party but as the patient's strongly committed advocate.

HOW DO YOU FIND SUCH A PERSON?

1. Concentrate first on who would be the primary doctor, the one who coordinates the team. This should be someone whose opinion you trust, to whom you can talk freely, and who is good at what she does.

2. Review the sections in Chapter 2 on finding and choosing a doctor.

3. Consult the sections that follow on what background material the physician should ask for and what your first meeting with her should be like. If the new physician does not seem to cover thoroughly all the points we mention, or if her judgments don't strike you as both thoughtful and confident, you should probably look elsewhere.

WHAT TO TAKE WITH YOU TO THE CONSULTANT'S OFFICE

Whether you are going for another opinion or seeking a new manager of your case, you will have to bring as much information as possible with you to the consultation so that the physician can fully understand your previous illness and how it was treated.

There is no doctor I know who doesn't get a twinge in whatever part of her anatomy her pride resides when a patient announces that she wants to consult someone else. But a competent and compassionate physician will recognize that when you are confronted with a serious medical problem, you should make as sure as possible that you are doing the right thing. The consultation may well result in your staying with your own doctor, reassured that the proposed plan of treatment makes sense. Perhaps the original medical team and the consultant may confer on your condition. Maybe you will decide to change physicians. What you should always remember is that it's your well-being that is at stake and your choice about how best to protect it.

Here are the things the consulting physician should ask for and that you should try to take with you to your first appointment:

1. A letter from your primary physician summarizing what has happened in your case up until the present. (Allow time for the letter to be prepared.)

2. A copy of the original surgery report, called an operative report. This detailed report of exactly what was done during the procedure is prepared by the surgeon and is part of the hospital record. Copies are kept in the surgeon's office.

3. Similar reports of any later operations or biopsies. These are available in the surgeon's office.

4. For each surgery and biopsy, there should be an accompanying pathology report. Many doctors will also ask you to bring them the actual slides of the tissue sections that were examined by the pathologist. The surgeon will have the pathology report, and his nurse can tell you how to get the slides if you need them.

5. If you had radiation therapy, ask the radiation oncologist for a radiation therapy report that summarizes the doses of radiation you received and the fields to which they were administered.

6. Sometimes the consulting physician will want reports on tests and treatments that were done in the hospital. Usually, the easiest way to get these is by using a request-for-records form. The consulting physician's office should send this form, signed by you, to the hospital's medical records department. The reports will then be sent to the consultant's office. You can also obtain such reports yourself at most hospitals, but the procedure is more complicated. In both cases, a fee may be charged.

7. The films of X-rays and scans may be at your radiologist's office or at the hospital. To get these from the hospital, the consulting physician's office must usually fill out another request-for-records form. Sign the form and have it marked with a statement that says, "Give material to patient or family member, please." Then you or someone you choose can pick up the material either from the file room of the hospital's X-ray department or from another file room to which X-ray department personnel can direct you. Again, there may be a charge for this service.

A COMPANION

It is a good idea to take someone with you when you discuss your recurrence with the doctors you consult. Refer to Chapter 6 for advice on choosing a personal advocate. Ask that person and others who are close to help you get all the material you need from previous doctors and the hospital. Try to spare yourself from having to do these chores on your own.

With the assistance of your companion and any others who may be of help to you, prepare a list of questions before your appointment. Give a copy of the list to the companion who accompanies you to the doctor's office, and ask her to take the responsibility for making sure all your concerns are covered.

Ask your companion to take notes during your office visits of what the doctor says and of any instructions she gives you.

THE FIRST VISIT TO THE CONSULTANT

1. The physician should carefully explore with you the discovery of the recurrence:

- Did you find a new symptom or sign of illness yourself?

- What was the symptom or sign? A new lump? Pain anywhere in the body? An inflammation of the skin?

- Did the recurrence show up on one of your follow-up tests? Which one?

- Since the discovery, has a biopsy been performed? What were the pathologist's findings? Have the new slides been compared to the original tumor?

- Have other tests been performed? What were their results?

2. The physician should now take a complete medical history (see Chapter 15).

3. A thorough physical examination should be performed, as described in Chapter 2.

4. Though the records you have brought with you may provide enough information for the consultant to recommend a treatment plan, there is the possibility that she may feel it necessary to order new tests in order to confirm the diagnosis of recurrence and to measure its extent. Good decisions will rely on answers to such questions as: Is the recurrence only in one area of the body? More than one?

5. With such information, the doctor will confirm the diagnosis, assess the extent of the disease, and establish a baseline, a summary of the current status of the illness, that can be used to evaluate how you respond to later treatment.

6. After the diagnosis, you and the consultant should be able to discuss tentative treatment options. The actual treatment plan may have to be taken up at a later visit, after all the information has been analyzed and when you have decided who will supervise your care.

7. At this time, the consultant will usually report her findings and treatment suggestions to your primary physician. It is at this point that you may have to decide whether to continue with your current primary physician or choose someone else to manage your treatment.

WHERE IS THE RECURRENCE?

When cancer cells leave their site of origin—that is, when they metastasize—they must find a hospitable environment. In order to survive, cancer cells require a type of tissue to which they can adhere and the formation of blood vessels that will bring them nutrition.

Because of their particular properties, breast cancer cells often establish themselves and produce a tumor recurrence in bone. Though any part of the skeleton may be affected, some bones are more likely to be involved than others. The bones of the spine, ribs, pelvis, and upper parts of the arms and legs are frequent sites; the bones of the arm below the elbow or of the leg below the knee are seldom affected.

Breast cancer may also spread into the skin and the lymph nodes. Among other organ systems, the lungs and liver are the most likely sites of recurrence.

In order to plan the treatment, we have to find out whether the recurrence is local or distant. A local recurrence is limited to the area of the previous surgery. Has the cancer come back in a breast previously treated with lumpectomy and radiation? In the chest wall at the site of a mastectomy?

A recurrence is considered distant if it is any place in the body other than the breast or the chest wall of the previously treated area. It is considered distant even if it is relatively close to the original site—above the collarbone, for example.

REVIEW OF PATHOLOGY

Because the cancer has come back, it is particularly important to compare its appearance under the microscope with the original cancer to make certain it is not a new and different malignancy. If possible, testing of the new biopsy should include an analysis for hormone receptors and HER-2/neu to see if the tumor has retained its original characteristics, since this may directly influence treatment. I find it best to have these slides reviewed at my own institution so that I can easily discuss findings directly with the pathologist. This is a pathology "second opinion."

PROGNOSIS

People with recurrences are sometimes told that though long-term control of the cancer is possible, there are no cures of recurrent breast cancer. *There are an increasing number of exceptions to this so-called rule.* There are also an increasing number of patients whose responses to the growing list of effective therapies are turning their breast cancer into a chronic disease.

The goal in each case should be to strive to make the particular patient who is being treated an exception to the rule. If it turns out that we cannot achieve that goal, then, after fighting the cancer with all our resources, we must see to it that every patient survives as long as possible.

I have seen many women go on, after a recurrence, to live a fulfilling life.

The wife of a childhood friend came to me many years ago with a local recurrence in the chest wall after a mastectomy. At that time she was at an extremely high risk for a series of increasingly serious recurrences. We had two choices: to use standard treatment and then wait for the inevitable, or to use the then relatively new combination chemotherapy in an all-out effort to achieve a cure. After discussion with the patient, the cancer was removed and the chest wall was treated with radiation. (We would now also prescribe tamoxifen, but since we didn't have the drug then, we removed the woman's ovaries.) I then began to treat her with chemotherapy, not knowing how long such treatment should continue. When the first year was over, I agonized over the risks of going on and of adding another group of drugs, and I finally decided to go ahead for another two years. It's twenty-one years later now, and she is still well.

Another patient had extensive recurrences in her chest wall. Surgery and radiation had been tried in the two years before she came to see me, and they had failed. The recurrences kept appearing, and she now had pain, suggesting a recurrence in bone. The family was told that she had less than a year to live.

CMFVP (see page 207) was still an experimental treatment at

the time, but we started using it, and to our joy, complete remission was achieved within ten months. To maintain the remission, I continued treating this woman for three years. She lived a full life, saw her children marry, and enjoyed her grandchildren before, still free of cancer, she died of another cause fourteen years later.

There are many more stories like these, some of them bittersweet but still important. For example, a young woman called me recently to tell me that her mother, whom I had treated many years before for breast cancer, had recently died of a cancer in the lung. The daughter had been only three years old when her mother came to the office with an inoperable, extensive recurrence of cancer at the mastectomy site. Radiation therapy and three years of chemotherapy kept her cancer-free for sixteen years. Then she apparently developed a tumor in the lung, was treated conservatively, and died two years later. I felt a great sadness at this news, but her daughter had another view: She was actually calling to thank me for "giving her a mother" during her childhood.

The point of these histories? Sometimes we don't understand why a patient with a serious diagnosis seems to defy the odds and go on living a good life. We don't always know why the disease may be in remission—that is, inactive for many years. Prognosis, as we learned in Chapter 10, is a prediction, one that is dependent on statistics and not necessarily applicable to any particular individual. And most important in considering recurrence—with vigorous, determined therapy, the odds can be made to tilt in your favor.

TREATMENT

LOCAL RECURRENCES

If the original breast cancer was treated with lumpectomy and it has reappeared only in the treated breast, this does not mean that the disease has spread. It indicates either a recurrence in that spot or a new cancer in another part of the breast. An MRI of the breast can show whether it is in a limited area. If so, it may be possible to do a second lumpectomy, particularly if the recurrence is in situ and not infiltrating. It is also useful to perform a sentinel node biopsy at the time of surgery, even though a sentinel node procedure or axillary dissection was previously done.

Surgery is the primary treatment. If the cancer has recurred in the orignal site, in most instances, the breast will now have to be removed in what you may hear referred to as a salvage mastectomy. Reconstruction is possible, but if radiation was used after the surgery, you may need one of the flap procedures described in Chapter 12, rather than an implant. Radiation therapy can sometimes be used in a localized approach if the recurrence is a new primary cancer in a separate quadrant of the breast.

Chemotherapy and/or hormone therapy is the next step. The regimen to be used will depend on the nature of the test findings and on whether or not you received adjuvant treatment the first time your breast cancer was treated.

If the recurrence is on the chest wall at the site of the mastectomy, it indicates regrowth of the original cancer and is associated with a higher risk of spread to other parts of the body. Though rare, a new breast cancer may grow in a remnant of breast tissue retained under the mastectomy flaps. This poses a lesser risk of spread but underscores the importance of a careful pathology examination before deciding on treatment.

In this situation, surgery is the first step: removal of the cancer. A margin of healthy tissue must also be removed. Depending on the size of the tumor and its location, this may involve removing underlying muscle and possibly bone, or it may require only a fairly limited excision.

To make sure that any microscopic disease in the area is destroyed, radiation is usually administered to the entire region of the mastectomy.

A course of hormone therapy or chemotherapy follows, though it has not been established whether this treatment should continue for limited or for prolonged periods of time. My own practice is to treat women with a recurrence in the chest wall as though they have had a recurrence in a distant part of the body. There have been enough women in my own practice who have fared well with this program that I consider this type of recurrence to be curable.

DISTANT RECURRENCES

I want to talk now about the word *palliate,* which the *Random House Dictionary* defines as "to relieve or lessen without curing." Palliation is the goal of many oncologists who treat recurrent breast cancer. They want to help their patients, of course, but because they believe that a recurrence is the signal that a patient will not survive, their goal is to palliate, to treat the disease as best they can without causing too many unpleasant side effects or discomfort.

Since there are now so many options for the treatment of breast cancer through hormone therapy and chemotherapy, almost all patients can expect palliation of their disease. But difficult as it may be, many of us do not automatically accept palliation as a goal. We consider each case individually and try to devise a strategy that achieves more than that. Sometimes, such a strategy may involve using a program likely to produce significant side effects. These must be measured against the risks of the disease and the potential benefits of the treatment.

Given this philosophy, which I share, how do we treat recurrences at distant sites? With the weapons now at our disposal: surgery, radiation, hormone therapy, and chemotherapy.

1. For disease that has spread, surgery is used to remove an isolated tumor or other cancerous tissue that gets in the way of normal function.

2. In cases where there is an isolated metastasis—a site in the lung or the brain, for example—we can at times provide a cure by removing it. Often, removal is required to confirm the diagnosis of recurrence and exclude the possibility of another—unrelated—primary cancer.

3. Radiation can reach otherwise hard-to-get-at locations, and it is particularly useful in relieving pain in bones where cancer has metastasized. It can destroy tumors in parts of the body

that you would not want to interfere with surgically, and it also works fairly quickly.

4. Hormone therapy can be used for women whose tumors are hormone receptor-positive (see page 98). It seems to work particularly well for women who have been free of cancer for a relatively long time since breast surgery, who have bone and soft tissue involvement rather than disease of the liver or lung, and who reacted well to previous hormone therapy.

5. For disease present in the inner organs of the body—the lung and particularly the liver—and where the tumor does not contain hormone receptors, chemotherapy can be used. An increasing number of drugs are available for this purpose.

HORMONE THERAPY

See Chapter 11 for descriptions of many of the drugs that are referred to below, including their side effects. Only drugs new to this chapter are described here.

Women with recurrent tumors that are both estrogen and progesterone receptor-positive respond to hormone treatment in almost 75 percent of cases. When only one type of hormone receptor is present, the response falls to 40 percent, and to 10 percent or less when both receptor levels are negative.

The first hormone-related drug used usually depends on whether the patient is premenopausal or postmenopausal. For premenopausal women, tamoxifen is generally the first drug given. Used alone, it can be very effective even in advanced breast cancer, but unfortunately it stops working, on average, in a little over a year. The physician can, however, usually switch to another drug and get a satisfactory response.

The drug often used next is anastrozole (Arimidex). Many tumors, particularly in premenopausal women, are stimulated to grow by estrogen. After the ovaries become inactive in postmenopausal women, their adrenal glands continue to produce estrogen precursors, which can serve as raw materials for the production of estrogen. These precursors are released into the bloodstream and then converted to estrogen by body tissues that produce the enzyme aromatase. Anastrozole stops aromatase from working and is therefore called an aromatase inhibitor. In premenopausal women, these drugs are effective only if the ovaries are removed or ovarian function is suppressed by drugs such as Lupron or Zoladex (see page 213).

In postmenopausal women aromatase inhibitors are more effective than tamoxifen, and they are generally used as the first hormone treatment, even before tamoxifen, when a recurrence is discovered. The dose taken is one tablet daily.

Another widely used aromatase inhibitor is letrozole (Femara). A third, related drug, Aromasin, may also be used. Aromasin is an aromatase inhibitor with a different chemical structure. It binds more tightly to the aromatase enzyme molecule than Arimidex or Femara does. It is a tablet taken once a day.

When an aromatase inhibitor fails to help postmenopausal women, however, tamoxifen will be given to block estrogen receptors. It can control tumors in both premenopausal and postmenopausal women.

When both tamoxifen and standard aromatase inhibitors are not effective, Faslodex (fulvestrant) may be used whether the patient is pre- or postmenopausal. This drug inactivates estrogen receptors more completely than tamoxifen, and may even work when tamoxifen, Arimidex, and Femara are no longer effective. Faslodex, which is given by injection once a month, permanently inactivates estrogen receptors, rather than blocking them by binding to them as tamoxifen does.

If aromatase inhibitors or Faslodex fail, an agent that resembles a male hormone, usually Halotestin, may sometimes be used. This drug is said to be particularly effective for treating bone metastases.

Megestrol (Megace), a progesterone-like substance, is also used in hormone therapy. It may be effective even when other hormones have failed. While it has few side effects, it increases appetite and therefore may cause weight gain. However, when appetite is poor, this may be an advantage; in fact, Megace is often used as an appetite stimulant.

Leuprolide (Lupron) mimics a natural hormone that decreases pituitary function when present in excessive amounts and thus reduces estrogen levels. It is well-tolerated by most patients, though a long list of side effects has been reported.

When two hormones are given together, they are *not* more effective than each given separately. In fact, as mentioned earlier, when tamoxifen and an aromatase inhibitor are given together they may be *less* active than an aromatase inhibitor alone. The one exception may be Faslodex and Arimidex, since the first drug inactivates estrogen receptors and the other suppresses estrogen formation.

Hormone treatment plays an important role in the treatment of recurrent breast cancer. Unfortunately, each drug has to be given in sequence, because in time it will stop being effective. It is for this reason that we prefer to combine hormone treatment with chemotherapy. In fact, even for patients whose disease is hormone receptor-positive and who respond to hormone therapy, there is some evidence that better results may be obtained when the two therapies are combined.

CHEMOTHERAPY

If the original tumor or the recurring tumor has no hormone receptors, chemotherapy is used from the start of treatment. If the patient's tumor is receptor-positive, many oncologists, myself included, often combine chemotherapy with hormone therapy. The first chemotherapy program used for a recurrence, in what is called first-line therapy, uses drug combinations containing Adriamycin, a taxane (Taxol or Taxotere), or methotrexate. If the tumor is HER-2 positive, carboplatin and Herceptin may also be used. (Refer to Chapter 11 for a full discussion of the drugs and drug combinations used in chemotherapy.)

If an Adriamycin-based program was used for the first line, the next regimen, the second-line therapy, will use a methotrexate- or taxane-based program, and vice versa. If one of these was used for adjuvant treatment before the recurrence, another will now be used. The term *third line* is used to describe the regimens that are used next.

Drug combinations are always in development, and research is likely to yield new programs at any time. Major advances have been made in recent years with the introduction of new second- and third-line treatments. They involve some of the drugs we've already discussed as well as others which are used only in this setting.

- **Abraxane** is a form of Taxol that has a unique formulation which permits it to be given without premedications such as Decadron, Benadryl, and Tagamet. It can, therefore, be used in higher doses.

- **Bevacizumab** (Avastin) is a targeted therapy, an antibody directed against VEGF, a protein that stimulates blood vessel growth in tumors. Combined with other drugs, it increases their effectiveness.

- **Capecitabine** (Xeloda) by itself has no direct effect on cancer cells. However, in the body it is converted by many tissues into 5-deoxy-5-fluorouridine and then into 5-fluorouracil. It acts in part as the equivalent of low doses of 5-fluorouracil given continuously, into a vein, over long periods of time.

- **Carboplatin** (Paraplatin) and the related **cisplatin** (Platinol) stop DNA function by cross-linking the two strands of which it is constructed.

- **Gemcitabine** (Gemzar) resembles a nucleoside, a building block of DNA. By introducing a false unit into the DNA, it prevents the cell from proceeding through the cycle of DNA reproduction that is necessary for cells to divide.

- **Irinotecan** (Camptosar) acts on an enzyme that assures proper assembly of DNA. Its action differs from that of any drug previously used for the treatment of breast cancer. It is used as a third or later line of treatment.

- **Lapatinib** (Tykerb), like Trastuzumab, which is described below, is directed against the surface proteins that are involved in growth stimulation. Unlike Trastuzumab it is a small molecule, not an antibody, and it blocks not only HER-2, but also the related HER-1 (EGFR).

- **Leucovorin** was at one time used primarily to limit the side effects of methotrexate. It is now also used to make 5-fluorouracil more effective.

- **Liposomal Adriamycin** (Doxil) is Adriamycin wrapped in a fatty envelope (liposome). It is designed to concentrate in the tumor, and therefore has less effect on the bone marrow, heart, and hair. It is sometimes effective even when Adriamycin treatment shows no benefit.

- **Mitomycin-C** (Mutamycin) is a natural product that interferes with DNA synthesis. It is most often used as a third-line treatment in combination with vinblastine.

- **Mitoxantrone** (Novantrone) works by a process that eventually inactivates DNA. It resembles Adriamycin in both therapeutic efficacy and toxicity.

- **Trastuzumab** (Herceptin) is a new category of drug, an antibody, that reacts with a specific protein, HER-2, found in large amounts on the surface of some breast cancer cells.

- **Vinblastine** (Velban) is related to vincristine, but it may be effective even if vincristine has already been used.

- **Vinorelbine** (Navelbine) is a semisynthetic product of the same plant that is the source of both vincristine and vinblastine. It interferes with the assembly of tubules needed for cell division.

HOW ARE THESE DRUGS USED?

Here is a summary of the principles that guide the use of chemotherapy for recurrent disease.

- When several treatment alternatives are available, the one selected should be the one that is likely to produce the greatest degree of tumor destruction.

- Since treatment benefits tend to diminish after a period of time, if two treatments produce equal levels of tumor destruction, the preferred treatment is the one that on average is able to maintain tumor control longer.

- For maximum benefit, whenever possible chemotherapy should be integrated with other forms of treatment, such as surgery and radiation, to reduce each patient's tumor burden to a minimum.

• Strategies to minimize and overcome side effects should be part of every treatment plan.

COMMONLY USED TREATMENTS

Some of the most commonly used first- and second-line treatments for recurrent breast cancer—such as CMF, CAF, and AC—have been discussed in Chapter 11 (see pages 204–08). The following are additional treatment programs:

• **Adriamycin/Taxol** is a combination given at various dose levels every twenty-one days. It combines the two most effective drugs for the treatment of recurrent breast cancer.

• **Camptosar** is a newcomer that, besides being useful in the treatment of breast cancer, is also useful against colon and lung cancer. Its unique action makes it a promising candidate for those who have not responded to other drugs.

• **Capecitabine** and **Taxotere** are two drugs that add to each other's effectiveness. Capecitabine, which is often used alone because it can be taken by mouth, is converted by the body into 5-fluorouracil and, when given daily, establishes low dose levels of fluorouracil in the bloodstream for long periods of time. Its advantage over standard fluorouracil is that it can be taken by mouth instead of given intravenously, using a pump, for many days. Capecitabine remains effective in a significant number of patients in whom other treatments have failed to work. Taxotere, while related to Taxol, may be effective even if Taxol does not work or has stopped working. Used alone, both Taxol and Taxotere can produce remission even when first-line programs that include Adriamycin and methotrexate have failed. When Taxotere is combined with Capecitabine, the two drugs provide longer-term benefit than when Capecitabine is given alone. Capecitabine has also been used in combination with Taxol, Navelbine, Adriamycin, and lapatinib.

- **Carboplatin, Taxotere, Trastuzumab (Herceptin)** Herceptin offers new options for treatment because of its unique targeted approach, specifically binding to the growth receptor HER-2 (see pages 182 and 331). However, it is effective only in cases where the tumor cells overexpress HER-2. Herceptin can be used alone or in combination with Carboplatin, Taxol, and Taxotere. It has been successfully combined with Adriamycin, but this combination has an increased risk of producing heart damage because of the Adriamycin. In laboratory studies the combinations of Taxotere and Herceptin, as well as Carboplatin and Herceptin, are synergistic—that is, more effective than the sum of either drug alone. This observation has encouraged the use of Carboplatin, Taxotere, and Herceptin for recurrent disease, often as first-line therapy. Taxol has been used to replace Taxotere in a similar combination.

- **CEF** is similar to FEC. However, unlike FEC, which is given every twenty-one days, CEF is given every twenty-eight days, with the cyclophosphamide (Cytoxan) given on days 1 and 14, and the epirubicin and 5-fluorouracil given on days 1 and 8.

- **5-fluorouracil** by continuous infusion requires placement of an Infus-a-Port or similar device (see page 196) to permit ready access to the venous circulation. 5-fluorouracil is then given intravenously through the Infus-a-Port, using a small pump that is worn in a pouch at belt level. Depending on the dose used, the drug can be given uninterruptedly for twenty-four hours a day for several days, weeks, or months. It has largely been replaced by Capecitabine (see above).

- **Gemzar/Taxol** is given every 21 days.

- **Herceptin** has been used against HER-2 positive tumors together with Taxol, Taxotere, Navelbine, and Gemzar.

- **Leucovorin, 5-fluorouracil** is a third-line treatment. The drugs are given in sequence, with leucovorin always first. Leucovorin is referred to as a 5-fluorouracil modulator, because it significantly increases the effectiveness of a drug that by itself has only a modest effect on breast cancer.

- **Methotrexate, 5-fluorouracil, and leucovorin** is another program that is useful in high doses. The high-dose methotrexate also acts as a modulator to enhance the effects of the 5-fluorouracil, but leucovorin must be taken eighteen to twenty hours later, to stop the methotrexate's action and limit its side effects. This program often works even after the leucovorin, 5-fluorouracil combination has failed.

- **Mitomycin-C, vinblastine** was at one time considered to be the standard third-line treatment. Though it is still in use, it is not likely to be effective in patients who have previously received large amounts of vincristine or Adriamycin.

- **Mitoxantrone, Thiotepa,** with or without methotrexate, is a drug combination that is useful for third-line therapy if only limited amounts of Adriamycin have previously been used.

- **Navelbine, Gemzar** is a relatively new combination that illustrates how the development of new drugs is expanding the number of available options for treating breast cancer. This combination is given on several schedules and it may afford long periods of remission.

- **Taxol or Taxotere** (both taxanes) with Avastin. This combination is more effective than either of the taxanes alone.

    Single drugs used against recurrent breast cancer include:

- **Abraxane** with or without Avastin

- **Doxil,** a unique Adriamycin preparation that is enclosed within a fatty envelope, which permits it to concentrate in tumors

- **IXEMPRA,** a member of the epothilone group of drugs, interferes with the tubules that form the skeleton of cells. While its action overlaps that of Velban and Navelbine, it can sometimes produce remissions even when these other drugs fail. The first epothilone has just been approved by the FDA and can be used alone or in combination with Xeloda.

SIDE EFFECTS

Side effects common to many forms of chemotherapy have been discussed in Chapter 11 (see pages 209–18). Here are details of specific side effects of the drugs and combinations we have mentioned:

- **Abraxane,** unlike the standard Taxol, can be given without premedication and at higher doses. However, it produces more nerve-related signs (neuropathy) than regular Taxol.

- **Bevacizumab (Avastin)** may cause moderate increases in blood pressure, bleeding (example: nosebleed), and perforations of the bowel wall.

- **Capecitabine (Xeloda)** has all the side effects of the drug the body converts it into: 5-fluorouracil. Much like 5-fluorouracil, when given at a high dose or for a long time intravenously, Xeloda may cause the hand-foot syndrome in which the palms of the hands and the soles of the feet become painful. These symptoms usually improve quickly, but if they persist, vitamin B_6 is a possible antidote. However, you should discuss its use with your doctor before taking the vitamin, because the benefits of vitamin B_6 have not been definitively confirmed by a clinical study.

- **Carboplatin** suppresses bone marrow function, causing anemia and a decrease in white blood cells and platelet numbers. (Platelets are small cell fragments present in the blood that help clots to form.) Moderate nausea is frequent and is prevented by pretreatment with antinausea drugs (see page 210). Nerve injury may occur, especially in the elderly.

- **Gemcitabine (Gemzar)** affects the bone marrow similarly to carboplatin. It may cause fever. Mild effects on the lung, liver, and kidneys have been observed. Overall, the drug is well-tolerated.

- **Irinotecan (Camptosar)** has significant side effects on the gastrointestinal system. While nausea is common, diarrhea is the most frequent toxicity and also the most difficult to manage. It is controlled with frequent doses of Imodium, and in many patients it can be markedly reduced or even eliminated by pretreatment with atropine.

- **Leucovorin** is a derivative of a B vitamin, folic acid. Leucovorin may produce an allergic reaction but otherwise has no major side effects.

- **Mitomycin-C (Mutamycin)** can injure the kidneys and lungs. It causes blood count changes that may persist. If it is accidentally released under the skin, it may cause major damage.

- **Mitoxantrone (Novantrone)** causes nausea, heart damage, and decreases in blood counts.

- **Taxol,** in addition to changes in blood count, may produce a severe allergic reaction at the time it is given. All patients must receive treatment with a combination of drugs before Taxol is administered, in order to prevent this response. Nerve damage, nausea, diarrhea, and/or arthritic pain may occur.

- **Taxotere** is similar to Taxol, but in addition causes fluid retention, increased tearing (it inflames the lacrimal ducts that normally drain tears into the nose), and thickening of the fingernails.

- **Thiotepa** causes fatigue, nausea, burning at times on urination, and dizziness.

- **Trastuzumab (Herceptin)** should be given with caution to anyone with a history of significant heart disease, because it can cause heart damage. About 40 percent of patients have fever and chills when they first receive the drug, but these side effects can easily be prevented with simple premedications. Diarrhea, usually mild to moderate, is also seen.

- **Vinblastine** produces more blood count suppression and causes less nerve damage than vincristine.

- **Vinorelbine** causes marked declines in white blood cell counts, which may require Neupogen (see page 212) to correct. Nerve damage, similar to that produced by vincristine, and nausea are other side effects.

- **Ixabepilone (IXEMPRA)** is associated with significant nerve-related symptoms (neuropathy), joint pains, tiredness, and nausea.

- **Capecitabine, Taxotere,** used together, may decrease blood counts and cause fatigue. Capecitabine may cause the hand-foot syndrome. Taxotere must be preceded and followed by the cortisone-like drug dexamethasone to prevent fluid accumulation in the legs.

- **Carboplatin, Taxotere, Trastuzumab (Herceptin)** causes fatigue, a drop in blood counts, and occasional allergic reactions to the Trastuzumab. Mild diarrhea may also occur.

- **Leucovorin, 5-fluorouracil** may cause burning in the mouth, hyperacidity, and diarrhea. This combination generally has fewer side effects than 5-fluorouracil alone, as long as dosage is carefully controlled.

- **Methotrexate, 5-fluorouracil, and leucovorin** has side effects similar to leucovorin, 5-fluorouracil, but the addition of methotrexate tends to produce greater fatigue.

- **Mitomycin, vinblastine** causes a fall in blood counts that may persist. Long-term administration can injure the kidneys.

- **Mitoxantrone, Thiotepa, with or without methotrexate,** causes fatigue, a fall in blood counts, burning mouth, and possible heart damage.

- **Navelbine, Gemzar** may produce severe pain along the vein used to administer the drug. This side effect is due to the Navelbine. It is often treated by putting in a port (see page 196), but it can be handled equally well by giving the Navelbine over a period of six minutes or less and then washing the vein out with additional intravenous fluids.

BISPHOSPHONATES

Bisphosphonates are antiresorptive agents, drugs that interfere
with the normal cycles of bone building and destruction (resorp-
tion) that permit the body to reshape the skeleton throughout life.
Because of this ability, they are widely used to treat osteoporosis.
Studies have shown that these drugs are also able to prevent or delay the spread of breast cancer to the bones. In the United States,
pamidronate (Aredia) and zoledronic acid (Zometa) are the most
widely used drugs of this group for the treatment of breast cancer.
They are given intravenously once every four weeks.

FOLLOW-UP DURING THERAPY

You should be carefully examined and tested during your treatment, for complications and side effects and also to keep track of
your general physical condition. (See Chapter 12 for the steps that
should be followed in a visit to the oncologist's office.) We also
want to know as precisely as possible whether the treatment is
working, whether it is beginning to fail, and when we feel safe in
stopping. Careful monitoring allows us to step in quickly to
change therapy should a particular program begin to fail. Blood
tests, particularly tumor marker tests (see pages 262–63), can
sometimes indicate whether the treatment is affecting the tumor,
but they are not always definitive. At intervals, imaging examinations such as X-ray, CAT scan, PET/CAT scans, and MRI (see
Chapter 4) may be performed for a more direct evaluation of how
you are doing.

IS THERE AN EFFECTIVE STRATEGY TO USE NOW?

The answer to that question depends on your goals. Is your aim to
prolong life? Assure a good life quality with limited drug side effects? Achieve cure?

Any sensible person would answer yes to all three questions.
The best approach to treating a recurrence of breast cancer is to

devise a strategy that reverses the order of those questions and puts the first and primary emphasis, wherever possible, on trying for cure. We attempt to accomplish that goal with a minimum of disruption of the life of the patient but with the understanding that when we are dealing with an aggressive cancer, we must act aggressively.

Let's now take up these goals one by one.

PROLONGING LIFE

Nearly everyone who has a recurrence of breast cancer can now expect that a strategy of treatment will be used that will arrest the illness for a significant period of time. The initial treatment after recurrence is more effective than treatments of the past, and if that treatment fails, there are, as you have seen in this chapter, many alternatives that can be used to restore control of the illness.

ASSURING THE QUALITY OF LIFE

The first thing to be said is that the use of chemotherapy is not inconsistent with preserving the quality of a patient's life. As we have seen, oncologists whose goal is palliation may delay giving chemotherapy to patients with recurrent cancer, so as to spare them what they consider "unnecessary suffering." Instead they may use hormone therapy alone—even when slow disease progression is evident—use an oral chemotherapy drug, even if it gives limited remissions, and they may also insist on using one drug at a time. While this is appropriate in some cases, my concern is that this approach gives chemotherapy a slimmer chance to be effective, because it is not being brought into play until the cancer has further progressed.

Chemotherapy, properly administered, need not cause patients anguish and suffering. The best quality of life, after all, comes from the lasting, complete remission that can be achieved by the early and creative use of chemotherapy.

CURE

Some patients with recurring breast cancer, particularly those with local recurrences, were cured in the past, but they were the exceptions. In most instances the disease eventually came back, despite the use of the best treatment then available.

But better strategies are now available. We do not have to accept the history of breast cancer recurrence as its future. The oncologist can examine the treatments currently available and devise a specific program that will give each patient her best possible chance for long survival.

Does this mean that everyone with recurrent breast cancer will be cured? No. But in my opinion a creative, intensive approach will certainly increase the length of remission and, at present, may actually cure some women. Over time, with more research, we hope to cure all of them.

SELECTING TREATMENT REGIMENS

Given the large number of treatments available for recurrent breast cancer it is important to select wisely which treatments should be given preference and in what sequence they should be used to get the best results. This, of course, depends on the goals of treatment. In Chapter 11 we focused on preventing recurrence. In that setting studies have shown that chemotherapy is best given in intensive protocols continued for periods of six months or less. On the other hand, to be effective hormone therapy must be given for long periods of time. The sequence is chemotherapy, radiation if needed, and then five or more years of hormone therapy.

In this chapter we are dealing with recurrence. Our goal is cure, but where that cannot be obtained, our focus is to extend life as long as possible. As you have heard, it is possible for someone to have a recurrence of breast cancer, and go on to live for many years. How is this best done? By selecting treatments that are not only effective in placing a patient's disease into remission, but also successful in maintaining remissions for long periods of time. In general, a few treatments that give extended remissions produce better results than a sequence of many treatments that produce a series of much shorter periods of disease control. The principles that seem to be the most important for you to remember are:

• Drug combinations tend to give longer periods of remission.

• Your doctor should start with a treatment that is likely to give you the longest possible remission.

• Your progress under treatment should be closely monitored, utilizing regular office visits and testing.

• Good responses to treatment take time. Both you and the doctor should be patient since it may take eight or more weeks to see the benefit of a particular therapy.

• The first treatment is not always the one that gives you the best results. As you can see from this chapter, there is a wide range of treatments available.

• If there is a problem, focus on finding a solution. A good oncologist has experience in solving problems.

• Sometimes changing to another treatment is the best solution.

• It is not enough just "being treated." Your oncologist should have an aggressive, long-term treatment plan.

• Don't quit because of a side effect. Instead keep calling it to the attention of your doctor. Controlling side effects is another skill essential for anyone who administers chemotherapy.

• Remember, this book has to be revised every four years, at which time one third of it has to be changed because of the impressive progress being made in the treatment of breast cancer.

Which treatment programs your medical oncologist chooses and in what sequence depends on the nature of your present tumor, what treatments for prevention you have received following surgery, the time from initial treatment to recurrence, the goals of your therapy, the minimization of side effects to optimize quality of life, and your oncologist's own experience as to which treatment pathways generally render the best results.

You may wonder why I don't offer you a set of tables of likely treatments like that in Chapter 8, listing the preventive (adjuvant) systemic treatments after surgery. The National Comprehensive Cancer Network, which outlines possible treatments for professionals, lists twenty-seven alternative initial treatments for recurrence (though there are many more possibilities). These treatments can be given in many different sequences depending on such considerations as those outlined above. The fact that there are so many choices is good for the patient, but it makes it difficult to outline the likely pathway your oncologist will choose in any comprehensible form.

As mentioned earlier, before any treatment is initiated the recurrent tumor should be biopsied to confirm its nature and at the same time to retest it for estrogen and progesterone receptors and the presence of HER-2. Some tumors that reappear may change from being receptor-negative to -positive and vice versa. Others, which were HER-2 negative, may now prove to be HER-2 positive. If you have previously received an Adriamycin-based treatment and less than a year has passed before your recurrence, you are unlikely to receive that drug again. On the other hand, if several years have passed since your first treatment, a drug used in the past may be used again. The treatments chosen will be more intensive when the goal is to eliminate all detectable tumor or to reduce the amount of tumor present to an absolute minimum, than when the focus is on suppressing disease so that it does not cause symptoms. Side effects of treatment may affect your quality of life, but there are very effective treatments that interfere relatively little in your day-to-day activities.

Clinical research is giving us an increasing range of options for treating recurrences and this is gradually changing recurrent breast cancer into a chronic disease with expectation of long-term survival. However, there is still much to be learned about which sequence of treatments is likely to give the best results in a specific case. This is where the oncologist's own experience becomes important; it is she who will be your guide as you proceed, and discuss with you what treatments she favors and why.

CHAPTER

15

PREVENTION

As we begin to talk about the prevention of breast cancer, we have to say that we don't know much about it. What we do know, however, is that there is no credible evidence to support the idea that women have done something to themselves to cause them to become ill. Your psychological attitude did not give you cancer. It is bad enough to develop cancer without having someone tell you that you have only yourself to blame. It's a burden no one deserves, and the blame really lies on the so-called experts who write books about "cancer personalities" or give simplistic advice about how you can cure yourself with good cheer.

As you will see in Chapter 16, a lot of research is now being done that may tell us within the next few years what causes breast cancer. One example of progress is that we can now discuss guidelines for prevention that are based on genetic information. This is the type of information we need before we can give definitive advice on how to prevent the disease.

If we knew more, for example, about why being born with a mutant gene places women at risk for developing breast cancer, we could work to find a strategy to correct the problem, perhaps through genetic engineering.

If we knew that the mutant gene triggers breast cancer only under certain environmental, nutritional, or other circumstances, we could work to protect women from those triggers.

If we knew why, when breast cancer spreads, it is often to the bone, the liver, and the lungs, and very seldom to the spleen, the kidney, or the skeletal muscle, perhaps then we could develop effective preventive measures.

In the meantime, all we can do is look at the data that are now available about the incidence of breast cancer and its various correlations with risk factors, and try to draw from them whatever lessons we can about prevention.

In this chapter we talk about what we know are risk factors, what we don't know, and about some of the real progress that has recently been made in learning about how to prevent this disease.

IS THE INCIDENCE OF BREAST CANCER INCREASING?

When the first edition of this book was written in 1992, there was strong statistical evidence showing a continuous increase in the incidence of new cases of breast cancer from the 1960s through the 1980s. The good news is that the increase stopped in the 1990s and the incidence became stable in 2000. Then in 2003 there was a 7 percent decline in women over 50. The most likely contributing factor was probably the almost 50 percent reduction in the use of hormone replacement therapy after 2002 (see pages 307–09).

Nonetheless, when the data are in, they are expected to show that there were 182,460 new cases of breast cancer in 2008, and 67,770 cases of in situ breast cancer. While this does indeed represent stabilization, it is still a high level of incidence. For the same year, deaths from breast cancer are anticipated to be 40,480. This reflects another important trend, a very slow but definite decrease in mortality in recent years. Nevertheless, breast cancer seems to be all around us now, near epidemic in proportion, if not by scientific definition. A woman said to me the other day, "I had breast cancer, my sister has it, and three or four people we grew up with are sick. We're all in our fifties, but this week I sent a friend who's thirty-six and about to get married to see you. I have another friend in her forties who has it, and someone in my office who's only twenty-five, and my neighbor's eighty-year-old grandmother. They come from all different backgrounds, and they're young and old, Asian and black and white. Why isn't someone doing something about it?"

WHY ARE THERE SO MANY CASES OF BREAST CANCER?

There are several risk factors that make individuals more vulnerable to developing breast cancer. What are they?

It's important to note here that we're not asking, "What can I do to avoid breast cancer?" in every instance. As you will see, several of the risk factors are beyond our control, such as being a woman and growing older. Nor can you change your family history. Still, studies have shown that 55 to 75 percent of women with breast cancer have no known risk factors. What we are exploring now are all the circumstances that have been shown to be related to the disease and whether you can take steps to lower your risk.

HEREDITY

Eighty-five percent of women who develop breast cancer have no family history whatsoever. Of the remaining 15 percent, about one third do seem to have a genetic connection, particularly when first-degree maternal or paternal relatives had breast or ovarian cancer or the relative was age forty or younger when her breast or ovarian cancer was first discovered.

Does that mean that if there is breast cancer in your family, you are certain to get it? No. As with the other risk factors and statistical odds we've been discussing throughout the book, this family history says nothing about any particular individual. Not every woman in such a family is fated for breast cancer. Until the breast cancer genes were cloned in 1995, we could be concerned only about an individual's risk based on her family history. Now we can identify many, though not all, of the women who have an inherited gene mutation that puts them in this risk category. More details about the significance of this information is given in the section later in this chapter headed "Recent Discoveries and New Options."

RACE

We begin with some numbers that are not, strictly speaking, concerned with the risk of developing breast cancer. They do, however, have a lot to do with the risk of not surviving the disease. While the incidence of breast cancer is a little lower for black women than for white, once they get the disease, African-American women do not do nearly as well. In fact, for the past thirty years the overall survival of younger black women has been consistently lower than that of white women.

Why? It probably has a lot to do with poverty. One-third of all Americans are, by common definition, poor, and one-third of the poor are black. Many African-Americans—as well as other economically disadvantaged women—cannot afford mammograms, professional physical examinations, and other health care measures, and are unaware of low-cost or free testing programs that are available to them. They therefore come in for treatment when the disease has advanced beyond the early stages. In addition, many of our public health facilities have a woeful record in treating poor women. Thus, the risk of developing breast cancer is not higher for black women, it is the chance of their surviving the illness that American society must begin to address.

In the past, Asian women had a lower breast cancer rate than Caucasians. Prior to World War II, for example, the disease was very uncommon in Japan. Then it was noticed that the rate began to rise in Japanese women who had immigrated to Hawaii. And when the daughters of these women were born and raised in Hawaii, their incidence of breast cancer was the same as that of the native-born Caucasian population. (And white Hawaiian women have among the highest breast cancer rates in the United States.)

Is there something about the air or water in Hawaii that causes breast cancer? Who knows? What we do know is that a similar generation of Japanese women, living in San Francisco, had a threefold rise in breast cancer over the women who stayed in Japan. Moreover, the sad development of recent years is that since 1975, the breast cancer rate has risen enormously in Japan as well. We can only speculate on the reasons for this phenomenon, but here are some of the possibilities:

- The Japanese diet has been "Westernized" to include a lot more fat than it had before, particularly animal fat.

- Japanese women have begun to menstruate earlier, and to enter menopause later, than they did before World War II.

- Japanese women now marry later and have their first child later than was customary in the past.

- The environment has changed a great deal in Japan, just as it has in the rest of the world. Greatly increased industrialization has brought with it sharply increased air pollution and other environmental hazards.

DIET

The most plausible culprit in the Japanese breast cancer mystery would seem to be the radical change in diet. The possibility that a high-calorie diet, and particularly a high consumption of fat, is connected to breast cancer has been supported by the kinds of studies we have been discussing, epidemiologic studies that compare large populations of people. It has also been supported by laboratory experiments with animals.

A "special communication" from the *Journal of the American Medical Association* in 1989 said, "Data from animal experiments and human correlation studies strongly support the dietary fat–breast cancer hypothesis. . . . Animals fed a high-fat, high-calorie diet have a substantially higher incidence of mammary tumors than animals fed a low-fat, calorie-restricted diet."

Additionally, we know that particularly in postmenopausal women, fat cells play a role in the production of estrogen. As we will see, there is reason to believe that a long period of estrogen stimulation is linked to breast cancer. Postmenopausal women who are overweight produce more estrogen and would therefore benefit from a lower-calorie diet.

Though not all population studies have supported this hypothesis about diet, there is a growing body of biological evidence of a relationship between breast cancer and body weight. By one estimate, a woman on a typical American diet could reduce her risk of getting breast cancer by:

• Lowering fat intake to less than 20 percent of the calories she consumes

• Lowering saturated fat intake to less than 10 percent

• Lowering intake of animal proteins to less than 6 percent

There are many people around the country who go further than this and advocate much more radical diet changes. A diet composed primarily of complex carbohydrates is said both to prevent cancer and to play a role in its cure. The same kinds of claims are made for macrobiotic diets.

All that can be said at this point is that there is no convincing evidence that such drastic regimens do what their proponents claim. A prudent diet rich in complex carbohydrates and fiber and low in fats is undoubtedly better for you than a diet rich in simple sugars and fats. But it does not seem sensible to eliminate from your diet other foods that may be useful to your body. Not enough is known about the effects of severely restricted diets for us to be able to say that they don't do more harm than good.

For example, while eating regular amounts of healthy soy products like tofu, soybeans, and soy milk would seem to be good for the body, these contain plant estrogens. There is no good proof that they are harmful or helpful, so you can enjoy these as part of your diet. However, you should avoid soy supplements.

For someone who has had breast cancer, diet may also play an important role in preventing recurrence. It does seem clear from various studies that a high level of obesity, weight gain, or both, after diagnosis is adversely associated with disease-free survival and overall survival itself.

EXERCISE

Women who exercise regularly, whether they are pre- or post-menopausal, have a decreased incidence of breast cancer. A study of 74,000 women published in 2003 showed that women who engaged in strenuous exercise starting at age thirty-five had a 14 percent decrease in their risk of breast cancer. Longer duration of exercise produced a greater decrease in risk. The benefits of exercise are particularly important in postmenopausal women, because for them obesity and weight gain are associated with an increased incidence of breast cancer. A regular program of exercise can help to avoid weight gain. No one is suggesting that you become an Olympic athlete, but the following are advisable:

• Choose activities you enjoy, like walking, bicycling, or swimming.

• Set a regular routine for exercises; work out in a gym with a trainer.

• Keep motivated by exercising with a partner.

VITAMINS AND MINERALS

As with the claims for radically limited diets, there is no evidence that megadoses of vitamins and minerals decrease the risk of breast cancer. In fact, it seems that the best-nourished women are at the greatest risk for breast cancer. While it is true that such women probably eat more fat than they should, their diets are also rich in vitamins and minerals.

Foods that are replete with vitamins and minerals are essential to your well-being. It may also be good for you to take moderate amounts of supplemental vitamins. Some of these supplements—calcium in postmenopausal women, for example—do seem to have beneficial effects. There is also a suggestion that folic acid may be helpful. But taking too much of a particular vitamin or mineral supplement can be dangerous, and there are documented cases of severe side effects. If you have been discovered through good, credible tests to have a deficiency, you should almost certainly use vitamin or mineral supplements, but self-medication can be harmful. Not all anemias, for example, are caused by iron deficiencies. In fact, the storage of excess iron in the body can lead to all sorts of unpleasant and even dangerous side effects.

Furthermore, some of the media "stars" among these supplements seem to perform poorly. The cancer protection afforded by selenium, for example, was widely touted in the press, but a very convincing study refuted these claims. And on the other side of the coin, there have been a few reported fatalities from taking contaminated selenium.

ALCOHOL

A clear relationship between alcohol consumption and breast cancer risk has been demonstrated in a number of studies. Alcohol raises the level of estrogen in the bloodstream of premenopausal women and has an even more pronounced effect after menopause. This is the most likely culprit. As little as one drink a day is estimated to increase a woman's risk of developing breast cancer by age seventy by about 7 percent compared to someone who never drank. The risk increases the more you drink. It does not matter whether the alcohol is consumed as wine, beer, or hard liquor. However, in deciding our personal course it is valid to consider the possible benefits of alcohol. We know that moderate amounts, one to two glasses of wine a day, raise the level of good cholesterol and is useful for maintaining a healthy heart. (It should also be noted that teenage drinking does not appear to have any effect later in life.)

So, what should you do?

• If you don't drink, don't start.

• One or two glasses of wine will probably raise your cancer risk only slightly.

• If you drink more than this, cut back.

There is evidence that the risk from alcohol may be lessened if it is accompanied by a large intake of folic acid. This is another good reason to eat your spinach, broccoli, corn, and vegetables rich in folates.

CAFFEINE

There is no indication at present that there is any link between caffeine and breast cancer. Coffee, tea, colas, and chocolate all contain caffeine, and though there was said to be some correlation between consuming these substances and developing breast cysts, the connection has not been proved. Some women whose breasts tend to become tender and lumpy during their menstrual periods report that limiting their intake of caffeine seems to help, but many more notice no link.

You don't need caffeine to be healthy, so if it makes you feel better to cut it out, there's no reason not to. But there is no evidence that it poses a cancer risk.

SMOKING

Lung cancer has become the number-one cancer killer of women in the United States, exceeding breast cancer. This is a maddening tragedy, because lung cancer, with its poor cure rate, is a disease that we do know how to prevent. If women would stop smoking, most of them would not get lung cancer. However, while smoking does not cause breast cancer, it does limit the ways in which we can treat the disease (see Chapter 12), because certain surgical reconstruction procedures cannot be used for women who smoke.

RADIATION EXPOSURE

Exposure to low or modest levels of radiation may sometimes cause breast cancer. (See pages 175–76 for a fuller discussion.) Young women who were exposed to radiation at Hiroshima were subsequently tracked by researchers and were found to have developed an increased number of breast tumors.

Women who were treated with upper-body radiation for Hodgkin's disease when they were young have also been found to have an increased risk of breast cancer. And though you are exposed to relatively little radiation in any single diagnostic X-ray, repeated X-rays over a long period of time may increase your cancer risk, particularly at the site of radiation.

As we saw in previous chapters, modern mammography requires very little radiation, so this should not be a concern. Make sure that the mammography facility you go to has been certified by the Food and Drug Administration (see page 61).

OTHER ENVIRONMENTAL CAUSES

We simply don't have any definite cause-and-effect conclusions to offer on this question. We do know that there seem to be geographic "hot spots" for breast cancer as there are for several other cancers; that is, there are certain areas of the United States where, for reasons we often don't completely understand, there is a higher incidence of an illness than would ordinarily be expected.

We have read, for example, of the high rate of blood cancers in parts of New Jersey and of breast cancer on Long Island, and one can hypothesize about the causes. PCBs and insecticides in the environment of these areas have been questioned and studied. Breast cancer activists have expressed appropriate concern and the CDC has supported studies. However, no correlation between these environmental factors and the incidence of breast cancer has been found. The only thing that can definitely be said about breast cancer and environmental hazards is that many more studies should be funded and carried out as soon as possible.

PERSONAL CARE

Both hair dyes and antiperspirants have been suspected of causing breast cancer, but no relationship has been found between the use of these products and the disease. Both the American Cancer Society and the National Cancer Institute have repeatedly stated that there is no scientific basis for this concern.

HORMONES

There seem to be some quite striking connections between breast cancer and hormones and, by extension, between breast cancer and the course of your reproductive life. This is an example of the type of risk factor we alluded to at the beginning of this chapter—one that is frustrating, because it may seem that there's not very much you can do about it.

Perhaps when more research is done we will better understand the link between breast cancer and estrogen. At the moment, all we can say is that there does seem to be a link. There is a higher breast cancer rate for women who begin menstruating at an early age, and also for those who reach menopause at a relatively late age. And women who have an early natural menopause or who are fairly young when they have their ovaries removed have a correspondingly lower breast cancer risk.

There are other aspects of a woman's reproductive life reflected by breast cancer statistics:

• Never having had a child increases your risk of breast cancer.

• The age at which you had your first child influences your risk. Women whose first child was born before they were eighteen have one-third the risk of developing breast cancer of those whose first child was born after they were thirty-five. Pregnancy before thirty appears to offer some protection against breast cancer.

• What seems to be at work here is the body's natural production of estrogen—and perhaps progesterone. Women who menstruate for a relatively long portion of their lives have estrogen stimulation regularly during that time, and this may be a factor in breast cancer development. About the pregnancy factor, we are less sure, but it may be that the high levels of progesterone during pregnancy offer some protection.

If there is such a connection, what about birth control pills, prescribed hormones, and hormone replacement therapy after menopause?

BIRTH CONTROL PILLS

Birth control pills used to contain large amounts of estrogen, sometimes alone, and sometimes in combination with small amounts of progesterone. In recent years, the two drugs have almost invariably been combined, and lower doses have been found to be effective. This has decreased any risk that may have existed in the earlier formulations. There is still a slightly increased risk of breast cancer, but these risks disappear after women stop taking birth control pills.

And there is evidence that women on birth control pills are actually protected from ovarian cancer even decades after they stop taking them. The pill also provides long-term protection against endometrial cancer which affects the lining of the uterus.

FERTILITY DRUGS

When women postpone their childbearing for career and other personal reasons, fertility becomes a problem and hormonal medications may be used to make pregnancy possible. These are also the years in which women become at increasing risk of getting breast cancer. Is there harm in using fertility medications such as Clomid, Pergonal, and HCG?

While these drugs do increase the level of circulating estrogen in the blood, evidence for a breast cancer effect has not been reported. Another way of looking at this is that risk factors do not translate into a certainty that you are going to get a cancer. Planning a family and helping to achieve conception are an important part of life. Before you embark on any program, though, make sure you:

• have a good clinical breast examination

• have a mammogram and sonogram

• perform monthly breast self-examination

• report any abnormal findings to your doctor.

HORMONE REPLACEMENT THERAPY

Estrogen, with or without progesterone, is frequently prescribed for postmenopausal women:

- to alleviate the symptoms of menopause, like hot flashes and vaginal dryness

- to help prevent osteoporosis, a condition that sometimes afflicts older women, causing their bones to become brittle and to fracture easily

For many years it was accepted that using estrogen replacement therapy over an extended period of time reduced a woman's risk for heart attack. Recent data have not supported this assumption.

Taking estrogen alone does not appear to be harmful to the breasts of postmenopausal women. But, it cannot be used alone unless there has been a hysterectomy because, without added progesterone, the continual stimulation of the uterine lining can cause tumors. On the other hand, when these drugs are used in combination, there is an increased risk of breast cancer. In 2002, a study was reported by the Women's Health Initiative that associated hormone replacement with an increased risk of breast cancer. This resulted in a precipitous decline in the use of hormone replacement therapy (HRT). In turn, there was a sharp decline in breast cancer incidence, beginning in 2003.

Thus, we must carefully consider when it is sensible for postmenopausal women to use hormone replacement.

- If you have very troublesome menopausal symptoms, there may be little harm in carefully monitored hormone replacement therapy.

- If in your particular situation there is an overwhelming risk of osteoporosis, you should consider the treatment.

You should, however, be cautious, because there is a higher incidence of breast cancer in women taking hormone replacement therapy. Estrogen does not cause breast cancer, but if cancer is present, estrogen may stimulate its growth. Be sure to have a thorough breast examination *and a mammogram* before beginning any hormone replacement therapy. Do not take hormones automatically, simply because you have reached menopause, and if you do take HRT, the lowest possible dose of progesterone should be used.

Though we don't have all the answers about the use of these supplements, the following factors should be considered:

• Women with a serious family history of breast cancer should try to avoid hormone supplements.

• Women who have breast cysts and find that more cysts develop when they start taking estrogen should stop.

• Unless they have had a hysterectomy (surgical removal of the uterus), women taking hormone replacement therapy are generally advised to use progesterone as well as estrogen because of the possibility of developing uterine cancer.

• The combination of progesterone and estrogen does appear to increase the risk of breast cancer.

In light of these facts, why should you take supplemental hormones at all?

• If you know, because of family history or for other reasons, that you are at significant risk for osteoporosis, the evidence is quite strong that estrogen replacement will act to protect you.

• If you have persisting, troublesome menopausal symptoms, as some women do, you will certainly get relief if you use hormone replacement therapy. However, you may wish to limit such treatment to the first few years after menopause, after which these symptoms tend to subside.

Up until now, we have talked about oral hormones. What about vaginal creams if you have already had breast cancer? Vaginal dryness can be a problem. There are a variety of moisturizers available that have to be used at least four days a week to maintain the proper moisture level in the vaginal walls. If these do not work, there are other vaginal creams that contain low-dose estrogens that should be used sparingly.

RECENT DISCOVERIES AND NEW OPTIONS

BREAST CANCER GENES BRCA1 AND BRCA2

If you have inherited a mutated BRCA gene, you have a markedly increased lifetime risk for developing a breast or ovarian cancer. Since this is a susceptibility gene, it does not mean you will *definitely* develop the disease. However, it does mean that you are up against high statistical probabilities. The following tables, based on several epidemiological studies, approximate the risk by decade for developing cancer.

Estimated Cancer Risks Associated with Positive BRCA1 Mutation

BREAST CANCER

RISK BY AGE	
30	3%
40	21%
50	39%
60	58%
70	69%
lifetime*	Up to 85%
contralateral breast cancer	5.6% per year

*General Population risk for breast cancer 12.5%

OVARIAN CANCER

RISK BY AGE	
30	<2%
40	3–5%
50	20%

60	40–50%
70	50–60%
lifetime*	62%

*General Population risk for ovarian cancer 1–2%

RISKS FOR MALE CARRIERS

Breast cancer lifetime risk*	Up to 6%
Prostate cancer lifetime risk**	Slight increase prior to age 65

*General Population risk for male breast cancer <1%
**General Population risk of prostate cancer (lifetime) 16%

Estimated Cancer Risks Associated
with Positive BRCA2 Mutation

BREAST CANCER

RISK BY AGE

30	0%
40	17%
50	34%
60	48%
70	74%
lifetime*	85%
contralateral breast cancer	4.2% per year

*General Population risk for breast cancer 12.5%

OVARIAN CANCER

RISK BY AGE

30	1%
40	≤2%
50	10%
60	18%

70	18%
lifetime*	18–27%

*General Population risk for ovarian cancer 1–2%

PANCREATIC CANCER

lifetime risks*	2–5%

*General Population risk for pancreatic cancer <1%

RISKS FOR MALE CARRIERS

Breast cancer lifetime risk*	7%
Prostate cancer lifetime risk**	20%

*General Population risk for male breast cancer <1%
**General Population risk of prostate cancer (lifetime) 16%

Fanconi Anemia Type D1 *Eastern European Jewish patients only.* Mutation carriers of childbearing age should consider having their spouses tested for a BRCA2 mutation, since two copies of the mutation (one from each parent) can result in a child with Fanconi anemia. This is a rare autosomal recessive cancer susceptibility syndrome characterized by congenital abnormalities, progressive bone marrow failure, and childhood leukemias.

Women with a BRCA1 mutation have an 85 percent lifetime risk for developing breast cancer—and the likelihood of developing another cancer in the same or opposite breast five years after a first cancer is discovered is 20 percent. At ten years this risk increases to almost 40 percent. With a BRCA2 mutation the lifetime risk is similar. The five-year risk of a new tumor in the opposite or same breast is about 12 percent. This doubles in the next five years.

While these are ranges, based on population studies, they are significant enough to encourage the recommendation of strategies, for prevention, whether medical or surgical. Since none comes with a 100 percent guarantee, probably the best term to use is "risk reduction" for both approaches.

TAMOXIFEN (NOLVADEX)

Until recently the best hope for "preventing" breast cancer was to discover the disease early through mammography and physical examination, thereby increasing cure rates. This approach, called secondary prevention, has extended and saved lives, but it has not diminished the incidence of the disease.

During the past eighteen years, as tamoxifen began to be taken as protection against the recurrence of treated breast cancers, it became apparent that those taking the drug also had fewer cancers in their other breast. This finding prompted several prospective studies of tamoxifen as a drug for stopping the disease process before it causes detectable invasive breast cancer. This approach is known as primary prevention. The largest of these studies was the Breast Cancer Prevention Trial, which started in June 1992 and whose results were reported in September 1998.

Altogether, 13,388 women entered this trial. To assure that the trial could be finished in a reasonable period of time and be statistically valid, only those with a defined increased risk of developing the disease were permitted to participate. The factors considered were age, number of first-degree relatives with breast cancer, absence of children or the age at which the first child was born, number of breast biopsies in the past, a finding at surgery of "atypical hyperplasia" (an increase in the number of cells within breast tissues, some of which appeared very abnormal, or atypical; see page 46), and age when first period occurred.

The final data analysis showed a 50 percent decrease in the risk of noninvasive breast cancer and a 49 percent decrease in the risk of invasive breast cancer.

On the basis of these findings, the Food and Drug Administration approved the use of tamoxifen for risk reduction in women who met the criteria of the completed study as determined by the Gail model, a computer program that uses personal and family history to estimate a woman's chance of developing breast cancer.

While we now finally have a drug that can reduce the risk of breast cancer, it is still not known conclusively that cancer is prevented forever by such treatment, rather than merely delayed—suppressed for a time, only to appear later. Further observation of those already in the current study should help to clarify this most important point.

Two other, much smaller studies in Italy and England have so far failed to confirm the American findings, but they are considered less reliable by virtue of their size and the nature of the population they studied.

As noted earlier (see page 214) tamoxifen is not without side effects. In the prevention study 2 percent of those taking the drug developed phlebitis. There was a very small but nevertheless twofold increase in the incidence of uterine cancer, particularly in women over the age of fifty.

The use of tamoxifen is an option for risk reduction for those women who have a mutation in their BRCA genes but have not yet had breast cancer.

RALOXIFENE (EVISTA)

No sooner had the promising news regarding the preventive effects of tamoxifen been announced than a second related drug, raloxifene, was put forward as another promising candidate for this purpose. Raloxifene is similar to tamoxifen but is claimed not to have any adverse effects on the uterus. Both belong to a new class of drugs called SERMs—selective estrogen receptor modulators. Current SERMs have antiestrogen effects on the tissues of certain organs, including the breast, and estrogenlike action on the tissues of other organs, such as bone. Research is in progress to find potent SERMs that have antiestrogen action alone. In a study of its use in osteoporosis, raloxifene was given to 5,100 women with this condition, while another 2,600 women with it remained untreated. When the incidence of breast cancer was studied in the two groups, those treated with raloxifene had a lower-than-expected rate of breast cancer. Side effects included phlebitis, but not uterine cancer.

Criticisms of the raloxifene study have included the fact that patients were treated and observed for a relatively short period of time. The study population has also been criticized, because the patients were admitted on the basis of their risk for osteoporosis, not breast cancer. Neither group had ever been assessed for its risk of breast cancer. Finally, only postmenopausal women were eligible for the trial.

However, the promise of raloxifene being more effective in reducing the risk of breast cancer with less risk of uterine cancer than the previously studied tamoxifen was sufficient to prompt the National Cancer Institute to undertake a five-year study, the STAR trial, comparing the preventive benefits of tamoxifen and raloxifene.

In this study a total of 19,747 postmenopausal women who were at an increased risk of developing breast cancer were enrolled in the trial. The results indicated that both drugs reduced the risk of developing invasive breast cancer by about 50 percent. There were one third fewer uterine cancer cases, and a similar reduction in blood clots, in the women assigned to raloxifene. However, tamoxifen was effective in reducing by half the incidence of both ductal and lobular carcinoma in situ, a feat that raloxifene could not accomplish.

While there is still much to be learned about which drugs should be used for primary prevention of breast cancer, the STAR trials do show that the strategy of using a SERM for at least preventing invasive breast cancer is a sound one. Currently, however, tamoxifen remains the preferred drug for this application.

AROMATASE INHIBITORS

When used for the treatment of recurrent breast cancer, aromatase inhibitors have been particularly effective in reducing the risk for breast cancer in the unaffected breast. As a result, studies are ongoing to see whether these drugs could provide greater protection against the development of breast cancer than either tamoxifen or raloxifene, at least in postmenopausal women.

In summary, a number of hormonal agents are likely to be available in coming years to reduce the risk of developing breast cancer among women who are BRCA1- and BRCA2-positive or have a strong family history of breast cancer. What remains to be discovered is how to identify a more complete spectrum of markers that identify who is at risk for breast cancer and to develop preventive drugs with many fewer side effects than current agents. This would enable them to be widely accepted by women who need such protection.

PROPHYLACTIC SURGERY

This very idea strikes most people as gruesome. Have a mastectomy or a bilateral mastectomy even before cancer is found? And remove *healthy* ovaries? But this is true *primary prevention,* an accepted method advised for women who are known to be at an extraordinary risk of developing breast and ovarian cancer. It has been proven to save lives.

Deciding to do this has to be an excrutiating decision. This approach, however, has been used over the years for women who have an extremely high risk of developing breast cancer and are very frightened by that possibility. Now, with the ability to detect genetic mutations with a blood test, we can identify the individuals who are carriers of mutated genes, more accurately assess their risks, and offer recommendations on how they can reduce that risk sharply. All this without forgetting that the BRCA genes are *susceptibility* genes. Not everyone who tests positive is going to get cancer.

Cancer can be prevented by removing both breasts. There is a 1 to 2 percent possibility that a microscopic island of breast tissue that remains after a mastectomy can develop cancer. However, this procedure offers good security for a woman whose family has been ravaged by breast cancer. Usually, women who elect to have double mastectomies choose to have breast reconstruction at the time of surgery.

Women who carry the BRCA genes also have a significant risk of developing ovarian cancer. I almost always recommend removal of the ovaries and Fallopian tubes because there is no good screening test for ovarian cancer. Annual pelvic examinations and ultrasound studies combined with a blood test for CA 125 are the best that can be offered, yet, when ovarian cancer is detected by this approach, it is almost always in an advanced stage. So when a patient is found to be BRCA positive, I use the risk tables on pages 310–11 as a guide, according to the type of mutation the patient has and her age, and advise early removal of the ovaries and Fallopian tubes. This can usually be accomplished through laparoscopic surgery, without opening the abdomen, a technique that markedly reduces trauma and essentially eliminates scarring from the surgery.

If the ovaries are removed in the premenopausal years, between ages forty and fifty, this surgery also reduces the risk of developing breast cancer by 50 percent.

So What Should I Do?

What do I tell my patients? For those whose histories are suggestive of familial breast cancer I advise genetic testing. If risk factors are present but the patient is not a carrier of a BRCA mutation, the advantages of risk reduction using tamoxifen are carefully considered.

For those who are found to have a BRCA gene mutation, there are difficult decisions to be made and no need to rush them. If you are in this position you should hear what your genetics counselor and your doctors—surgeon, oncologist, and internist—have to say. You will also need to discuss the situation with your family, since this is a family matter, and it may be wise for other members of the family to be tested, too, to see whether they are positive or negative for BRCA mutations.

As noted, there is no good screening for ovarian cancer, and removal of the ovaries and Fallopian tubes (bilateral salpingo-oophorectomy, or BSO) is usually recommended. If a patient chooses bilateral prophylactic mastectomies, hormone replacement therapy can, of course, be safely given. When BSO only is carried out in a premenopausal woman, hormone replacement therapy can be used to alleviate menopausal symptoms until a normal menopause would occur.

For a woman who is a carrier who does not already have breast cancer, I am more likely to initially advise BSO than bilateral mastectomies, since the berasts can be screened with mammography, sonography, and MRI. There is the expectation that if a cancer appears, it will be detected at an early and curable stage. However, this cancer will need to be treated, and this frequently involves surgery, possibly radiation therapy, and systemic therapy. Because even heightened screening will not always find early breast cancer, the only true prevention and thus the most effective strategy is prophylactic mastectomy.

And I also tell these patients—and all of my patients—not to smoke. Not because it has much to do with breast cancer but because there's not much point to breast cancer precautions or any other lifesaving techniques if you're going to die as a result of smoking—from lung cancer or heart disease or emphysema.

There is, of course, one recurrent theme in this chapter, as you have no doubt noticed. While we are beginning to discover drugs that can either prevent or delay the occurrence of breast cancer in those who are at highest risk, we do not know enough about the causes of breast cancer to develop a comprehensive program for its eradication. We therefore continue to be cautious in giving you specifics about what you should and should not do to keep yourself free of breast cancer. Keep an open mind about participating in clinical trials that may be helpful to you (see pages 333–40), because what we need most is research to learn more about fighting breast cancer, both its onset and the disease itself.

CHAPTER

16

NEW DIRECTIONS

T hose of us who are old enough remember when years ago the March of Dimes campaign turned the search for a cure for polio into an annual national crusade. The imagination of the entire country was engaged. People went door-to-door soliciting contributions, and the scientists who worked in the field and eventually found a vaccine were national heroes. And the effort worked! In a surprisingly short time, the polio epidemics that had been so dreaded came to an end.

Why isn't there a comparable fervor about finding cures for cancer? In part, perhaps it is because the man who was president of the United States, Franklin D. Roosevelt, was a victim of polio and a constant, visible symbol of its devastating effects. Also, infantile paralysis—as it was often called—struck down large numbers of children, thus evoking a special sympathy.

But I think that something else is going on as well. Despite the valiant efforts of the American Cancer Society and other organizations, we just don't have the optimism that prevailed when the country was marching against polio. Most people don't seem to believe that cancer can be cured. They are wrong. We are making progress in the laboratory in unraveling the puzzle of what unleashes uncontrolled cell growth. We are also making progress in treating the disease. Since this book was first published, in 1992, women's advocacy groups have succeeded in making the public and Congress aware of the urgency of solving the breast cancer problem (see Chapter 18). Funds for cancer research have increased significantly, but there is a great deal more research that has to be completed to stop this national tragedy. To conquer breast cancer, we need to rally the nation more than ever.

Ralph Waldo Emerson said, "Enthusiasm is one of the most powerful engines of success. When you do a thing, do it with all your might. Put your soul into it ... and you will accomplish your object. Nothing great was ever achieved without enthusiasm."

In the field of cancer research, there is already a lot to be enthusiastic about in the findings of those who do laboratory research as well as of those who study patients.

MOLECULAR BIOLOGY

This branch of science is concerned with cell structure, and function and their control by genetic information. It is extremely important in cancer research. A most promising area of that research is the burgeoning exploration of the nature of genes. Almost every week we learn more about normal genes, as well as those implicated in cancer. This research is moving so fast that its results are already being translated into techniques of cancer prevention and treatment.

In order to understand what is going on, it may be helpful to review the nature of cells, chromosomes, and genes, if only enough to be able to interpret the many reports of new discoveries in this field and their application to cancer.

CELLS AND COMPUTERS

We want to concentrate here not on the use of computers in research but on the computer as a good model for understanding how the human cell works.

For a computer to function, it must rely on stored instructions that can be called upon for solutions to specific problems. These instructions are written in a language the computer can "read." The human cell also works from stored instructions, but they are written in another sort of language—the genetic code. Computer instructions are stored in programs, each with a specific task. The equivalent units in the cells, complex and efficient programs, are called genes.

The computer stores its information on a disk. The coded information of the human cell is stored in meticulously organized structures called chromosomes. Despite its microscopic size, each human cell contains more stored instructions than the largest supercomputer now in use.

To use a computer, you first have to instruct it to call upon a specific program. In order to do that, you double-click, for example, on an icon or menu line labeled "Word," "Excel," or "WordPerfect." To receive program instructions, cells have receptors on their surface, each capable of receiving a single message. Once the message is received, it is transmitted to the center, or nucleus, of the cell, where it is processed and its order then conveyed to the specific gene that does the job being called for. For this system to work, the right gene must be found, which means that the gene for this function has to have a fixed location in all cells.

There are estimated to be 30,000 genes, and while we have learned a great deal about their location on specific chromosomes through the Human Genome Project, the function of most of these genes remains to be discovered. And as to how these genes work together to account for the complex and sophisticated functions of a human cell, even less is known.

THE BIOLOGY OF BREAST CANCER

To go back to our computer analogy, we know that you can introduce into a computer "viruses" that give unwanted and often destructive instructions. In the 1960s and 1970s we learned that there are actual viruses that can do the same thing in human cells, producing genetic instructions that cause cells to grow abnormally. Once such viruses infect a cell, the instructions—contained in *viral oncogenes*—override the genes that regulate normal growth and cause rapid, uncontrolled growth.

Sometimes the normal controlling genes, called *proto-oncogenes,* will themselves become corrupted because of exposure to dangerous chemicals or radiation. If this happens, they will come to resemble viral oncogenes and may also stimulate abnormal growth. The presence of oncogenes is one of the prerequisites for the conversion of a normal cell to a cancer cell.

Certain viruses that can cause cancer may be defective themselves, in the sense that they may not carry their own oncogenes. When these viruses infect cells, they fuse with chromosomes next to existing growth-regulating genes and stimulate their otherwise quiet neighbors to become uncontrollably active.

A second kind of gene involved in cancer has also been identified. Called *suppressor genes,* these normally produce substances that slow or suppress abnormal cell growth. If they are damaged, cancer begins to appear. This discovery is particularly important because normal suppressor genes appear to act like an off-switch and thus may be useful in stopping further growth of cancer.

New cells are produced by the division of existing cells into two equal parts. For this to be accomplished, a new set of chromosomes must first be manufactured so that both progeny cells have a full complement of genes. Since chromosomes are composed of DNA, one way to tell whether a cell is preparing to divide is to measure the amount of DNA it contains (see Chapters 5 and 10). Growing cells have been found to go through stages in their life cycle of DNA production. The recognized sequence is rest, DNA manufacture (synthesis or S phase), rest, cell division. This sequence is referred to as the "cell cycle." There are control points between phases of the cell cycle, and in recent years the genes that determine whether a cell will continue to cycle have been identified. Many of these genes are controlled by suppressor genes.

When chromosomes are copied, mistakes can occur. Such mistakes are called mutations, which, if they are permitted to persist, most often cause biochemical changes that kill the cell in which they are found. To limit such damage, cells have mismatch repair genes that correct such errors. However, there can be mutations in the mismatch repair genes themselves, which means further mutations will occur, causing a higher risk of cancer. In fact, such gene defects are being identified in human cancers.

The substances that bind to cell surface receptors to initiate cell growth are called *growth factors*. Abnormal growth factor production may stimulate the growth of cancer cells. Cancer cells can sometimes manufacture their own growth factor and thus empower themselves to reproduce endlessly. And sometimes cancer cells produce receptors that are abnormal and behave as if they have been stimulated by growth factors, though there are none present.

Although both oncogenes and suppressor genes have been identified for some time, manipulation of these genes alone does not appear to cause cancer. A final line of defense against uncontrolled growth may be special sections of DNA called *telomeres*. These cover the two ends of each chromosome. When cells replicate their DNA to manufacture new chromosomes, each copy is a little shorter than the original chromosome. The telomeres are there to permit this shortening without affecting the functioning of the genes of the chromosome. However, after a given number of cell divisions, the telomeres become so short that the chromosomes can no longer be copied. Cell growth then stops, and the cell eventually dies. This natural limit on cell life is independent of the activity of oncogenes or suppressor genes. But cancer cells regenerate their telomeres, permitting long-term cell growth.

While most cells have a limited life span, there is a small percentage that represents the cell of origin of all other cells. These special cells, called *stem cells,* have a relatively long life span, divide less often, generally have no biologic function other than reproduction (maintaining their own species), and are much more resistant to environmental influences than other cells. There is increasing evidence that *rogue* stem cells, originating from normal stem cells that have acquired new mutations in their chromosomes, are responsible for many, if not most, breast cancers. This may explain in part why simply reducing tumor bulk does not necessarily cure the tumor. As a result of this research, abnormal stem cells are becoming a new target for breast cancer therapy.

EPIGENETICS

However, abnormal cell growth is not always due to abnormal genes. Genes are regulated by a variety of regulatory pathways that determine whether or not their messages can be expressed. There are three different ways in which their behavior can be altered: methylation, histone-acetylation, and excessive actions of the ubiquitrone/proteasome system that regulates protein levels within the cell. The science relating to these pathways is referred to as epigenetics.

Epigenetic pathways are more likely to be affected by environmental factors than are genes themselves. One of the most important of these pathways determines whether a gene is or is not *methylated*, the process in which the carbon molecule *methyl* binds to a gene. When methylated genes are inactive, their message cannot be read and converted into instructions. Gene methylation is an important event when a living being is first created; it permits organs to focus on their own specialized functions. For example, it prevents kidney genes from acting in the liver, or liver genes from acting in the kidney. As a person ages, however, the methylation controls may be impaired, so that certain genes that are necessary for growth regulation and normally are active, such as suppressor genes, may become inactivated by methylation. This can lead to the development of cancer.

Histones are proteins that surround genes and may in some cases determine whether they are expressed. The degree to which histones do this is determined by their interaction with the proteins of a chemical group referred to as acetyl. When a histone binds to an acetyl group, it is *acetylated*. This step generally leads to the activation of a gene. When the acetyl group is removed, the gene can no longer act. Cancers can be caused when this system malfunctions because it may prevent growth-regulating genes from performing their important roles.

A third example of nongene changes that may alter the intended function of genes is the influence of the ubiquitin/proteasome system. Since the late 1950s we have known that proteins are manufactured according to the instructions of genes, which determine the sequence in which the building blocks of genes, called amino acids, are strung together to make a specific protein. What has not been known until recently is what happens when a particular protein is no longer needed. For instance, as soon as you eat a piece of chocolate cake, the pancreas prepares additional insulin to permit digestion of the sugar that it contains. But when you have finished the cake and additional insulin is no longer needed, what happens to the extra insulin? When all that new sugar has been processed, the ubiquitin/proteasome system is turned on. Ubiquitin binds to the extra insulin, which then enters a proteasome that acts as a chemical furnace, taking the insulin apart and making its amino acids available for the manufacture of new proteins. When this system malfunctions, the proteins needed for regulating cell growth may be prematurely inactivated, possibly leading to cancer.

BREAST CANCER GENES

Above, we discussed two genes, BRCA1 and BRCA2, which together account for up to 75 percent of all familial breast cancers. Additional mutated genes are being identified that account for some of the remaining inherited cases of this cancer. These genes include p53, PTEN, CHEK2, ATM, NBS1, RAD50, BRIP1, and PALB2. They have been discovered because they are more frequently found in families with a higher incidence of breast cancer than in the general population; that is, in family-based "linkage" studies. Those who inherit abnormal forms of these genes have a high risk of breast cancer because the genes are *high penetrance*, meaning that they not only increase risk but often actually cause the disease. Typically these cases of cancer occur at an earlier age than most "nonfamilial" cases of breast cancer.

Most cases of breast cancer are said to be sporadic in nature—

that is, without a known inherited cause. Some of these cases may in fact be due to inherited gene abnormalities that are difficult to identify by the classic family-linked approach because they increase the risk of developing breast cancer only modestly. Such genes are referred to as moderate- to low-penetrance genes. In most cases, however, breast cancer is considered to originate from a noninherited (somatic) genetic mutation that may be related to an incidental exposure to a chemical, radiation, or virus. Major research efforts are now under way to identify which genes, when injured, are responsible for such sporadic breast cancer.

METASTASIS

Uncontrolled growth is characteristic of cancer cells, but it is not their only property. Cancer cells also have the ability to travel from one part of the body to another—that is, to metastasize. They accomplish this by breaking through the supporting tissue and entering lymphatics or blood vessels.

We are continually learning about the biology of metastasis. One aspect we have discovered is that a cell that will metastasize seems to develop the ability to produce enzymes that digest proteins and enable the cell to invade normal tissue.

There is another group of genes whose role is very different. These genes seem to have the ability to inhibit metastasis. When these genes are inactivated, the cancer can spread.

THE RESULTS OF RESEARCH

If ever there was a time to ask "What does it all mean?" this is it. From an extremely complex group of findings, we are trying simultaneously to understand the cause of cancer and also to treat it. Molecular biologists and biochemists are hard at work on the former task, and from their still incomplete findings, pharmacologists are working to come up with drugs that will save people's lives.

Current research aims to attack uncontrolled cell growth on many fronts:

- By inactivating abnormal oncogenes or their products, which include growth factor receptors that are present on the cell surface

- By preventing growth factors from attaching to receptors

- By interrupting the message of "turned-on" receptors before they reach the cell nucleus

- By introducing new genes to replace abnormal suppressor genes

- By inhibiting specific factors that control the cell cycle, in order to stop cells from growing

- By encouraging tumor cells to undergo natural cell death (apoptosis)

- By interfering with the enzyme that preserves telomeres, and therefore permits cells to divide without limit

- By interfering with the inactivation of genes that prevent abnormal cell growth

- By stopping the destruction of proteins that normally prevent tumor development

- By stopping production of the enzymes cancer cells use to invade normal surrounding tissue

- By preventing the growth of new blood vessels into tumors

One tactic being worked on is to try to manufacture copies of cell-surface receptors for growth factors and give them intravenously. The growth factors would then "make the mistake" of attaching themselves to this injected material before they reached the receptors on the cells themselves.

Since there are many types of receptors, the goal is to develop drugs against as many of them as possible. The first of these, Herceptin (see page 202), is already being used.

Another line of research concentrates on the activity within the cell *after* the growth factor has reached it. When a particular receptor on the outside of a cell is activated, this sets off a chemical reaction on its other end, inside the cell. If you can interfere with this reaction deep in the cell, then growth will not take place. New drugs are being developed to accomplish this.

Genes such as p53, when normal, prevent abnormal cell growth; therefore, p53 is a *suppressor gene*. About 60 percent of breast cancers have abnormal p53 genes. There are other suppressor genes such as PTEN that also play an important role in the development of breast cancer. Studies are under way about how these genes can be replaced to assure a return of normal cell-growth regulation.

The cell cycle that makes cell division possible is often abnormal in cancer cells. Specific steps have been identified in breast cancer that may account for an increase in cell growth rates. Cell cycle abnormalities are also common in other forms of cancer, and drugs are being developed to regulate cell cycle functions. Cells that cannot enter the cell cycle can no longer produce DNA, and so cannot continue growing.

All cells, including breast cells, have a built-in mechanism for self-destruction. This process is referred to as apoptosis. For instance, when a baby is born, the mother's breasts enlarge; after she stops breast-feeding, they get smaller. Because they are no longer needed, the extra cells in the breast receive a signal to undergo apoptosis. As we continue to define this process, we will have new targets for treatment. For example, specifically designed drugs may encourage tumor cells to destroy themselves.

Telomeres (see page 323) are extensions of both ends of each chromosome that are needed to permit the chromosomes to be copied in preparation for cell division. They themselves are copied for the new chromosome, but as noted, with each copy the telomeres grow shorter, until no more copies (and therefore no more new cells) can be made. Cancer cells have an enzyme, telomerase, that overcomes this block to their reproduction rebuilding and extending telomeres. Drugs against telomerase are being developed.

Methylation (see page 324) is the process by which unneeded genes are permanently inactivated. The abnormal methylation of the genes needed to regulate cell growth may occur in tumor cells. A demethylating drug was recently approved by the FDA for use in a disease known to develop leukemia in some patients. New drugs in development may have direct benefit in the treatment of cancer.

The proteins needed for cell growth control may be inactivated prematurely if the ubiquitin/proteasome system described earlier is damaged. Drugs to counter this effect are being developed. The first of these, Velcade, is proving to be of importance in the treatment of the blood-related cancers lymphoma and myeloma. Future drugs of this sort may be important for the treatment of breast cancer as well.

Cancers rely on certain enzymes, not found in normal cells, that have the ability to digest proteins and thus infiltrate and spread into other tissues. Drugs that interfere with the work of these enzymes are being tested.

Another avenue that is being pursued is to starve the cancer by cutting off its blood supply. The drugs that are being developed for this purpose are called *antiangiogenesis* agents. The term derives from *angio* (blood vessel) and *genesis* (creation). The first drug approved by the FDA for this purpose is Avastin. Another drug, which combines antiangiogenesis with anti–growth factor receptor activity, sunitinib (Sutent), is currently being tested.

Poisoning the enemy—so to speak—is yet another technique that is already in use. In order for genes to duplicate themselves and for cells to divide, a finely tuned orchestration of many genes must take place. One approach is to let cells manufacture genes but to feed them the wrong nutrients—antimetabolite drugs, such as 5-fluorouracil—so that the new genes are inactive. There is a problem with this treatment however; it is only moderately selective, and so may interfere with gene manufacture in healthy as well as cancerous cells.

We are now looking for drugs that will be "smarter," that will turn off only the specific genes related to uncontrolled growth. The effects of these drugs will be so focused that they will be able to pinpoint cancer cells and avoid damaging normal cells. Most of these new approaches depend on determining what has gone wrong in the cancer cell. This is how the targets of "targeted therapy" (see page 196) are identified.

IMMUNOLOGY

Although molecular biology is the field in which the most important advances are being made in cancer research, scientists involved in immunology also have an important role to play. This is true despite the fact that a great deal of the work that was done in immunology and cancer in the 1970s turned out to have disappointing results. The drugs that were used to "increase immunity" did not accomplish that goal, for various reasons:

• Perhaps immunity does not play as significant a role in cancer as in other diseases.

• Immunity may be suppressed by the tumor in ways we don't yet understand.

• While there may be functions of the immune process that do work to suppress cancer growth, there may be other functions that are actually used by tumors to facilitate such growth.

There are, however, some areas in which progress is being made. In work with what are called biological response modifiers, the goal is to selectively stimulate aspects of the patient's immune system as well as to treat the illness. We have been able to identify substances, such as interferon and interleukin 2, that are part of the body's natural immune system. Isolating the genes that manufacture these substances allows us to use genetic engineering to produce them in large quantities.

When these substances have been given to patients, the results have been mixed. Interferon has not been found to be useful in the treatment of breast cancer. Though interleukin 2 has been shown to be helpful in treating cancer of the kidney, it has not yet been proven effective for people with breast cancer. However, there are additional regulators of immunity available, and any of them, singly or in combination, may prove to be effective against breast cancer.

Progress is being made in the manufacture of antibodies,

proteins that attack specific targets, or antigens, by binding to them. We have known for a long time, for example, about the effectiveness of an antitoxin in preventing tetanus. What we actually do is to give a large dose of the antibody against the poison produced by tetanus bacteria.

Antibodies are part of the natural defenses of all animals, including humans. Antibodies produced by the progeny of a single cell are called *monoclonal antibodies*. These antibodies have the ability to detect one specific chemical on the surface of a cell. Because of this skill, they are able to distinguish between cells that even under a microscope look identical.

An effort is now being made to use monoclonal antibodies against cancer by having them:

• Isolate targets that are unique to the surface of a cancer cell

• Destroy the target on their own or carry a drug or radioactive substance that will destroy it

• Bind to receptors on the surface of the cancer cell to prevent the attachment of growth factors

Herceptin, a monoclonal antibody to the protein product of HER-2/neu (see page 202), a breast cancer–associated gene produced by molecular methods and made to resemble a human antibody, is being used with outstanding success (see page 208) together with chemotherapy to prevent the recurrence of breast cancer in the 25 percent of breast cancer patients whose tumor is HER-2 positive. It has shown more modest success in the treatment of women with advanced breast cancer. In these more advanced cases it can be used alone or in combination with chemotherapy.

Avastin, already mentioned as an antiangiogenesis factor, and in use for the treatment of recurrent breast cancer, is now being studied in combination with chemotherapy for its effectiveness in the prevention of a recurrence of breast cancer when it is given immediately after surgery. This drug is a monoclonal antibody directed against the blood vessel growth factor VEGF.

There is renewed interest in tumor vaccines. Most testing is at an experimental stage, directed toward seeing whether patients are able to develop an immune reaction to substances on the surface of breast cancer cells.

NEW PROCEDURES

New procedures for early diagnosis are being studied. Among these are *ductal lavage* and *ductoscopy*. Because most breast cancer starts in ducts, efforts are under way to investigate the interior of these ducts to find early signs of malignancy. Ductal lavage is a procedure used to examine asymptomatic women who have an increased risk of breast cancer. The ducts at the nipple are entered with a small catheter and washed (lavaged) to secure cells from the duct linings. Such cells are then examined by the pathologist to see if there is any malignancy present. Fine scopes have also been developed to look directly into ducts. If ductoscopy proves effective, for instance, in finding papillomas (see page 47), the scopes may also be able to remove these tiny lesions without surgery. The American Cancer Society states that there are at present "insufficient data to recommend the use of ductal lavage either as an independent screening modality [method] or in combination with screening mammography."

As part of the current effort to limit the amount of tissue removed at the time of breast surgery and to reduce scarring, *cryosurgery,* and the destruction of a tumor by *radiofrequency ablation* are being investigated. For both procedures, the tumor is first evaluated with a core needle biopsy (see Chapter 4). If cancer is found, a needle is then placed in the lesion to be destroyed, and it is subjected either to freezing conditions (cryosurgery) or to heat (radiofrequency ablation). An area of normal tissue around the target mass is also destroyed. Studies of the effectiveness and safety of this approach are in progress. Since this procedure is still experimental, a standard lumpectomy usually follows.

PATIENT STUDIES

We have been talking up to now about what is sometimes called bench research—the laboratory bench, that is. Now we will consider what can be learned from studying patients through clinical research.

HOW ARE CLINICAL STUDIES PUT TOGETHER?

In order to tell whether a drug or a treatment method is effective and safe, it has to be tried on enough people and under circumstances that are controlled well enough to give us reliable evidence. Sometimes you can find these conditions at a single very large institution, but in actuality most of this work is done by cooperative groups that have been organized specifically to conduct such studies, usually with funding from the National Cancer Institute.

The largest of these groups include the Eastern Cooperative Oncology Group (ECOG), the National Surgical Adjuvant Breast and Bowel Project (NSABP), the Cancer and Leukemia Group B (CALGB), and the Southwestern Oncology Group (SWOG). Each group has many separate medical institutions affiliated with it, so if you decide to participate in a clinical trial, it will probably be at one of these institutions.

To begin with, a study must be designed so that all participating researchers use a uniform approach in seeking answers to particular questions about chemotherapy, surgical treatment, causes of the disease, and other areas of investigation.

Preliminary planning includes answering questions such as these:

• What is the reason for this investigation?

• Who should be treated?

• Age range?

• Sex?

• Patient's condition?

• Stage of disease?

• Previous treatment?

• What treatment will be given?

- Specific surgery?

- Specific adjuvant treatment?

- Drug regimen, including combination, dosage, frequency, schedule?

- How will patients' progress be measured?

- How will information be gathered?

- How will information be analyzed?

If several different treatments are going to be considered, patients are often selected randomly to receive one or another of them. Sometimes, in order to ensure impartial and clear results, a study is designed so that some patients receive the drug that is being tested and others receive a placebo, a substance that has no pharmaceutical effect.

Patients are treated and carefully followed by means of regular tests and visits. For uniformity and reliability, particularly complex tests may be performed by specially designated laboratories. Records are kept of the specific information the study was designed to gather, and the results are analyzed by study statisticians.

Often, if patients getting a particular treatment do especially well, the study will be stopped so that all patients can be given what has been shown to be the more effective treatment.

THE PHASES OF DRUG TESTING

When a new drug is being tested, the study is usually conducted in several stages, or phases, to ensure the safest possible conditions for the patients and the most rigorous gathering of information.

PHASE I

- Before any drug is tested on human beings, it must be shown, through animal testing or preclinical testing, to be safe and potentially effective.

- An application is filed with the Food and Drug Administration (FDA) to begin clinical studies using the drug on human beings.

- The treatment and the possible risks are carefully explained to patients who may wish to participate. Patients also must sign an informed consent form.

- The plan must be approved by the institutional review board (IRB) of each participating facility.

- Initially, the drug is given to participating patients in low doses.

- Dosages are gradually increased to determine effectiveness, side effects, and toxicity.

Should you join a Phase I drug test? It all depends. If you have already had an unsuccessful course of treatment that you think was as vigorous as possible, you may welcome the chance to try something new. There is certainly reason to believe it may work, because to get to a Phase I study, a drug has to have shown promise in preclinical trials. Only a few drugs a year ever get to this point.

On the other hand, a Phase I drug should not be used if you have not yet tried an already established treatment that is known to be effective. The potential side effects that are already known from animal studies should be thoroughly reviewed, and it should be explained to you that there may only be a small chance that the drug will help you.

PHASE II

By the time a drug gets to this point, we already know quite a lot about its potential benefits, side effects, toxicity, and appropriate dose levels. The Phase II study explores the drug's benefits for patients with a particular form of cancer.

- Only the drug being studied is given to participating patients.

- One or more fixed dose levels, adjusted for your height and weight, are administered.

Before you join a Phase II study, you should be assured that there are already data that suggest it will be helpful in your particular situation. You should be sure that there is not an already established treatment that might benefit you and that potential side effects have been thoroughly explained to you.

PHASE III

A Phase III drug has been shown to have good potential as a treatment for a particular condition. The questions that remain are: Is it better than treatments already in use? How does it measure up against other drugs or combinations of drugs? In order to answer these questions, some patients participating in the study will be given the new treatment, and some will be given treatments already in use.

Consider these factors carefully as they relate to your own case, and bear in mind that when a new treatment is being tested in a Phase III study, you won't necessarily get it, even if you are participating in the study. Patients in the study are randomly selected to receive the new treatment so that established and new therapies can be compared. You may turn out to be in a control group, which does not receive the new treatment.

Phase III studies are the least problematic for participating patients, in the sense that we know a great deal about the treatment, its side effects, proper dosages, and so forth, by the time we get to this point.

PHASE IV AND ACCELERATED APPROVALS

Phase IV studies are those done after the FDA has approved a drug for release. These are also known as post-marketing studies. They are entirely voluntary, except in the case of accelerated approval, which is a process for the more rapid approval of drugs for patients with life-threatening illnesses. Drugs being considered for accelerated approval fill an urgent need and do not have to meet the strict criteria for effectiveness that the FDA usually demands before giving a drug company permission to begin distribution. However, at the time of approval, the drug manufacturer must outline the clinical trials that it will undertake to complete in the future. Many of the newer cancer drugs first became available through accelerated approval.

PERSONALIZED THERAPY

PHARMACOGENETICS

Medicines are selected because of their proven effectiveness. Sometimes, however, they don't seem to work as well as expected. We have learned that not everyone handles a drug in the same way. Tamoxifen is converted (metabolized) in the liver to endoxifen, the active form. If there is an alteration in the enzyme CYP2D6, metabolism may be slower or faster than expected, depending on the genetic form of the enzyme. Patients who are poor metabolizers get the least benefit from tamoxifen and ultra-rapid metabolizers do best with it. They also seem to suffer the most side effects. Furthermore, drugs such as Prozac, which are used to counter side effects, are also affected by the same pharmacogenetic pathways that affect tamoxifen and may interfere with the activation of tamoxifen itself. Other antidepressants such as Paxil have a lesser effect.

As we learn more about genetic differences among individuals we are also discovering how to use this information to tailor drug treatments and doses to each patient. When you take a drug, your body processes it and converts it to a variety of molecules using enzymes. Some of these molecules account for the benefits of the drug. All are eventually excreted, mostly into the urine or the intestinal system via the liver. Many of the body's drug-processing enzymes are present in different amounts in different patients. The targets the drugs are directed against also vary somewhat in structure from individual to individual. These differences in drug processing and in the nature of the targets they bind to can affect the safety and effectiveness of drugs we use. This can be of particular importance when we are dealing with antitumor drugs that provide low margins of safety and require relatively high doses. In progress are studies intended to choose drug treatments for each individual that are tailored to his or her own genetic characteristics.

THE ETHICS OF CLINICAL TRIALS

It used to be that people would say they didn't want to be "guinea pigs"; they wanted to be sure of a drug's effectiveness before they tried it. In recent years, however, many gravely ill patients have been eager to try whatever is available and relatively safe, if it shows promise of helping them.

In terms of advances in medical treatment, a great deal of what we know about breast cancer has come from such clinical trials.

It was an NSABP trial that established that lumpectomy and radiation are as effective in treating Stage I and Stage II breast cancer as mastectomy.

A group of researchers at the National Tumor Institute in Milan established that if cancer has spread to the lymph nodes near the breast, using adjuvant CMF chemotherapy after surgery was better at preventing recurrence than no further treatment at all. This set the stage for the broad use of preventive hormone therapy and chemotherapy.

Several groups have demonstrated that even in patients with localized breast cancer and negative lymph nodes, chemotherapy can push cure rates up.

In addition to the studies related to basic science research that we have discussed, clinical studies now under way include investigations of:

• Whether there is need for a complete axillary node dissection in women if a sentinel node contains microscopic malignancy

• Whether limited, short-term radiation therapy can safely replace the current standard of five to six weeks of radiation treatment for patients undergoing a lumpectomy.

• Whether radiation therapy can be safely omitted for women over seventy years of age following lumpectomy.

• Whether a gene profile such as Oncotype can be relied on to determine what type of preventive therapy a patient should receive after surgery

- The length of time patients should be treated with tamoxifen

- Whether prolonged treatment with an aromatase inhibitor will prevent late recurrences of breast cancer

- The comparative benefit of different hormonal drugs in preventing breast cancer and the sequence in which they should be given

- Whether Adriamycin should be given as adjuvant therapy to patients whose tumors are HER-2 negative

- New drug combinations, doses, and schedules for chemotherapy

- Drugs that reduce the toxicity of already existing treatments

- The use of chemotherapy for patients whose tumors are 1 centimeter or less

- The use of chemotherapy to reduce tumors to a size that permits breast-conserving surgery

- Whether Avastin will add significantly to the benefits of preventive chemotherapy

- Which of the two drugs that are now available against HER-2 positive breast cancer, Tykerb (lapatinib) or Herceptin, will be more effective? If used together will they be even more successful?

Obviously these studies have great potential value. You should consider participating under the following circumstances:

- Established therapy to help you has been exhausted, or the new treatment is likely to produce benefits just as good as or better than established therapy.

- You are fully informed about what the study is intended to accomplish.

- You understand why this treatment offers you a special opportunity.

• You have been told the range of possible side effects and have been assured that every effort will be made to limit them.

HOW DO I FIND OUT ABOUT CLINICAL TRIALS?

If you have decided that you want to look into the possibility of participating in a clinical trial, there are several ways you can proceed:

• Start by talking to your physician. Many breast cancer specialists trained at cancer research centers and regularly participate in their clinical studies.

• Research centers around the country enlist the help of local physicians. Your doctor may be taking part in a study by one of these centers, or she may be able to refer you to someone else who is.

• You can call (800) 4-CANCER, the Cancer Information Service of the National Cancer Institute. This phone number gives you access to PDQ, a computer service that will produce a printout of all ongoing breast cancer trials, with the names and phone numbers of the principal investigators.

MEDIA

Everyone is interested in the results of clinical trials. These are published as articles in scientific journals. Before publication each article is reviewed by a number of expert physicians in the relevant area of research, who carefully examine both the study methods used and the way conclusions were reached, in order to ensure the validity of the results. This is called "peer review." Because of their importance to the public, the results are often presented on the front pages of newspapers or on nightly television news shows before the issue of the scientific journal is printed. If you have read such accounts, don't be disappointed if your doctor asks you to wait until she has read the article in the journal; she cannot provide appropriate advice until she has seen the findings and has considered their significance with respect to *your* case.

CONSENSUS CONFERENCES

Despite all the studies and analyses, serious questions sometimes remain as to how to proceed in the treatment of cancer. The National Cancer Institute has tried to deal with such thorny questions by calling Consensus Conferences of clinical investigators, supporting professionals, and patients.

Their purpose is to evaluate available scientific information, to resolve safety and effectiveness issues, to advance the understanding of technology or of a medical question, and then to provide information that will be helpful to health professionals and to the public. In practical terms, these conferences are a way of consolidating what we know and of recommending what ought to be done in day-to-day practice.

The conferences have helped crystallize certain treatment standards, they have aroused useful debate, and they have stimulated research and analysis that may prove useful in finding the causes of and the cure for breast cancer.

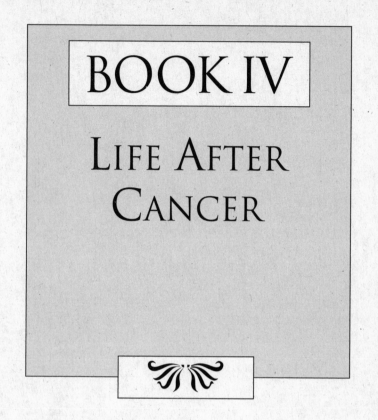

BOOK IV

LIFE AFTER CANCER

CHAPTER

17

LIFE AFTER BREAST CANCER

❧

There is no particular program for coping emotionally with breast cancer, no regimen that I as a doctor can prescribe with assurances to you that, taken twice daily, you'll be all right. This chapter, therefore, relies heavily not on advice but on the experiences of the women I've known and heard about who have had this illness.

No sane person would choose to have breast cancer or, having had it, would say that it was an ennobling experience. Nobody who has had a grave illness, or who has lived through the experience of surgery, or who has worried about the effects of powerful treatments, would mouth such a platitude.

One of my patients whose breast cancer was only one of a series of terrible life events described a time she completely lost her temper when a self-avowed "religious" neighbor advised her, "Be thankful, dear. God doesn't give us more than we can bear."

And yet, difficult though it is to live through, many patients who have recovered say that having had breast cancer does eventually recede into their past. One woman, seven years after her surgery, said, "I think about it when I go for my yearly mammogram, and I sometimes scare myself when I read about recurrences in the paper, but it's just not part of my daily agenda anymore. Life goes on, the good stuff and the bad."

Another woman said, "I remember that when I found out, my first reaction was 'Oh, my God, I'll lose my breast!' Then I realized that wasn't the issue. I was afraid I would die, and because I couldn't talk about that, I focused on my breast. Later on, each treatment made me feel safer, and—believe it or not—I was afraid to stop chemotherapy. Now every year that goes by, I worry a little less."

That is not to say that this is by any means a trivial matter or that it does not leave its mark on you, as these two women report: "I've become much more of a health nut than I ever was before. I listen to my body more. . . . Sometimes I even feel I'm being a little hypochondriac. But the good side is, I read a lot about taking care of yourself and I watch my diet more—hardly any fats at all— and I'm religious about going for physicals and mammograms right on schedule."

"I can go for months feeling great, and I don't even think about cancer. Even though I see my mastectomy scar every day, I've just gotten used to it, and it doesn't make any difference. But the week I have to see my doctor, I'm a wreck. I never can figure out what the problem is until the visit is over and he tells me I'm okay."

The period after surgery, just after they have come home from the hospital, is the time when most women experience their highest level of depression and anxiety. There has been an enormous amount to get through from the time they first realized something was wrong, through the period of evaluating their choices and making decisions, through the surgery itself. Now they must face picking up their lives again and also coping with whatever further treatment has been decided upon.

"When I first got out of the hospital, I was afraid I wasn't going to be able to manage everything that was waiting for me. You know, even though you wish the nurses wouldn't wake you at six in the morning to take your temperature, and the residents wouldn't keep asking you the same questions over and over again, still those are signs you're being taken care of. You get a little infantilized in the hospital, as if you don't have to take care of yourself; you have all these nursemaids to do it. And then—boom! You're home, and people expect you to be a responsible grown-up again."

Women have various ways of dealing with the issues of self-image, relationships, career, and continued treatment after they have had breast cancer. One woman said, "I've always got a list for everything—food shopping, my kids' schedules, what I want to tell my boss the next time I accidentally on purpose meet him at the coffee shop. After my breast surgery there were so many things to worry about, I decided to make a list. It had some pretty ridiculous items, like '1. Afraid to walk the dog. Maybe he'll hurt my arm,' followed by '2. Hire a dog walker for a few weeks.' It sounds sappy, but I even had on there when I thought my husband and I could start having sex again. Just putting it there gave me the sense that everything has a chance of falling into place if I cross each item off one at a time."

The unknowns that women face after breast cancer lie in many corners of their lives, and some of them, as we'll see in the following pages, quite naturally cause a great deal of concern. But after a while, when the "tincture of time" has had a chance to do its work, there seems to be a universal ebbing of anxiety.

"The first few weeks, that's all I could think about—my cancer, my mastectomy, my reconstruction. It's as if I had to give all my energy to that. I was pretty depressed, I guess, but then those dark periods would alternate with normal times, when I'd be laughing with my kids and getting it all together. Gradually, there were more good times than bad."

Getting Through the Crisis

WHERE DOES HELP COME FROM?

Though there are variations in their reactions, most women who have breast cancer go through the crisis without long-lasting psychological or sexual problems. Some of them use short-term professional therapy to help them manage, but many accomplish this by becoming actively involved in their treatment, as well as by accepting the support of family and friends and other women who have had breast cancer. They also find groups such as Reach to Recovery, Cancer Care, the nurses or social service workers at the hospital, the American Cancer Society, and other individuals and organizations in the community of great practical as well as emotional support.

Very often, not only you but also your life partner and other family members can avail themselves of such services. It may be helpful to remember that you're not the only novice in this game. So are your family and friends. They are often frightened for you and for themselves, and they may be worried about whether they'll be able to give you the care you need. They may not know what to say or how to say it. Particularly during the sometimes long haul of extended chemotherapy, when you may need more help than usual, children can forget why their mother is not as available to them as she ordinarily is.

One woman who was suffering from nausea during her chemotherapy said, "I don't know why, but washing out the bathtub made me feel sick. It became a real issue with my sixteen-year-old son, your typical teenage slob. Eventually, I explained to him that—irrational or not—this was a time in our lives when he was going to have to go more than halfway. He did try harder after that, and luckily my medication was changed and I didn't have the problem anymore."

Another woman, in speaking of her friends' concern, said, "Sometimes the sympathy of my friends and family was a burden for me. Everyone was so sad. I could see how worried they were, and in a way it scared me even more. I used to enjoy being with people once in a while who didn't know about my cancer, so I could forget about it myself for a couple of hours. But those feelings weren't really important. In spite of a twinge like that once in a while, what kept me going was the support I got from the people around me."

That last is the recurring theme from women who have had breast cancer: being able to accept the support and practical help of friends and family is what got them through.

To become seriously ill, whatever the disease, often carries with it an element of shame or guilt that is irrational but no less real. There is a part of us that believes that being less than the picture of radiant health portrayed everywhere around us means that we've somehow failed as human beings, that we're inadequate. As an extension of that attitude, some women seem to feel that they have let their husbands down by getting breast cancer.

One woman expressed those feelings on a recent television report on breast cancer. Asked whether she was upset about losing her breast, she said something like "I guess I don't mind so much, but I feel bad for my husband."

Her husband, without missing a beat, replied, "I don't care about that. You and me and the kids, we're a family. That's the important thing."

What was impressive about this man was not only his loyalty but also his ability to express it. That, for all concerned, seems to be of primary importance. Being able to talk about your illness is key to your well-being. In general, I have found that it is not psychiatrists who seem to be of the most help in this instance, but other women. They may have been trained in counseling, as social workers, nurses, or physical therapists, or they may not be in the helping professions at all. Women who have had breast cancer can often be especially useful to those who now have the illness, both in terms of practical advice based on their experience and as a source of emotional support.

Women who have recovered say they frequently get telephone calls from "friends of friends" who have heard they had breast cancer and want advice. "I feel like there's a powerful underground network of women helping each other," one of them said. One patient who had recently learned she had breast cancer said, "People I never knew had breast cancer are just coming out of the woodwork. It almost seems like every other person I know has had it, or her sister did. And most of them want to help."

Group sessions led by a woman experienced in counseling can be helpful, as can counselors with special experience with the issues of breast cancer. I work with one counselor who is so good that I consider her my greatest resource. She'll talk to women anytime, even on the telephone before formally meeting them. It's not only her professional training that makes her so good, but also the fact that she has had mastectomies and chemotherapy herself.

Her view is that "women need short-term support to take them through what they have to do, and then they have to go on with their lives." She's right. Cancer doesn't make your life better, but it shouldn't take it over.

DON'T I HAVE A SAY?

STAYING INFORMED

Staying informed about one's health is obviously important in the long run to help assure the best possible outcome. But there may be times when too much is being said for you to be able to absorb or deal with it all at once—or so much may be happening that you can't be confident the choices you will make will be the right ones. At this point it is probably best to say, "Stop. Let me deal with one thing at a time." Constructive participation in your care not only means that you are involved in decision making; it also means that you must be able to understand what the issues really are. If pressures are preventing you from focusing on these issues, say so, but make it clear that if in the future you want those details, that information will be readily available.

CHOOSING WHICH TYPE OF SURGERY TO HAVE

As discussed in Chapter 8, detection of breast cancer at an early stage has made it possible for most women to have a tumor removed without losing a breast. For other women, their age, being pregnant, the size of the tumor or its location within the breast, or the presence of a gene mutation makes mastectomy the safer alternative. Sometimes both approaches are equally good as regards potential cure. If that happens to you, as you consider the advantages and disadvantages of each type of surgery, it may be helpful to know that research has shown that reconstruction after mastectomy, very much like breast conservation, helps a woman to achieve a more positive self-image and increased sexual satisfaction. Studies have also shown that the type of surgery performed has a surprisingly small effect on a person's overall psychological health and ultimate sexual functioning. When you meet with your surgeon, if you don't quite understand what he is telling you about the pros and cons of the various types of surgery, ask and continue asking until you feel you know enough to make an informed decision—one that will be right for you.

WORRYING ABOUT SIDE EFFECTS OF OTHER TREATMENTS

The side effects of radiation therapy were reviewed in Chapter 9. They tend to be mild and short-lasting. However, anticipation of receiving what we have often heard described as a dangerous treatment, in an unfamiliar environment, can be a frightening experience. Furthermore, radiation treatments may last as long as six or seven weeks. What of the disruption that can cause in a person's life? Becoming informed and planning ahead are particularly helpful in allaying such fears. The most reassurance will come from the radiation oncologist. He will tell you about the nature of the treatments, how they are planned and given, and what procedures are in place to assure your safety. He may discuss with you whether partial or accelerated radiation may be an alternative for you. In addition, most radiation oncologists will arrange for a tour of their facility so that you can meet those who will help him take care of you and see the setting in which radiation therapy is given. Preparing questions ahead of time about things that concern you the most will prove helpful. Some of your questions should deal with the length of each treatment and how you can arrange to schedule them so that they are most convenient for you. An important advantage may be that radiation therapy following surgery for breast cancer does not have to be given immediately. A delay of several weeks is safe. Often, such treatments are first administered five or six months after surgery, in programs that include chemotherapy. Since you will have time to plan ahead, discuss with the radiation oncologist how to schedule appointments at the times you prefer. You may want your treatments early in the morning so that they do not interfere with your day's schedule, or perhaps later in the day, after work. Setting this up well in advance will let you choose what is best for you.

What of chemotherapy? There is evidence that adjuvant chemotherapy can improve survival rates for most women who have had breast cancer. But knowing that a certain treatment is helpful and needed does not necessarily provide peace of mind. What about the side effects? What of the horror stories we are bombarded with in the press—uncaring doctors, bald women, nausea and vomiting? No wonder many women report being both depressed and very frightened before they start their treatments. The good news, as discussed in Chapter 11, is that a lot of attention has been given to devising ways to limit side effects. Studies have shown that once chemotherapy is under way, the levels of tension and concern are quickly reduced. Make sure your oncologist is readily available to you so that if something unexpected happens, you can quickly find out whether it has anything to do with your treatment—as well as what to do about it. Staying informed before and during treatment is the key to peace of mind.

Be prepared for emotional reactions that overwhelm any rational analysis. Anticipatory stress before treatments may make it difficult for you to work, pay attention to others, even eat. If you are receiving a drug such as Adriamycin or Taxol, you may be told that you will lose your hair for a time, but only for a time. You say to yourself, "I can take that, as long as the hair comes back after the treatments are over." During the first few days when your hair actually falls out, however, you will find it extremely difficult to console yourself. If you prepare yourself beforehand for this emotional letdown, it will provide you with a measure of reassurance. You can also take heart from the fact that reactions like these tend to ease as treatments proceed, and clear away once they are over.

HOW DO I HANDLE MY JOB?

Let's begin this section with the good news and then go back to the practical questions and the strategies that seem to have suc-

ceeded best in this crucial area of breast cancer's impact on a job
or a career. The first thing to be said is that having had breast cancer and then returning to work has not had a negative long-term
impact on the careers of most women. That is not to say there are
no problems. As we will discuss, there are practical considerations, like insurance coverage, getting time off for adjuvant treatment, and the physical demands of the job. There are also more
abstract questions that have to do with the attitude of coworkers
and of company executives toward your illness and their percep-
tion of your ability to do the job well.

HEALTH INSURANCE

"I'm pretty new on this job, and I'm afraid they'll be so mad
about these medical bills I'm submitting to the insurance company, I may be fired."

This not uncommon worry has a straightforward answer: You
can't be fired for being sick. Your health insurance can't be termi-
nated if you get cancer, as long as you're able to do your job. The
information you or your doctor provides in connection with an
insurance claim is confidential. If you do leave your job, you are
entitled to coverage at a group rate for a period of time until you
can make other arrangements.

Unfortunately—and surely society must very quickly address
the problem that over forty-seven million Americans do not have
health insurance—these new insurance arrangements can be very
hard to make and also are very expensive. Insurers often make it
difficult for people who have "expensive" illnesses to get new coverage, especially when they are applying on their own and not as
part of a group. Even with group coverage, there may be excessive
waiting periods before the costs of treatment for a preexisting illness are reimbursed. If you are concerned about your insurance
coverage, you should consult the hospital social worker. These
professionals are often very knowledgeable and can refer you to
specialists in the field of health insurance or give you advice themselves. There are, for example, professional and social organizations throughout the country that offer health insurance to their
members and that accept new members quite readily. In many

instances, there is an open period once a year, a time when unaffiliated people can apply to health insurance companies and be accepted without meeting the usual eligibility requirements. Again, however, the coverage offered may be expensive.

If you are employed at the time of your illness and are covered by your company's medical insurance policy, it probably makes sense to stay at your job, at least for the period that you are receiving treatment. I have seen some patients and their families beside themselves with worry about health insurance. (It probably makes sense to stay on your job for other reasons, too. You are undergoing enough difficulties at the moment without adding another stressful change.)

WHOM SHOULD I TELL AT WORK?

The question of how open you are going to be about your illness, especially at work, is an extremely personal one. Some women talk freely about having breast cancer and seem not to suffer any unpleasant consequences. Others have what appear to be legitimate reasons for not wishing their private affairs to become public, particularly in the workplace. They may have a very strong sense of privacy. They don't even want the word *cancer* to be written on their health insurance forms lest other people find out about it. (This is not possible. The diagnosis must be noted in order for you to receive insurance benefits and any disability pay.)

Such women don't want to "cope with their coworkers," in the sense of having to talk about their treatment and other aspects of their illness. They may also worry that their careers will suffer: "I'm in a really competitive field. One word of my having the big C and I'm right off the fast track."

You may indeed be in a work situation where it is simply not a good idea to discuss the details of your illness. There are certain highly competitive or cutthroat businesses and professions where the "fast track" doesn't make accommodation for serious illness. In those situations, taking time off—and being discreet about what was wrong—may serve you best. It is worth repeating that filing an insurance claim does not automatically trigger disclosure of what is wrong with you. In most situations, the insurer and the company's benefits department are specifically enjoined from such disclosure. Many companies also have a system under which you can send your claim directly to the insurer.

A problem sometimes arises for women in jobs that require a lot of physical effort. They usually can manage sick time for their illness, but they are concerned that if word gets around that they had cancer, their employers and coworkers will incorrectly conclude that they'll never again be able to work hard. They are particularly worried that they may not get time off for adjuvant radiation or systemic therapy or that they may be fatigued after those treatments. In these situations, it may be best to figure out who among your supervisors is likely to be the most sympathetic. Take that person into your confidence and ask him or her to help you devise a plan that will work best for the company and for you. If you are a member of a union, talk to the shop steward or some other union official about what benefits and time off you can expect.

But ... there is no reason to assume that people will act badly. As we have seen, the breast cancer rates in this country are unfortunately high enough that the majority of your colleagues will have people close to them who have had the illness. Furthermore, enough well-known women—Olivia Newton-John and Sandra Day O'Connor among them—have made no secret of their breast cancer and have helped those who don't have personal experience with the disease to understand it.

As a result, most people will react helpfully and sympathetically, as this woman describes: "I talked to the head of our personnel department when I first found out about my cancer. She told me that she'd be of whatever help she could, but she also went out of her way to drop some remark like, 'Of course, none of us have any way of knowing what's on your medical claims.' "

However, the most important point here is that even if the information becomes known—either because you yourself talk about it or by some other means—it does not seem to have long-term detrimental effects on the careers of most people. Whatever its initial impact in the workplace, once the original crisis of the illness is over, any shock to your colleagues your cancer has caused seems to wear off.

That also seems to work out when eventually women do make job changes (and this seems to be true of both women and men, whether they have had breast cancer or other cancers). People forget. They see what you are doing in your career today, and many of them assume that what's past is past.

That obviously is not true in every case. There are some stories about women who were passed over, particularly for a new job, because of their illness. Nevertheless, if a potential new employer does know you have had cancer, there is no point in denying it. There are laws in most states against discrimination in hiring, and you may want to avail yourself of them.

It is an unfortunate reality that a certain number of misguided conceptions and unsympathetic attitudes about cancer are out there in the workplace. They are cruel and ignorant, and we should be doing everything we can to eliminate them. In fact, as noted, most states and localities have legislation on their books against overt discrimination, and you should utilize the law's protection in the unlikely case that it may become necessary.

Fortunately, that kind of drastic action is rarely necessary. Many women with breast cancer report that they shared with their colleagues everything that was going on and that they had no reason to regret that course of action. Though there might have been some awkwardness on the job when they first became sick, after a while, when they were back at work, most people seemed to have forgotten about the problem.

HOW DO I HANDLE MY PERSONAL LIFE?

SEXUALITY

We talked earlier in the book about how important the breast is to many women and men as a symbol of sexuality. After breast surgery, couples need to work out their private lives, striking a balance between rushing back into sexual relations, to "prove" everything is the same as ever, and allowing unspoken fears and inhibitions to build up and make it difficult to resume a fulfilling physical relationship. The old signals may not serve: The husband may have doubts about whether his wife is ready for lovemaking, and she may mistake this for aversion. Or the woman who had breast surgery may feel quite fragile and need time to slowly reaccustom herself to making love.

One woman described an even subtler problem: "In our relationship, when one or the other of us is in some trouble, we tend to cuddle a lot and get comfort from being physically close. That often leads to sex—except now I'm just ready for the cuddling and not the next step. I need some time to get used to my body again."

We have learned over the years how important it is in a good physical relationship for partners to tell each other what they need and want. This is especially important now, after breast cancer.

One patient had a funny revelation when she talked to her longtime lover about how worried she was about her appearance. She said, "When I was a girl, we walked around with a tape measure to keep checking that our dimensions were right, and girls went through all sorts of agony, especially if their chest wasn't big enough. Well, after my mastectomy, mine sure wasn't, but when I said something like that to Jim, he looked at me as if I was crazy. 'Listen, I've always loved the way you looked because you're so elegantly slim—like a model or one of those '20s pictures of some woman golf star.' "

After breast cancer, single women who are seeking a new relationship may worry about how a new person will react, and they may be reluctant to mention their illness: "I'm not dating anyone now, and I'm afraid that if this gets around, I'm doomed to spending my life alone."

However, as discussed several times earlier in the book, the good stories seem to be at least as numerous as the bad. A forty-year-old patient told of meeting the "man of her dreams" only about six weeks after breast surgery: "All the time we were getting to know each other, I was thinking either 'Why didn't this happen last year?' or else 'Why couldn't this happen next year, when the scars will look better?' "

Certainly for most women the best course of action seems to be to give yourself time after the surgery to make peace with all you have been experiencing before beginning a new relationship. But this woman said, "Rushing into a relationship with Fred at that point in my life was probably foolhardy. But it turned out to be the best psychological medicine I could take. It made me feel that I was still a desirable woman."

Not every story of a new relationship turns out so well. Some people may shy away from what they see as the added responsibility of becoming involved with someone who has been ill. They may have fears about illness in general. Obviously, you won't want to share the facts of your illness with everyone you meet, but as you become close to new people, you will probably find it most comfortable to tell them about what is, after all, a major event in your life.

A new attitude has been emerging lately: Young women, especially, have been writing and saying that they don't want to go "into the closet" about breast cancer. They are proud of their bodies, breast cancer or no; they want to be able to talk about their experiences as women, including their illnesses, without the shame that women commonly used to feel about their physical lives: about menstruation, or the details of childbirth—or breast cancer.

GETTING PREGNANT

Getting pregnant is not high on the list of priorities of many women after breast cancer, but if you are young, it may be something you fervently want. Systemic treatments after surgery do interfere with fertility, but less so in younger women. I have a patient whom I first saw in her twenties. She received one year of CMFVP, a program that includes Cytoxan, which is thought to particularly affect fertility. After completing therapy, she had five children. Recently, she called me to invite me to her first daughter's wedding.

About eight years ago I saw a woman with a strong family history of breast cancer who two months earlier had bilateral mastectomies. Now she was pregnant and had a recurrence. She was advised to have an abortion before starting chemotherapy. On examination I realized that the apparent recurrence was really a residual tumor that had not been removed by the previous surgeon. With my coauthor, Dr. Pressman, as surgeon, the residual tumor and all remaining breast tissue was removed. No abortion was needed. Recently, this patient, who is quite soft-spoken, visited my office for a follow-up examination. When I examined her abdomen, I found her to have a seven-month pregnancy and thanked her for the nice surprise. When she delivered two months later, she called my office to let me know, a call I returned a few days later. At the time, only the patient's husband was home. He thanked me for calling and then told me that they just had a baby boy, adding: "I want you to know that from the day we first came to your office we have had five sons." Wow!

Other former patients have had one or two children. It is still not a common event, but for those who want a child, it is reassuring to know that it does happen. At one time it was thought that pregnancy might reactivate a previous case of breast cancer. There is no evidence that this is true.

FAMILY AND FRIENDS

"My marriage wasn't that strong before all this happened. I just don't think it will survive so much trouble, but I'm in no condition right now to take on another big upheaval."

"It's so strange; we used to have a lot of rocky times before, but it feels like this breast cancer thing has brought us closer together. I think when you have hard times, both people come to realize how much they rely on each other."

There seems to be a surprisingly low incidence of divorce among my patients. Perhaps that is due to a reordering of priorities; perhaps both partners are unlikely to make changes during a stressful time; perhaps having been through such a crisis together strengthens the relationship thereafter. Though everyone has heard or read about husbands and lovers who do not come through in a crisis, the overwhelming majority of them do. And, whether married or single, heterosexual or homosexual, women who had rewarding social and sexual lives before their breast cancer seem to take up where they left off and build those good lives again.

The need for honesty with your husband or partner is pretty straightforward, but it is also important to be forthcoming with your children. Even young children need to be told why you are going to the hospital or for treatment, and they also need to have some idea of what's going on with your body. There's a good analogy between frankness about this and giving your kids information about sex. You tell them as much as they can understand and absorb, without overwhelming them, being evasive, or making them think there's some terrible secret.

One man, whose wife was ill with breast cancer when their daughters were twelve and fourteen, said that one of the girls, who is now twenty, recently expressed great anger that she had been neglected during the illness, that no one in the family had seemed to care about what was happening to her and her sister. Her father said, "But Joan, your mother was really sick. We had to put all our effort into taking care of her." And Joan replied, "You should have tried. We could have died or something, too, and nobody would have noticed."

The problem is painful and complex. To say that more communication was probably needed is much too facile a comment. When you are gravely ill, you put all your energy into fighting the illness. To also be an especially sensitive and participating parent at this time is extremely difficult. Even so, it would be helpful if the parent who is not ill would bear in mind that the children may be frightened or even angry at what is happening to their mother and to their normal family life. Talking about the course of treatment and what their mother will be doing and feeling can alleviate some, if not all, of their anxieties.

Dealing with older children, especially girls and young women, may be harder, since they may very well fear that what has happened to you is going to happen to them. Refer them to Chapter 15 in this book on risk factors. Explain that the information we have is statistical. It does not mean that they are doomed to develop breast cancer. If one of the doctors who has taken care of you is particularly compassionate and helpful, ask your daughter if she would like to talk to her.

IN SOCIAL SITUATIONS

After surgery, when they are busy working on reestablishing their own identity, some women choose to "stay private" because they don't want to concern themselves with other people's reactions. They want to do their own adjusting before they cope with others'. One woman said, "I don't want people looking at my chest, trying to figure out which breast I lost, and then my having to make them feel less embarrassed when I catch them at it."

Other women seem to have a great need to talk about it, to discuss what they are learning about their illness as well as the emotional impact of the disease.

"It felt good for me to air my feelings. I called my friends and family right away, and people really rallied round. I needed to talk about it a lot and to get a lot of feedback. It gave me confidence that people cared about me, and that was important, especially right before I went into surgery."

"I couldn't bring myself to cook the first day or two after every chemotherapy treatment. One of my friends kept track of when I had to go, and she'd bring some tasty little meal over to tempt me. Am I glad she was in on what was going on!"

These women and many others like them were able to accept help and support from the community around them. They gained a great deal from being able to let other people know about their illness.

Above all, women say that they do not want to be pitied. "I'm used to being the one who helps other people, and I take pretty good care of my own affairs besides. I almost wish I'd kept my mouth shut about this, because now I can't stand it when people are so obvious about feeling sorry for me."

If you have friends who are so ignorant as to think they'll catch breast cancer from you or so unfeeling as to let your illness make a difference in your relationship—well, they are not friends worth having. Most women with breast cancer say that their family and friends were so helpful and sympathetic that they could not have come through without them. They also tell stories of the occasional individual who could not seem to cope with their troubles. "Fair-weather friends," they used to be called, and no great loss.

THE ELDERLY

"My forty-five-year-old son talks to the doctor as if I'm not in the room. Does he think having breast cancer has affected my IQ? The other day he even asked the doctor, right in front of me, 'Is she going to die?' "

Older people who have any serious illness often feel that they are being treated condescendingly or that they are being bypassed when the time arises to make care and treatment decisions. That does in fact sometimes happen. Recently, a doctor friend and his wife were outraged that his mother-in-law consulted with a surgeon and oncologist "on her own" and made a decision to have a lumpectomy and radiation therapy against their wishes. My friend was equally annoyed that his mother-in-law's physician did not call to tell him what was going on. He might have been talking about a teenager and not a seventy-six-year-old woman who is still a practicing attorney, albeit one with breast cancer.

Unless a person's age has rendered her mentally incompetent— not a common event—she deserves the same right of self-determination as anyone else. That does not mean that you should not ask for help if you need it. If you are of advanced age and have worked hard to maintain your independence, it can seem a terrible defeat to admit that at least for a few weeks, you are going to have to stay with someone, or else arrange for someone to come to your home to be with you for a while after breast surgery.

One woman expressed it well. She said, "I've had to face up to the fact that by the time you're my age—I'm eighty-one—not only is your energy level way down, but you don't have quite the same capacity to cope with troubles. I guess it's that you've had your share by this point in your life. So, even though having a mastectomy isn't the big deal for me it would have been when I was younger, I still need a helping hand—and I asked my children for it."

You should get all the help you need, and if it is necessary, you should ask for it, either of family and friends or of the social services available to you. On the other hand, your family should not take the authority for your care away from you as if you were a minor child. In their effort to "protect" you, your friends and family may talk to your doctors in your place or make arrangements for your care that may not suit you. This kind of behavior can damage your relationship with your doctors and make you feel distrustful of what you are being told.

Most elderly Americans use Medicare as their primary health insurance. You may find that the government reimbursement for the various treatments you must undergo for breast cancer is far less than the actual fees you are being asked to pay. If you do not have supplemental health insurance, you should discuss the matter of payment with the staff of each doctor and facility you are dealing with so that anxiety about bills is not added to the strain of your illness. Here is one more place in this book where it is unfortunately necessary to say that our society must quickly turn its attention to ensuring excellent health care for all its citizens. Affordable medical care for the elderly should be an important priority.

DEALING WITH A HIGH-RISK CANCER

Though you may be in a situation where you have had a recurrence or perhaps extensive metastases, you can still help yourself by making a determined effort to get the very best available treatment.

That most definitely does not mean that your life has to be devoted to breast cancer. As we have seen, even women with advanced-stage cancer can, with vigorous treatment, live a long time. Think of yourself as having a chronic illness. Take good care of yourself. Be diligent in going for your examinations and treatment. But leave your disease in the doctor's office. That's the proper place for it.

There are examples every day of women who have done this. One patient, for example, had a very important position on the board of education of a large city school system. She came to my office with a widespread cancer and very little hope. Yet after a year of chemotherapy, she was so much better that before scheduling her next appointment, she'd take out her calendar to see if she "could squeeze me in." This woman went on to have a rewarding career for many years after her initial grave diagnosis.

This is not a question of denial, of refusing to admit that you are ill. It is a practical acknowledgment that women with breast cancer are living much longer than what used to be considered their "expected time" and are living full and productive lives.

CAN I GET ANYTHING POSITIVE OUT OF THIS EXPERIENCE?

The fact is, many women do. A patient who is an actress always felt that being young and beautiful was crucial to her career. She's had a mastectomy and a reconstruction and is still young and beautiful, but she said, "Now I look forward to getting older. Every year that passes since I had cancer is a year gained, not lost."

Women frequently become much more interested in their personal appearance after having breast reconstruction by a plastic surgeon. It is never a surprise when I see a patient looking particularly well a year or so later, and she tells me she has had a face-lift or cosmetic eye surgery. I think that's just fine, because it contributes to her sense of well-being.

Having had cancer can be for some people a powerful incentive to reorder their priorities. One woman who had breast surgery two years ago said, "I don't sweat the small stuff so much anymore. I used to be a total workaholic on my job and a compulsive neatness freak at home. I still enjoy working and I still like things to be orderly, but I'm more likely to spend Saturday in the park with my pals now and worry about what's in my briefcase some other time."

Many patients seem to have an understanding of the uncertainty of life that people who have not had cancer may not have. A woman who had a mastectomy when her baby was only six months old kept saying, "I only hope I live long enough to bring her up." Well, it's twenty-three years later and that patient is now a grandmother, babysitting for her grandchild.

It would obviously be dishonest to say that every occurrence of breast cancer has so happy an ending. And in a larger sense, none of us knows with any certainty what life will bring. But I see in many of my patients a special appreciation of family and friends, as well as new gusto for the pleasures of life. Some of them seem to have a renewed religious feeling. Some become active in trying to help other people or in working on the medical and social issues they came to understand through their own illness.

Everyone reacts differently to trouble. There is no "correct" way to cope with or get over an experience as trying as breast cancer. But from what I have observed, women are in fact coming through it with intelligence, sensitivity, and a very moving gallantry.

18

THE SOCIAL ISSUES OF BREAST CANCER

I f, as we have learned, one out of eight women in America will develop breast cancer during her lifetime, why aren't we doing more about it? Why isn't this a primary national concern? Why aren't more effort and more money being put into the problem?

RESEARCH

Breast cancer is now reported as striking 182,460 women a year. That figure, however, does not include the additional 67,770 women a year who have preinvasive (in situ) cancers but who are not part of these statistics.

In 2008, 40,480 women were expected to die of breast cancer.

The good news is that after years of rising, the incidence of invasive breast cancer began to level off and now has actually started to fall. Between 1980 and 1987 the incidence of breast cancer increased by 3.7 percent a year. The increase fell to 0.5 percent a year from 1987 to 2001. The latest figures show that between 2001 and 2004 the yearly incidence of breast cancer has fallen to 3.5 percent. The diagnosis of in situ disease rose rapidly in the 1980s and 1990s. This was particularly true for women above fifty years of age and was attributed to the increase in the number of women having mammography. Since 2000 the incidence of in situ cancer has leveled off among women over fifty but is still rising in younger women. Most encouraging, death rates from breast cancer fell an average of 2 percent a year from 1990 to 1997. Between 1999 and 2003 there was an additional decrease of nearly 10 percent in the number of women dying each year of breast cancer, from 44,000 to 40,000, and it is now stable. It is becoming clear that after years of pessimism and talk of our losing the battle against cancer, our efforts are beginning to succeed. We can now see what Congress has always demanded: that the dollars spent on research can be translated into lives saved.

After years of stagnation, the United States government's breast cancer research budget began to expand after 1992 as the result of efforts by advocacy groups who were inspired by the methods of those who fought for AIDS research funding. Funding for basic research into the causes of breast cancer, and clinical research directed to early detection and to finding optimal treatments, has increased and is being supplemented by a broader range of investigations into risk factors, prevention, and the impact of breast cancer on the quality of life of breast cancer survivors and their families.

Among the most important programs made possible by increased research funding are those related to clarifying the role of hormonal treatments in preventing the development and recurrence of breast cancer. Thanks to these efforts, we now know that in those at highest risk for developing breast cancer, treatment with tamoxifen can reduce the incidence of breast cancer by up to 50 percent. Furthermore, a reduction in risk of recurrence, of similar magnitude, can be achieved with tamoxifen in the nearly 67,700 women in the United States each year who are diagnosed with in situ breast cancer, and the reduction may be even larger with aromatase inhibitors. For women with invasive breast cancer, tamoxifen used for five years after surgery reduces the recurrence rate by 47 percent and Arimidex, an aromatase inhibitor, reduces the remaining risk by another 24 percent.

The possible role of environmental exposure to cancer-producing agents is an area of research that has attracted scientific interest and funding. Among the wide range of causative factors being reinvestigated is a possible link between breast cancer and insecticide residues that may have entered the food chain and water supply. The National Institute of Environmental Health Sciences is funding studies of genetic factors that may influence a woman's susceptibility to environmental factors.

In 1990 the government's breast cancer research budget at the National Cancer Institute (NCI) was $77 million. The first major expansion of that funding came in 1992, when NCI support for such research was increased to $132 million. The following year the pressure of expanded advocacy groups, unwilling to take no for an answer, had its full impact. NCI support grew to $196 million, and a new source of funds, the Department of Defense, was identified. As one of the most visible aspects of the "peace dividend," Congress assigned $210 million of defense funds to cancer research. In 2003, NCI was supporting $536 million of breast cancer research, and the Department of Defense allocation was $150 million. Since then the annual NCI budget for cancer research has increased slightly and the Department of Defense allocation has decreased modestly.

Despite the significant funds that are being allocated to breast cancer research, many feel that cancer research in general, and breast cancer research in particular, remain underfunded. This is particularly true now that the benefits of research are evident and the additional gains that can be made with additional funding are clear. Furthermore, delay also has direct consequences, an increase in needless loss of lives.

From 1998 to 2003, Congress doubled the budget of the National Institutes of Health, ending with the 2004 budget. Recent increases have been very small. Each year, innovative research proposals are submitted to the National Cancer Institute for approval. All are reviewed by impartial panels of scientists. Of those accepted as worthy of support, there is at present only enough money to fund 20 percent. Each grant not funded represents an opportunity lost. The National Cancer Legislation Advisory Committee has in the past recommended to Congress that it raise the budget of the National Cancer Institute to a level that would permit 40 percent of approved grants to be funded. Such an increase would significantly accelerate progress in all aspects of cancer research, including prevention, finding the causes of this disease, developing methods for earlier detection, and discovering new, more effective methods of treatment.

DIAGNOSIS AND TREATMENT

Mammograms cost from $90 to $425, and the cost is often doubled by the addition of sonography. The Middle Atlantic states, with New York in the forefront, are the most expensive for medical care. Cost remains an important consideration in efforts to encourage screening mammography for all women who would benefit. For women over sixty-five and for those disabled women who are eligible, Medicare allows annual screening mammograms and pays 80 percent of an allowed cost. The patient is responsible for the balance.

In 1970 there were few drugs available for the treatment of cancer. For pharmaceutical firms, research in this area was usually considered low priority, because it was perceived as a relatively small market with low profit margins. At that time, the cost of sixty Cytoxan tablets, a typical month's supply, was $19.

This situation changed with the introduction of Adriamycin in the mid-1970s. The cost of a single treatment with this new drug usually exceeded $100, and was often considerably higher, depending on the dose used. The price of drugs introduced later was at approximately the same level, and even the cost of older drugs, such as Cytoxan, rose to meet this new standard. By 1995, the monthly cost of Cytoxan was about $180 and in 2008, the generic version cost $285.

Taxol, an important new drug originally obtained from a rare source, the bark of the Pacific yew tree, became available in 1992. The high costs of development and testing resulted in a price of over $2,000 per treatment. Taxol's price once again changed the standard of cost for anticancer drugs. In a few instances generic alternatives have become available, and when that happened the prices of some of these drugs have fallen. However, the addition of new drugs such as Herceptin is again increasing the overall cost. The cost of a typical year of weekly Herceptin is about $60,000. Avastin, recently approved by the FDA for use in mestastic breast cancer, costs $100,000 a year.

A typical course of chemotherapy after surgery, which includes chemotherapy drugs, antinausea medications, and the costs of drug administration is about $92,000. When Herceptin is also needed for one year, this cost rises $60,000. Generic tamoxifen given daily for five years adds $1,080/year to the cost. Only women who have pharmaceutical insurance are covered for drug expenses, and some policies have a co-pay of 20 percent. These increases in drug costs are causing significant concern both to the insurance industry and to policymakers.

A course of radiation therapy after lumpectomy costs up to $25,000. The average cost of a modified radical mastectomy is anywhere from $1,200 to $6,000, depending on where in the country it is performed. Medicare pays about $1,100 for the procedure.

Breast reconstruction after mastectomy, a procedure that many women consider essential for their general well-being, costs from about $3,500 to $24,000, depending on which procedure is performed and where. Medicare pays about $2,500. Many private insurance companies pay a flat fee, and many do not compensate surgeons for more complicated operations.

INSURANCE

More than ever, a person's insurance coverage may determine the care he or she receives. Managed care plans now cover the majority of Americans under age sixty-five. They offer the advantage of lower initial cost and smaller co-payments, but the need to control costs restricts the services available to those who have this insurance. For instance, when an insured patient is required to choose from a closed panel of surgeons, that panel may not include a surgeon who specializes in breast surgery. Hospitalization has at times been denied to patients after breast surgery, including mastectomy. Access to tumor-marker blood tests, bone scans, and especially to CAT scans and MRIs often require special permission, resulting in significant delays and sometimes arbitrary denials. Increasingly, the use of certain drugs is being limited or requires special approval. At this writing, managed care companies have been protected from legal action for denial of care, although this may be changing under the new attention being given to the issue of patients' rights by state and federal legislatures.

At the same time more attention is being directed to care for the poor and uninsured. Under the Breast and Cervical Cancer Mortality Prevention Act of 1990, free mammography has been offered to those unable to afford such testing. By 2006, over 3 million women had been tested under this program, with 31,000 cases of breast cancer and over 100,000 cases of premalignant cervical lesions and invasive cervical cancers discovered.

GENETIC TESTING

As noted earlier, genetic testing may save lives by identifying women who are at higher risk of getting breast and ovarian cancer. Prior experience with genetic testing for other diseases has shown that if such information becomes available to other parties, it can be used to discriminate against tested individuals and their families, affecting that individual's ability to buy insurance or find a job. At this time none of my patients has had any benefits or procedures denied to her because she is known to have inherited a gene for breast cancer. In fact, in cases where women have requested a prophylactic mastectomy and have a positive gene, insurance companies have approved the procedure based on this information.

The Genetic Information Nondiscrimination Act (GINA), which was passed by the House of Representatives by a wide margin in 2007 and by the Senate in a unanimous vote in 2008 and signed by the president, prohibits insurers from using genetic information to deny benefits or raise premiums for both group and individual policies based on that information. The act also bans employers from collecting genetic information or using it to make decisions about hiring, firing, or compensating employees.

THE CONSEQUENCES

The need for more research, better and more affordable care, fewer insurance hassles, and affordable drugs are among the most important issues facing our society. All these elements affect the future health of women in this country. We are beginning to recognize that such issues can be resolved only if we give them high priority and the sense of urgency they deserve.

What are the practical results when we add up these needs? While we are further along than we were a decade ago, there are still a growing number of women whose well-being and quality of life are being threatened by breast cancer. We can do better and must continue to mobilize support for a growing effort to determine how to prevent this disease and how to treat it more effectively.

People talk so much about "reordering our national priorities" that the phrase has come to seem a cliché, and one that could have a divisive national impact. Who would want to decide that we should, for example, cut back on funds for heart research when so many of our people die of cardiac problems? Or that we should take the dollars allocated for AIDS research and funnel those monies into breast cancer research? Surely we have to do everything we can to fight an epidemic like AIDS, which has destroyed so many thousands of lives so quickly and so terribly.

But the women who suffer from breast cancer need help. They need it also, not instead of. Watching the response to the AIDS epidemic, they were inspired to form their own national movement to eradicate breast cancer through increased research, improved access to care, and extended involvement in decision making. Breast cancer advocates have not argued that current medical research is misplaced—rather, that AIDS *and* breast cancer, as well as other health concerns, should have higher government priorities for funding.

The National Breast Cancer Coalition, an organization

headquartered in Washington, D.C., has been particularly effective in articulating the need for public action. Also important have been the efforts of the Susan G. Komen Foundation in Dallas, which has become a major nongovernment source of breast cancer research funding.

In 2000 Congress appointed the National Cancer Legislation Advisory Committee (NCLAC) to review what had been accomplished since the National Cancer Act of 1971, when the nation first declared a "war on cancer," and then present its findings and recommendations for the future to Congress. In October 2001, on the thirtieth anniversary of that act, the NCLAC Report was issued. It confirmed that a concerted effort against cancer had produced significant progress but recognized that a great deal more had to be done. The recommendations included:

- Continued strong support for the National Cancer Institute budget to permit a significant expansion in its research effort

- Funding to increase the pool of well-trained biomedical researchers and health care professionals involved in patient care

- Expanded cancer research centers to permit them to more rapidly translate research findings into new preventive and treatment approaches to cancer

- Increased support for the National Institute for Environmental Health Sciences and the National Cancer Institute for research into the interaction between genes and the environment

- The founding of a national cancer screening initiative in an effort to achieve the highest possible rates of early detection

- A streamlined Food and Drug Administration drug approval process

- Additional public and private partnerships to mobilize funds for developing new cancer treatments

- Adequate health insurance coverage for all Americans concerned about or diagnosed with cancer

While far from a complete list, these recommendations deserve strong support and remain to be implemented.

There are some specific problem areas also in need of our attention. Among them are the aging of the U.S. population, the increase in the minority population, changes in patterns of health care delivery, disparities between states in cancer-related infrastructures, and the need for more rapid communication of health information.

We will soon see a rapid growth in the number of women over sixty-five. In 2001, 12.7 percent of the population was sixty-five or older. That figure is projected to be 20 percent by 2030. Since the risk of breast cancer rises sharply with age, it is estimated that the number of new cases diagnosed each year will more than double in the next twenty-five years. Research directed toward prevention and early detection is therefore particularly important.

As minority populations increase, more is being learned about the unique aspects of the disease for them. Breast cancer in younger black women is particularly aggressive. There are few studies under way to deal with special problems like these.

The rise of managed care in an effort to control health care costs has also meant a change in the interaction between physicians and patients. There is less time for patient education and for supportive interchanges between a worried patient and a caring physician. When costs rise, specialty-care rationing is seen. Tests require preapproval, which may delay diagnosis and treatment. As treatment improves, the importance of individualizing breast cancer care has become an issue, but individualizing requires more time. What will this mean in the context of cancer workforce shortages, physician education, and the response of payers such as insurers?

Much of what we know about breast cancer in the U.S. comes from state cancer registries and the SEER (Surveillance, Epidemiology, and End Results) program of the National Cancer Institute. State registries vary greatly in quality. Only 26 percent of the U.S. population is being monitored by SEER, yet it is on the basis of the statistics from these sources that the national strategy against cancer is being planned. Similar disparities between states exist with regard to Medicare. It is therefore not surprising that Medicare's response to changing needs has been consistently slow.

Finally, the enhancement of communication that has come with the introduction of cable, the Internet, cell phones, and DVDs offers great promise for a better exchange of health information, more effective implementation of public health policies, better patient-physician interaction, and more direct communication with our government representatives. However, we are still learning how best to use these opportunities. For instance, tentative steps toward developing a common repository for each patient's medical history are being taken, but there is matching concern about the dangers of loss of privacy. While the Internet offers a great deal of information, too much of it is unreliable. Electronic billing was intended to reduce paperwork, but privacy concerns are making implementation difficult. While e-mail is a very effective means for communicating with patients, it is not yet a secure medium, which discourages its use by physicians. A focused effort is needed to convert the promise of new technologies into tools for expediting progress.

In June 1991 a bipartisan coalition of senators and representatives responded to the newly formed breast cancer advocacy movement with a "Breast Cancer Challenge." They called upon the National Cancer Institute and the medical community to join in the fight so that by the year 2000 we would:

• Understand the causes of and find a cure for breast cancer

• Reduce the incidence of breast cancer

• Reduce the breast cancer mortality rate by 50 percent

• Ensure that all women over forty get regular mammograms

• Ensure that all mammograms are of the highest quality

As the fifth edition of this book is completed, where do we stand on meeting these goals? The causes of breast cancer are under intensive investigation. Advances in genetics continue to lead the way in this research. The entire human genome has been mapped, so we have a much better idea of how many genes there are and where they are located. At least two genes that play a major role in the development of breast cancer have been identified.

But do we *know* what causes breast cancer? Not really. How can we find out? We are much closer to the answer than we were a decade ago, but only through research will we find it. The progress already made should encourage us to press ahead, though this can be achieved only with adequate funding and incentives for such research. How are we doing in our efforts to find a cure? We are making progress but the problem is far more complex than planners imagined and unless there is full commitment on the part of society to proceed as rapidly as possible, the cure is unlikely to be found for quite some time. On the other hand, if we are really determined to proceed, and if Congress is willing once again to expand the funds committed to this cause, we have in our hands a much broader range of tools than we ever had before and may indeed find the answers we need in our own lifetimes.

As for reducing the incidence of breast cancer, the best strategy we now have to achieve this goal is to identify high-risk women early. We have learned that tamoxifen can reduce the number of such women who develop breast cancer, and that aromatase inhibitors may be even more effective. Prophylactic surgery can prevent breast cancer. Progress in our understanding of the genetic changes that underlie the development of breast cancer should help us to develop new strategies to this end. When treating postmenopausal symptoms, avoiding the combinations of estrogen and progesterone where possible may also be of considerable benefit.

We have also discovered how to prevent the recurrence of breast cancer by treatment with chemotherapy, hormone therapy, and targeted agents directly after surgery. The result is a continuing decrease in breast cancer mortality. But much of this progress has come at the cost of a considerable decrease in the quality of life over what often is an extended period, and while the results of treatment are improving, for too many there is ultimately no cure. We can take heart that we are beginning to see this change. As we learn more about the way each cell normally controls growth, we are starting to understand what goes wrong in the cancer cell. This knowledge allows the design of drugs specifically engineered to correct errors as they are found. That is the basis for the new *targeted therapy* that was only a concept when this book first appeared.

Breast imaging continues to play an important role in lowering the risk of disease once it is discovered. More women than ever are aware of the importance of following an early-detection screening plan: regular mammograms supplemented by breast self-examination and an annual examination by a physician. To this has been added a growing contribution from improved sonography. The proportion of women over forty who get regular mammograms has increased, but we still have not reached all women who should be screened. New technology is also playing a role. For women with a strong family history of breast cancer or known to be carriers of either the BRCA1 or BRCA2 genes, breast MRIs have now been established as an important new means for early breast cancer detection.

The greatest progress has been made in ensuring that mammograms are of the highest quality. The Mammography Quality Standards Act, passed in 1992, and the Mammography Quality Standards Reauthorization Act of 2003 led the Food and Drug Administration to create a program that assures that all facilities performing mammograms meet federal standards for quality (see page 61). The 2003 act also added a provision requiring that each patient receive a summary of the mammography report from the facility in which the study was done in terms a layperson can easily understand. Together, these provisions have not only enhanced the quality of mammograms but also helped see to it that any finding leads to early follow-up and, if necessary, treatment.

As gratifying as this progress has been, we have a long way to go before the fight against breast cancer is fully won. We need the same determination that has taken us this far if we are finally to eradicate this terrible disease. Former Colorado Congresswoman Pat Schroeder has said, "We have in America all the ingredients needed to beat breast cancer: political will, grassroots activism, and the medical brainpower."

The question is whether we have the commitment. Certainly women have it—those vast numbers of women who have had breast cancer or who have faced its prospect, or whose close friends or relatives have had it. And if we add to that number the men whose wives and sisters and girlfriends and mothers have had the disease—and those of us who are physicians working with those women—it means that a very large proportion of our population has a stake in a national determination to beat breast cancer.

Whether we can mobilize to achieve this goal remains to be seen.

RESOURCES

NCI-DESIGNATED CANCER CENTERS

(Updated as of March 2008. For more information, visit each center's website. For the most recent version of this list, go to NCI online at cancercenters.cancer.gov, or call the NCI at 800-4-CANCER.)

ALABAMA

UAB Comprehensive Cancer Center
University of Alabama at Birmingham
1802 Sixth Avenue South, NP 2555
Birmingham, Alabama 35294-3300
Tel: (205) 934-5077
Fax: (205) 975-7428

ARIZONA

Arizona Cancer Center
University of Arizona
1515 North Campbell Avenue
P.O. Box 245024
Tucson, Arizona 85724
Tel: (520) 626-7685
Fax: (520) 626-6898

CALIFORNIA

City of Hope National Medical Center
Beckman Research Institute
1500 East Duarte Road
Duarte, California 91010-3000
Tel: (626) 256-HOPE
Fax: (626) 930-5394

Salk Institute Cancer Center
10010 North Torrey Pines Road
La Jolla, California 92037
Tel: (858) 453-4100 X1385
Fax: (858) 457-4765

The Burnham Institute
10901 North Torrey Pines Road
La Jolla, California 92037
Tel: (858) 646-3100
Fax: (858) 713-6274

Rebecca and John Moores UCSD Cancer Center
University of California at San Diego
3855 Health Sciences Drive, Room 2247
La Jolla, California 92093-0658
Tel: (858) 822-1222
Fax: (858) 822-1207

Jonsson Comprehensive Cancer Center
University of California at Los Angeles
10833 Le Conte Avenue
Los Angeles, California 90095-1781
Tel: (310) 825-5268
Fax: (310) 206-5553

**USC/Norris Comprehensive
Cancer Center**
University of Southern California
1441 Eastlake Avenue
Los Angeles, California 90089-9181
Tel: (323) 865-0816
Fax: (323) 865-0102

**Chao Family Comprehensive
Cancer Center**
University of California at Irvine
101 The City Drive, Building 56
Orange, California 92868
Tel: (714) 456-6310
Fax: (714) 456-2240

UC Davis Cancer Center
University of California at Davis
4501 X Street, Suite 3003
Sacramento, California 95817
Tel: (916) 734-5800
Fax: (916) 451-4464

**UCSF Helen Diller Family
Comprehensive Cancer Center**
University of California at San
  Francisco
2340 Sutter Street, Box 0128
San Francisco, California 94115-0128
Tel: (415) 502-1710
Fax: (415) 502-1712

COLORADO

**University of Colorado Cancer
Center**
University of Colorado at Denver &
  Health Sciences Center
P.O. Box 6508, Mailstop F434
13001 E. 17th Place
Aurora, Colorado 80045

Tel: (303) 724-3155
Fax: (303) 724-3162

CONNECTICUT

Yale Cancer Center
Yale University School of Medicine
333 Cedar Street, Box 208028
New Haven, Connecticut 06520-8028
Tel: (203) 785-4371
Fax: (203) 785-4116

DISTRICT OF COLUMBIA

**Lombardi Comprehensive Cancer
Center**
Georgetown University
3970 Reservoir Road, NW
Research Building, Suite E 501
Washington, D.C. 20057
Tel: (202) 687-2110
Fax: (202) 687-6402

FLORIDA

**H. Lee Moffitt Cancer Center &
Research Institute**
The University of South Florida
12902 Magnolia Drive
Tampa, Florida 33612-9497
Tel: (813) 615-4261
Fax: (813) 615-4258

HAWAII

Cancer Research Center of Hawaii
University of Hawaii at Manoa
1236 Lauhala Street
Honolulu, Hawaii 96813
Tel: (808) 586-3013
Fax: (808) 586-3052

ILLINOIS

University of Chicago Cancer Research Center
5841 South Maryland Avenue
Chicago, Illinois 60637-1470
Tel: (773) 702-6180
Fax: (773) 702-9311

Robert H. Lurie Comprehensive Cancer Center
Northwestern University
303 E. Superior Street, Suite 3-125
Chicago, Illinois 60611
Tel: (312) 908-5250
Fax: (312) 908-1372

INDIANA

Melvin and Bren Simon Cancer Center
Indiana University
Indiana Cancer Pavilion
535 Barnhill Drive, Room 455
Indianapolis, Indiana 46202-5289
Tel: (317) 278-0070
Fax: (317) 278-0074

Purdue University Cancer Center
Hansen Life Sciences Research
    Building
South University Street
West Lafayette, Indiana 47907-1524
Tel: (765) 494-9129
Fax: (765) 494-9193

IOWA

Holden Comprehensive Cancer Center at the University of Iowa
200 Hawkins Drive
Iowa City, Iowa 52242
Tel: (319) 353-8620
Fax: (319) 353-8988

MAINE

The Jackson Laboratory Cancer Center
600 Main Street
Bar Harbor, Maine 04609-0800
Tel: (207) 288-6041
Fax: (207) 288-6044

MARYLAND

Sidney Kimmel Comprehensive Cancer Center
Johns Hopkins University
401 North Broadway
Baltimore, Maryland 21231
Tel: (410) 955-8822
Fax: (410) 955-6787

MASSACHUSETTS

Dana-Farber/Harvard Cancer Center
Dana-Farber Cancer Institute
44 Binney Street
Boston, Massachusetts 02115
Tel: (617) 632-2100
Fax: (617) 632-4452

Center for Cancer Research
Massachusetts Institute of
   Technology
77 Massachusetts Avenue
Cambridge, Massachusetts 02139-4307
Tel: (617) 253-8511
Fax: (617) 253-0262

MICHIGAN

**University of Michigan
Comprehensive Cancer Center**
6302 Cancer Center
1500 East Medical Center Drive
Ann Arbor, Michigan 48109-0942
(800) 865-1125

**The Barbara Ann Karmanos
Cancer Institute**
Wayne State University School of
   Medicine
4100 John R
Detroit, Michigan 48201
Tel: (800) KARMANOS
Fax: (313) 576-8630

MINNESOTA

**University of Minnesota Cancer
Center**
420 Delaware Street, SE
Minneapolis, Minnesota 55455
Tel: (612) 624-8484
Fax: (612) 626-3069

Mayo Clinic Cancer Center
Mayo Clinic Rochester
200 First Street, SW
Rochester, Minnesota 55905
Tel: (507) 266-4997
Fax: (507) 284-1544

MISSOURI

Siteman Cancer Center
Washington University School of
   Medicine
660 South Euclid Avenue, Campus
   Box 8109
St. Louis, Missouri 63110
Tel: (314) 362-8020
Fax: (314) 454-1898

NEBRASKA

**University of Nebraska Medical
Center/ Eppley Cancer Center**
600 South 42nd Street
Omaha, Nebraska 68198-6805
Tel: (402) 559-4238
Fax: (402) 559-4652

NEW HAMPSHIRE

Norris Cotton Cancer Center
Dartmouth-Hitchcock Medical Center
One Medical Center Drive, Hinman
   Box 7920
Lebanon, New Hampshire 03756-0001
Tel: (603) 653-9000
Fax: (603) 653-9003

NEW JERSEY

**The Cancer Institute of New
Jersey**
Robert Wood Johnson Medical
   School
195 Little Albany Street
New Brunswick, New Jersey 08903-
   2681
Tel: (732) 235-8064
Fax: (732) 235-8094

NEW YORK

Albert Einstein Cancer Research Center
Albert Einstein College of Medicine
Chanin Building, Room 209
1300 Morris Park Avenue
Bronx, New York 10461
Tel: (718) 430-2302
Fax: (718) 430-8550

Roswell Park Cancer Institute
Elm & Carlton Streets
Buffalo, New York 14263-0001
Tel: (716) 845-5772
Fax: (716) 845-8261

Cold Spring Harbor Laboratory
P.O. Box 100
Cold Spring Harbor, New York
  11724
Tel: (516) 367-8383
Fax: (516) 367-8879

NYU Cancer Institute
New York University Medical Center
550 First Avenue
New York, New York 10016
Tel: (212) 263-6485
Fax: (212) 263-8210

Memorial Sloan-Kettering Cancer Center
1275 York Avenue
New York, NY 10021
Tel: (212) 639-2000 or (800) 525-
  2225
Fax: (212) 717-3299

Herbert Irving Comprehensive Cancer Center
College of Physicians & Surgeons
Columbia University
1130 St. Nicholas Avenue
New York, New York 10032
Tel: (212) 851-5273
Fax: (212) 851-5236

NORTH CAROLINA

UNC Lineberger Comprehensive Cancer Center
University of North Carolina at
  Chapel Hill
102 Mason Farm Road, CB 7295
Chapel Hill, North Carolina 27599-
  7295
Tel: (919) 966-3036
Fax: (919) 966-3015

Duke Comprehensive Cancer Center
Duke University Medical Center, Box
  2714
Durham, North Carolina 27710
Tel: (919) 684-5613
Fax: (919) 684-5653

Wake Forest Comprehensive Cancer Center
Wake Forest University
Medical Center Boulevard
Winston-Salem, North Carolina
  27157-1082
Tel: (336) 716-7971
Fax: (336) 716-0293

OHIO

Case Comprehensive Cancer Center
Case Western Reserve University
11100 Euclid Avenue, Wearn 151
Cleveland, Ohio 44106-5065
Tel: (216) 844-8562
Fax: (216) 844-4975

Comprehensive Cancer Center
The Ohio State University
310 West 10th Avenue
Columbus, Ohio 43210
Tel: (614) 293-7521
Fax: (614) 293-7522

OREGON

OHSU Cancer Institute
Oregon Health & Science University
3181 S.W. Sam Jackson Park Road
Portland, Oregon 97239-3098
Tel: (503) 494-1617
Fax: (503) 494-7086

PENNSYLVANIA

Abramson Cancer Center
The University of Pennsylvania
16th Floor of Penn Tower
3400 Spruce Street
Philadelphia, Pennsylvania 19104-
4283
Tel: (215) 662-6065
Fax: (215) 349-5325

The Wistar Institute
3601 Spruce Street
Philadelphia, Pennsylvania 19104-
4268

Tel: (215) 898-3926
Fax: (215) 573-2097

Fox Chase Cancer Center
333 Cottman Avenue
Philadelphia, Pennsylvania 19111
Tel: (215) 728-3636
Fax: (215) 728-2571

Kimmel Cancer Center
Thomas Jefferson University
233 South 10th Street
Philadelphia, Pennsylvania 19107-
5799
Tel: (215) 503-5692
Fax: (215) 503-9334

University of Pittsburgh Cancer Institute
UPMC Cancer Pavilion
5150 Centre Avenue, Suite 500
Pittsburgh, Pennsylvania 15232
Tel: (412) 623-3205
Fax: (412) 623-3210

TENNESSEE

St. Jude Children's Research Hospital
332 North Lauderdale
Memphis, Tennessee 38105-2794
Tel: (901) 495-3982
Fax: (901) 495-3966

Vanderbilt-Ingram Cancer Center
Vanderbilt University
691 Preston Research Building
Nashville, Tennessee 37232-6838
Tel: (615) 936-1782
Fax: (615) 936-1790

TEXAS

Dan L. Duncan Cancer Center
Baylor College of Medicine
One Baylor Plaza
Houston, Texas 77030
Tel: (713) 798-1354
Fax: (713) 798-2716

M.D. Anderson Cancer Center
University of Texas
1515 Holcombe Boulevard
Houston, Texas 77030
Tel: (713) 792-2121
Fax: (713) 799-2210

San Antonio Cancer Institute
University of Texas Health Science
   Center at San Antonio
2040 Babcock Road, Suite 201
San Antonio, Texas 78229
Tel: (210) 567-5286
Fax: (210) 567-5292

UTAH

Huntsman Cancer Institute
University of Utah
2000 Circle of Hope
Salt Lake City, Utah 84112-5550
Tel: (801) 581-4485
Fax: (801) 581-2175

VERMONT

Vermont Cancer Center
University of Vermont
89 Beaumont Avenue
Burlington, Vermont 05405-0110
Tel: (802) 656-4414
Fax: (802) 656-8788

VIRGINIA

UVA Cancer Center
University of Virginia Health
   Sciences Center
MSB West Complex
Jefferson Park Avenue, Room 6171 E
Charlottesville, Virginia 22908
Tel: (434) 243-6784
Fax: (434) 982-0918

Massey Cancer Center
Virginia Commonwealth University
P.O. Box 980037
Richmond, Virginia 23298-0037
Tel: (804) 828-0450
Fax: (804) 828-8453

WASHINGTON

**Fred Hutchinson Cancer
Research Center**
P.O. Box 19024, D1-060
Seattle, Washington 98109-1024
Tel: (206) 667-4305
Fax: (206) 667-5268

WISCONSIN

**UW Paul P. Carbone
Comprehensive Cancer Center**
University of Wisconsin
600 Highland Avenue
Madison, Wisconsin 53792-0001
Tel: (608) 263-8610
Fax: (608) 263-8613

AMERICAN CANCER SOCIETY DIVISIONS

California Division, Inc.
1710 Webster Street
Oakland, CA 94612
Tel: (510) 893-7900
Fax: (510) 835-8656

Eastern Division, Inc.
(NJ, NY)
6725 Lyons Street
East Syracuse, NY 13057
Tel: (315) 437-7025
Fax: (315) 437-0540

Florida Division, Inc.
(including Puerto Rico operations)
3709 W Jetton Avenue
Tampa, FL 33629-5146
Tel: (813) 253-0541
Fax: (813) 254-5857

Puerto Rico
Calle Alverio #577
Esquina Sargento Medina
Hato Rey, PR 00918
Tel: (787) 764-2295
Fax: (787) 764-0553

Great Lakes Division, Inc.
(MI, IN)
1755 Abbey Road
East Lansing, MI 48823-1907
Tel: (517) 332-2222
Fax: (517) 664-1498

Great West Division, Inc.
(AK, AZ, CO, ID, MT, ND, NM,
NV, OR, UT, WA, WY)
2120 First Avenue North
Seattle, WA 98109-1140
Tel: (206) 283-1152
Fax: (206) 285-3469

High Plains Division, Inc.
(HI, KS, MO, NE, OK, TX)
2433 Ridgepoint Drive
Austin, TX 78754
Tel: (512) 919-1800
Fax: (512) 919-1844

Illinois Division, Inc.
225 N. Michigan Avenue, Suite 1200
Chicago, IL 60601
Tel: (312) 641-6150
Fax: (312) 641-3533

Mid-South Division, Inc.
(AL, AR, KY, LA, MS, TN)
1100 Ireland Way, Suite 300
Birmingham, AL 35205-7014
Tel: (205) 930-8860
Fax: (205) 930-8877

Midwest Division, Inc.
(IA, MN, SD, WI)
8364 Hickman Road, Suite D
Des Moines, IA 50325
Tel: (515) 253-0147
Fax: (515) 253-0806

New England Division, Inc.
(CT, ME, MA, NH, RI, VT)
30 Speen Street
Framingham, MA 01701-9376
Tel: (508) 270-4600
Fax: (508) 270-4699

Ohio Division, Inc.
5555 Franz Road
Dublin, OH 43017
Tel: (614) 889-9565
Fax: (614) 889-6578

Pennsylvania Division, Inc.
Route 422 and Sipe Avenue
Hershey, PA 17033-0897
Tel: (717) 533-6144
Fax: (717) 534-1075

South Atlantic Division, Inc.
(DC, DE, GA, MD, NC, SC,
VA, WV)
2200 Lake Boulevard
Atlanta, GA 30319
Tel: (404) 816-7800
Fax: (404) 816-9443

BREAST CANCER INFORMATION RESOURCES*

ORGANIZATIONS

American Cancer Society's nationwide toll-free hotline provides information on all forms of cancer, and referrals to local Reach to Recovery and many other support programs. The ACS also offers numerous brochures and educational materials for patients and health care professionals. Their website is an increasingly valuable source of information. Contact the ACS at (800) ACS-2345 or www.cancer.org.

The Breast Health Access for Women with Disabilities Project (BHAWD) provides direct services and public and professional education to increase access and utilization of breast screening by women aged 20 and older with limitations in mobility, vision, or development. Contact BHAWD at (510) 204-4866; www.bhawd.org; or c/o Alta Bates Medical Center, Herrick Campus Rehabilitation Services, 2001 Dwight Way, 2nd Floor, Room 2362, Berkeley, CA 94704.

CancerCare, Inc. offers support, education, information, referrals, and financial assistance for diagnostic and support services through the AVONCares Program for Medically Underserved Women. CancerCare's

*The information in this section, used by permission, is based on materials developed and published by the National Alliance of Breast Cancer Organizations (NABCO) prior to its closing in June 2004.

staff of oncology social workers assist cancer patients nationwide through their toll-free counseling line, and telephone support groups and education programs are available on many topics. Contact CancerCare at (800) 813-HOPE, info@cancercare.org, or www.cancercare.org.

The Cancer Information Service (CIS) of The Canadian Cancer Society (CCS) is an information service where callers can receive accurate and up-to-date information in English, French, or Chinese on all aspects of cancer, from medically approved and complementary therapies to programs and services across Canada. The CCS's CIS is open Monday through Friday, 9:00 A.M. to 6:00 P.M. CST, at (306) 566-5700 outside Canada. This organization can also be reached by e-mailing info@cis.cancer.ca or by visiting their website at www.cancer.ca.

The Cancer Information Service (CIS) of the National Cancer Institute (NCI) is a national telephone and web-based information and education network composed of regional offices that offer resources and direction on all aspects of cancer. The CIS provides the NCI brochures indicated in this list without charge, and refers callers to medical centers and clinical trial programs. Spanish-speaking staff members are available to answer calls and questions. Contact the NCI's CIS at (800) 4-CANCER (Monday through Friday, 9:00 A.M. to 4:30 P.M. EST) or by visiting their website at www.cancer.gov. Deaf and hearing-impaired callers with TTY equipment can call (800) 332-8615.

Judges and Lawyers Breast Cancer Alert (JALBCA) offers a confidential hotline for judges, lawyers, and law students who have been diagnosed with breast cancer. Contact JALBCA at (212) 289-9720; home@jalbca.org; www.jalbca.org; or 1369 Madison Avenue, PMB 424, New York, NY 10128.

The National Breast Cancer Coalition (NBCC) advocates on both national and local levels to support legislation, regulation, and funding that benefits breast cancer patients, survivors, and women at risk. NBCC facilitates Project LEAD, an intensive training course that provides breast cancer advocates with scientific concepts and knowledge for active participation in public policy and breast cancer research processes. Contact NBCC at (800) 622-2838; www.stopbreastcancer.org; or 1707 L Street NW, Suite 1060, Washington, D.C. 20036.

The National Coalition for Cancer Survivorship (NCCS) raises awareness of cancer survivorship through its publications, quarterly newsletter, education programs, and advocacy for insurance, employment, and legal rights for people with cancer. NCCS also facilitates networking among cancer programs, serves as an information clearinghouse, and encourages the study of cancer survivorship. On a national level, NCCS provides public policy leadership on legislative, regulatory, and financing matters and promotes responsible advocacy among national cancer organizations. For more information, contact the NCCS at (877) NCCS-YES or (301) 650-9127; www.canceradvocacy.org; or 1010 Wayne Avenue, Suite 770, Silver Spring, MD 20910-5600.

Pregnant with Cancer Support Group is a national organization created to offer hope and support to women who are facing a diagnosis of cancer while pregnant. Through a network of women across the country, this group will match a new patient with someone who once faced cancer while pregnant. Contact Pregnant with Cancer Support Group at (800) 743-4471; www.pregnantwithcancer.org; or P.O. Box 1243, Buffalo, NY 14220.

SHARE is a national nonprofit organization of breast and ovarian cancer survivors who offer hotlines, support groups, educational activities, and advocacy activities for women suffering from either of these diseases. Contact SHARE at (866) 891-2392; www.sharecancersupport.org; or 1501 Broadway, Suite 704A, New York, NY 10036.

Sharsheret is a national nonprofit organization of cancer survivors which is specifically tailored to aid young Jewish women with breast cancer. One of the many services they offer is genetic counseling for Jewish women who have a strong family history of breast and ovarian cancer. Contact Sharsheret at (866) 474-2774; www.sharsheret.org; or 1086 Teaneck Road, Suite 3A, Teaneck, NJ 07666.

Sisters Network is a national organization that works to increase local and national attention to the impact that breast cancer has in the African-American community. Contact Sisters Network Inc. at (713) 781-0255 or (866) 781-1808; www.sistersnetworkinc.org; or 8787 Woodway Drive, Suite 4206, Houston, TX 77063.

The Susan G. Komen Breast Cancer Foundation seeks to eradicate breast cancer as a life-threatening disease. In addition to funding research, the foundation supports education, screening, and treatment projects in communities around the world and delivers the lifesaving message of early detection to millions of women and men. Contact Komen at (877) 465-6636 or (972) 855-1600; www.komen.org; or 5005 LBJ Freeway, Suite 250, Dallas, TX 75244.

The Young Survival Coalition is an international organization that focuses on the issues and challenges faced by women aged 40 and under who are diagnosed with breast cancer. Contact the Young Survival Coalition at (877) YSC-1011 or (212) 206-6610; info@youngsurvival.org; www.young survival.org; or Box 528, 52A Carmine Street, New York, NY 10014.

Breast Cancer Network of Strength (formerly known as Y-Me National Breast Cancer Organization) offers breast cancer information and peer support twenty-four hours a day through their national hotline, (800) 221-2141, and Spanish-language hotline, (800) 986-9505. Network of Strength also offers support to male partners of women with breast cancer through their national hotline. Their website is also a useful source of information. Contact Network of Strength at (312) 986-8338; www.networkofstrength .org; or 212 West Van Buren Street, Suite 500, Chicago, IL 60607-3908.

WEBSITES

www.breastcancer.net is a web-based newsletter offering daily e-mail updates for a yearly subscription of $20.00.

www.breastcancer.org is a nonprofit Internet resource that offers information on breast cancer risk, early detection, treatment, and support.

www.cancer.gov is the website of the National Cancer Institute, which provides information on breast cancer treatment, screening, genetics, clinical trials, and supportive care.

www.cancer.org is the website of the American Cancer Society, which provides information on all forms of cancer and offers numerous brochures and publications for patients and health care professionals.

www.bespoke-books.com/wordpress/?cat=1 offers easy access to a wide variety of breast cancer resources on the Internet.

www.komen.org is the website of The Susan G. Komen Breast Cancer Foundation and covers such topics as risk factors, diagnosis, staging, treatment, after-treatment care, and breast cancer financial and insurance issues.

www.plwc.org is the patient information website of the American Society of Clinical Oncology (ASCO), which provides information on various types of cancer and their treatments, clinical trials, and side effects.

www.networkofstrength.org is the website of Breast Cancer Network of Strength (formerly known as Y-ME National Breast Cancer Organization). It offers breast cancer information, publications, and links to their ten affiliate chapters.

CHOICES ABOUT TREATMENT

UNDERSTANDING CHOICES

A Breast Cancer Journey: Your Personal Guidebook (American Cancer Society, Second Edition—2005, $18.95). Written for the newly diagnosed, this clear and comprehensive resource provides information on treatment options as well as practical tips on managing the emotional and treatment side effects of breast cancer. Includes insights from breast cancer survivors. 416 pages. Contact the ACS at (800) ACS-2345 or www.cancer.org.

A Patient's Guide: Understanding Tumor Markers for Breast and Colorectal Cancers (American Society of Clinical Oncology, 2007). This patient guide explains the role of tumor markers in diagnosing, treating, and following cancer. Contact ASCO at (888) 273-3508 or www.ascocancer foundation.org (look under "Patient and Survivor Resources," and then "Patient Guides").

Be a Survivor: Your Guide to Breast Cancer Treatment by Vladimir Lange, MD (Lange Productions, Fourth Edition—2007, $24.95). The latest edition to this series, which includes a video and CD-ROM, offers information on all aspects of breast cancer. Includes diagrams, pictures, charts, and personal reflections. 158 pages. Contact Lange Productions at (888) LANGE-88, langeinfo@langeproductions.com, or www.langeproductions .com.

Breast Cancer Treatment Guidelines for Patients (American Cancer Society and National Comprehensive Cancer Network, July 2007, Version IX). These guidelines were developed by a diverse panel of experts to provide a clear and understandable source of currently accepted approaches to treatment for the breast cancer patient. Includes a glossary. Also available in Spanish. Call the ACS at (800) ACS-2345 or contact the NCCN at (888) 909-NCCN or www.nccn.org to download the guidelines in both English and Spanish.

CancerCare, Inc. offers seminars, telephone education programs, and CancerCare Briefs on many treatment-related topics. Contact CancerCare at (800) 813-HOPE, info@cancercare.org, or www.cancercare.org.

Dr. Susan Love's Breast Book by Susan M. Love, MD, with Karen Lindsey (DaCapo Press, Fourth Edition—2005, $22). This general reference discusses all conditions of the breast, from benign to malignant. The author's viewpoint on treatment options and controversies is clearly presented in a friendly, accessible style. 620 pages. Bookstores or visit Da Capo Press at www.perseusbooksgroup.com/dacapo.

FINDING A BREAST CANCER SPECIALIST: The American Board of Medical Specialties, (866) ASK-ABMS or www.abms.org, can verify a physician's board certification by specialty and year, and will refer callers to local board-certified doctors who are members. The National Cancer Institute's (NCI) Cancer Information Service Physician Data Query (PDQ) contains a directory of physicians whose practices center on cancer treatment. This list can be accessed by contacting the NCI's CIS at (800) 4-CANCER. Visit your state's department of health "Consumer Information" section of their website for an updated alphabetical listing of state physicians who have been cited for professional misconduct.

FINDING A CANCER CENTER: To locate a major cancer center in your state, see the listing of NCI-affiliated treatment centers at the beginning of this section. Additional community centers are members of the NCI's Community Clinical Oncology Program (CCOP); a current list is available online at www.cancer.gov. If no NCI-affiliated center is conveniently located, call the department of surgery at the nearest one to ask for a local referral.

FINDING A RECONSTRUCTIVE SURGEON: For referrals to a plastic surgeon for corrective or reconstructive breast procedures, contact the American Society of Plastic Surgeons—(888) PLASTIC or www.plasticsurgery.org—for a list of local board-certified plastic surgeons.

HER-2: The Making of Herceptin, a Revolutionary Treatment for Breast Cancer by Robert Bazell (Random House, New York, NY, 1998, $15.00). Written by NBC's chief science correspondent, this book tells the story of the creation of Genentech's Herceptin, the monoclonal antibody that is the first gene-based therapy for breast cancer. 240 pages. Bookstores or contact Random House at (800) 733-3000 or www.randomhouse.com.

Informed Decisions: The Complete Book of Cancer Diagnosis, Treatment and Recovery by Harmon Eyre, MD, Dianne Lange, and Lois Morris (American Cancer Society, Atlanta, GA, Second Edition—2001, $29.95). A resource on cancer risk, screening, diagnosis, and treatment as well as diet, pain relief, and sexuality. Includes an extensive resource section. 784 pages. Bookstores or contact the ACS at (800) ACS-2345 or www.cancer.org.

Making Informed Medical Decisions: Where to Look and How to Use What You Find by Nancy Oster, Lucy Thomas, and Darol Joseff, MD (O'Reilly and Associates, Sebastopol, CA, 2000, $17.95). An overview of the tools necessary for health-information seekers either to become fully informed or to build a network of information and support for making tough medical decisions. 364 pages. Bookstores or visit www.patientcenters.com.

Now You Have a Diagnosis: What's Next? (Agency for Healthcare Research and Quality, 2000). This booklet explains how and where to find reliable health care information and how to use that information to evaluate the benefits and risks of available treatments. Call the AHRQ at (800) 358-9295.

Questions to Ask the Doctor About Breast Cancer (Susan G. Komen Breast Cancer Foundation, 2007). This booklet of fourteen topic cards offers suggestions of important questions to discuss with your doctor regarding a specific topic. Also available in Spanish. Contact Komen at (877) SGK-SHOP or www.komen.org.

Talking with Your Doctor (American Cancer Society, 2006). This booklet offers suggestions for effective doctor-patient communication. Also available in Spanish. Call the ACS at (800) ACS-2345 or visit their website at www.cancer.org.

Teamwork: The Cancer Patient's Guide to Talking with Your Doctor (National Coalition for Cancer Survivorship, Fourth Edition—2006, $2.00 shipping or download PDF from the Internet). Useful suggestions on how best to begin and maintain a working relationship with a physician that is constructive for both the doctor and the patient. Also available in Spanish. Contact the NCCS at (877) NCCS-YES; www.canceradvocacy.org/resources/publications; or 1010 Wayne Avenue, Suite 770, Silver Spring, MD 20910.

Breast Cancer—Treatment Guidelines for Patients (National Comprehensive Cancer Network [part of the American Cancer Society], 2007). This NCCN booklet addresses the common questions that new patients may have about breast cancer and the therapies that are available to them. The topics covered include early detection, diagnosis, treatment, adjuvant therapy, and breast cancer in pregnancy. Call (888) 909-NCCN, or access the booklet online at www.nccn.org.

Understanding Your Pathology Report (Breast Cancer Network of Strength [formerly Y-ME], 2004). This brochure outlines the purpose of a pathology report and defines the different elements that are included. Also available in Spanish. Contact the Network of Strength at (800) 221-2141 or www.networkofstrength.org.

Your Breast Cancer Treatment Handbook by Judy C. Kneece, RN, OCN (EduCare Publishing, Columbia, SC, Sixth Edition—2004, $24.95). This easy-to-use book contains information about managing treatment decisions and addresses sensitive emotional issues in an insightful manner. 230 pages. Contact EduCare Publishing at (800) 849-9271 or www.cancer help.com.

Your Guide to the Breast Cancer Pathology Report (breastcancer.org, 2007). This brochure explains the different sections of a pathology report. Available at www.breastcancer.org.

WEBSITES

www.fda.gov/cder/cancer is the oncology tools website of the Food and Drug Administration and offers information on approved oncology therapies, what drugs are approved for what diseases, and how to obtain access to unapproved drugs.

www.oncolink.org is ONCOLINK, one of the first online cancer resources. It provides comprehensive information for cancer patients, families, health care professionals, and the general public about specific types of cancer, updates on cancer treatments, and news about research advances. Also offers a clinical trials matching service.

www.ibcresearch.org is the website of the Inflammatory Breast Cancer Research Foundation (IBC), which offers information, support resources, updated listings of clinical trials for inflammatory breast cancer, treatment information, and more. Visit their website or contact IBC at (877) STOP-IBC. If your telephone call has not been returned within forty-eight hours, please call again.

Accessible at http://sis.nlm.nih.gov/outreach/womenshealthoverview.html and http://orwh.od.nih.gov/nat_lib_med.html is a website jointly created by the National Library of Medicine (NLM) and the National Institutes of Health's Office of Research on Women's Health (ORWH). This resource contains up-to-date information on a number of topics in women's health, all of which is peer-reviewed.

CLINICAL TRIALS

Cancer Clinical Trials: Experimental Treatments and How They Can Help You by Robert Finn (O'Reilly and Associates, Inc., Sebastopol, CA, 1999, $14.95). This book is targeted at cancer patients to guide them through the clinical trials process, from defining a clinical trial to insurance and other financial issues. 216 pages. Visit www.oreilly.com to buy the book.

Clinical Trials Q & A (National Cancer Institute, 2006). This fact sheet describes the types of clinical trials that are available, who sponsors them, how the doctors who conduct them keep patients safe, et cetera. It can only be accessed online, at https://cissecure.nci.nih.gov/ncipubs/.

Community Clinical Oncology Program (CCOP) is a network of the sixty-one medical centers in thirty-four states, the District of Columbia, and Puerto Rico that have been selected by the National Cancer Institute to introduce new clinical protocols and to accrue patients to clinical trials at the community level. To receive contact information for CCOP institutions in your area, call the NCI's Cancer Information Services at (800) 4-CANCER.

If You Have Cancer ... What You Should Know About Clinical Trials (National Cancer Institute, 2001). This brochure offers basic information about clinical trials and offers suggestions of questions to ask before agreeing to participate in a clinical trial. *Only* available in Spanish. Contact the NCI's Cancer Information Services at (800) 4-CANCER or https://cissecure.nci.nih.gov/ncipubs/.

Physicial Data Query (PDQ) is the computerized cancer database of the NCI that provides information on treatment, organizations, doctors involved in cancer care, and a listing of clinical trials that are open to patient accrual. Contact the NCI's Cancer Information Services at (800) 4-CANCER or www.cancer.gov/cancerinfo/pdq.

Taking Part in Cancer Treatment Research Studies (National Cancer Institute, 2007). A booklet designed for patients who are trying to decide whether to participate in cancer trials. It discusses how patients are chosen for these trials, and what they can expect if they are chosen and they agree to participate. Contact the NCI's Cancer Information Services at (800) 4-CANCER for a copy, or read it online at http://www.cancer.gov/clinicaltrials/.

WEBSITE

www.cancer.gov/clinicaltrials is an up-to-date NCI online resource for information about cancer clinical trials. It is easy to navigate and was designed to help users find and choose a treatment trial. It also posts news about research discoveries.

TYPES OF THERAPY

Chemotherapy and You: A Guide to Self-Help During Treatment (National Cancer Institute, 2007). A booklet, in question-and-answer format, addressing concerns of patients receiving chemotherapy. Emphasis is on explanation, self-help, and participation during treatment. Includes a glossary. Also available in Spanish. Contact the NCI's CIS at (800) 4-CANCER or https://cissecure.nci.nih.gov/ncipubs.

Chemotherapy: Your Weapon Against Cancer (Chemotherapy Foundation, 1998). An explanation of the benefits and side effects of chemotherapy. Includes a glossary. Contact the Chemotherapy Foundation at (212) 213-9292; www.chemotherapyfoundation.org; or 183 Madison Avenue, Suite 403, New York, NY 10016.

Consumer's Guide to Cancer Drugs by Gail M. Wilkes, RN, MS, AOCN; Terri B. Ades, RN, MS, AOCN; and Irvin Krakoff, MD (Jones & Bartlett Publishing, 2003, $24.95). A clear and quick reference for the essential facts about chemotherapy and symptom management drugs. A glossary of cancer treatment terms is included. 535 pages. Contact the ACS at (800) ACS-2345 or purchase from Internet vendors.

Coping with Lymphedema by Joan Swirsky, RN, and Diane Sackett Nannery (Avery Books, New York, NY, 1998, $15.95). This book is a practical guide to understanding, treating, and living with lymphedema (swelling and inflammation of the arm or chest area), a side effect of some types of breast cancer treatment. 304 pages. Bookstores or contact Penguin Putnam Publishing Group at (800) 788-6262 or www. penguinputnam.com.

Lymphedema: A Breast Cancer Patient's Guide to Prevention and Healing by Jeannie Burt and Gwen White, PT (Hunter House Publishers, Alameda, CA, Second Edition—2005, $14.95). This book describes the options women have for treating lymphedema. 245 pages. Bookstores or contact Hunter House Publishers at (800) 266-5592 or www.hunterhouse.com.

The National Lymphedema Network is a nonprofit organization providing information about the prevention and treatment of lymphedema to patients and health care professionals, as well as information on support groups. Contact the National Lymphedema Network at (800) 541-3259 or (510) 208-3200; www.lymphnet.org; or Latham Square, 1611 Telegraph Avenue, Suite 1111, Oakland, CA 94612.

Radiation Therapy and You: Support for People with Cancer (National Cancer Institute, 2007). This booklet clearly explains the external beam and internal (implant) forms of radiation therapy. Also available in Spanish. Contact the NCI's CIS at (800) 4-CANCER or https://cissecure .nci.nih.gov/ncipubs.

Tamoxifen: Questions and Answers (National Cancer Institute, 2002). A fact sheet on tamoxifen and its side effects. Also available in Spanish. Read it online at cancer.gov/cancertopics/factsheet/therapy/tamoxifen.

Understanding Chemotherapy (American Cancer Society, 2006). This booklet provides an introduction to chemotherapy and explains its benefits and side effects. Also available in Spanish. Contact the ACS at (800) ACS-2345 or www.cancer.org.

Understanding Radiation Therapy (American Cancer Society, 2007). This booklet provides an introduction to radiation therapy and explains its benefits and side effects. Also available in Spanish. Contact the ACS at (800) ACS-2345 or www.cancer.org.

Insurance and Financial Issues

A Cancer Survivor's Almanac: Charting Your Journey edited by Barbara Hoffman, JD (John Wiley and Sons, New York, NY, Second Edition—1998, $18.95). This reference volume from the National Coalition for Cancer Survivorship includes thorough and understandable information about public and private health insurance, survivorship issues, disability benefits, employment rights, and legal and financial concerns. 384 pages. Contact the NCCS at (877) NCCS-YES; www.canceradvocacy.org/resources/publications; or 1010 Wayne Avenue, Suite 770, Silver Spring, MD 20910.

The American Federation of Clinical Oncologic Societies has identified fifteen basic criteria for choosing a health insurance plan to ensure coverage of high-quality cancer care. Available in the "Policy and Practice" section of www.asco.org.

The Center for Medicare Advocacy, Inc. is a nonprofit organization that provides education, advocacy, and legal assistance to help Medicare beneficiaries obtain necessary health care. Contact the center at (860) 456-7790; www.medicareadvocacy.org; or P.O. Box 350, Willimantic, CT 06226.

Guide to Indivdual Disability Income and Insurance (Health Insurance Association of America, 2007). A comprehensive guide to understanding disability insurance. Contact the HIAA at (800) 828-0111 or www.hiaa.org.

Questions and Answers About Health Insurance (Health Insurance Association of America, 2007). A comprehensive guide to understanding health insurance. Available online at www.hiaa.org.

Medicare and You (CMS, frequent updates). This government publication for Medicare beneficiaries can be obtained free of charge from the Centers for Medicare and Medicaid Services (CMS). For the most current available edition visit www.medicare.gov, or if you would like a printed edition, call (800) MEDICARE or write to CMS at 7500 Security Boulevard, Baltimore, MD 21244.

Medicare Rights Center provides a hotline service for individuals with Medicare questions or problems, and educational brochures about

Medicare benefits and rights. Many brochures are available in both English and Spanish. Call (800) 333-4114, ext. 1. For Medicare HMO members who are appealing HMO denials of care or coverage, call (888) HMO-9050. For free brochures or for more information visit their website, www.medicare rights.org.

The Patient Advocate Foundation is a national nonprofit organization that serves as a liaison between the patient and her insurer to resolve insurance matters related to her diagnosis. Offers several resources, including the Patient Pal, a guide to help patients needing assistance with insurance issues. Contact the PAF at (800) 532-5274; www.patientadvocate.org; or 700 Thimble Shoals Boulevard, Suite 200, Newport News, VA 23606.

U.S. Department of Labor, Employee Benefits Security Administration describes the Health Insurance Portability and Accountability Act (HIPAA) of 1996 and the Women's Health and Cancer Rights Act (WHCRA) of 1998. This service also publishes *FAQs About the HIPAA's Nondiscrimination Requirements*, regulations that were issued in January 2001. Contact (800) 998-7542 or www.dol.gov/ebsa/faq_hipaa_ND.html.

What Cancer Survivors Need to Know About Health Insurance (National Coalition for Cancer Survivorship, 2007). Provides a clear understanding of health insurance and how to receive maximum reimbursement for claims. Contact the NCCS at (877) NCCS-YES; www.canceradvocacy .org; or 1010 Wayne Avenue, Suite 770, Silver Spring, MD 20910.

Women's Health and Cancer Rights Act of 1998 states that women who are eligible for mastectomy benefits under group medical coverage, and who elect breast reconstruction in conjunction with surgery, are eligible to receive coverage for reconstruction on the breast on which the mastectomy has been performed, surgery and reconstruction on the other breast to produce a symmetrical appearance, and prostheses and treatment for any physical complication, including lymphedema. For a copy of this law, contact the U.S. Department of Labor, Employee Benefits Security Administration at (866) 444-EBSA or www.dol.gov/ebsa/publications/ whcra.html.

Your Guide to the Appeal Process (Patient Advocate Foundation, 2000). This brochure offers suggestions and advice to help patients navigate the appeal process. Also available in Spanish. Contact the PAF at (800) 532-5274; www.patientadvocate.org; or 700 Thimble Shoals Boulevard, Suite 200, Newport News, VA 23606.

WEBSITE

www.iii.org is the website of the Insurance Information Institute. It answers consumer questions about insurance and offers problem-solving support, including information on life, business, auto, and property casualty insurance. The information is also available in Spanish.

FINANCIAL ASSISTANCE

CancerCare, Inc. has a toll-free counseling line staffed with trained oncology social workers who can suggest referrals for financial assistance. The AVONCares Program for Medically Underserved Women at CancerCare provides financial assistance for diagnostic and support services. Contact CancerCare at (800) 813-HOPE, info@cancercare.org, or www.cancercare .org.

Be Prepared: The Complete Financial, Legal and Practical Guide for Living with Cancer, HIV, and Other Life-Challenging Conditions by David S. Landay (St. Martin's Press, New York, NY, 2000, $19.95). Although not cancer specific, this easy-to-understand book offers practical guidance for the many financial, legal, and practical issues for people living with a life-challenging disease. 480 pages. Bookstores or contact St. Martin's Press at (888) 330-8477 or www.stmartins.com.

Getting to Know Your Entitlements (CancerCare, Inc., 2000). This patient brief provides an overview of the various entitlement programs for which individuals with cancer may apply. Contact CancerCare at (800) 813-HOPE, info@cancercare.org, or www.cancercare.org/get_help/pwc.php.

National Association of Hospital Hospitality Houses, Inc. (NAHHH) has more than 150 hospitality houses throughout the U.S. that provide family-centered lodging and support services to families and their loved ones who are receiving medical treatment far from home. Contact NAHHH at (800) 542-9730; www.nahhh.org; helpinghomes@nahhh.org; or P.O. Box 18087, Asheville, NC 28814.

The National Financial Resources Guidebook for Patients (Patient Advocate Foundation, 2003). This valuable resource provides listings of federal and state resources for obtaining financial assistance for a broad range of needs, including housing, transportation, utilities, medical payments, and insurance deductibles. 257 pages. Contact the PAF at (800) 532-5274;

www.patientadvocate.org/patient.htm; or 700 Thimble Shoals Boulevard, Suite 200, Newport News, VA 23606.

Social Security Handbook (Social Security Administration, March 2008). A comprehensive overview of social security, including a description of disability benefits. Access it online at www.socialsecurity.gov/OP_Home/handbook/SSA-hbk.htm.

COPING AND EMOTIONAL RECOVERY

I Am Not My Breast Cancer: Women Talk Openly About Love and Sex, Hair Loss and Weight Gain, Mothers and Daughters, and Being a Woman with Breast Cancer by Ruth Peltason (William Morrow, New York, NY, 2008, $25.95). Organized in three sections—Diagnosis, Living with Breast Cancer, and The Big Picture—this book shares the combined knowledge and experiences of eight hundred women who have breast cancer. 400 pages. Bookstores or contact William Morrow at www.william morrow.com.

The Association for Cancer Online Resources (ACOR) offers different types of online cancer support resources. One popular list serv (discussion group) is the Breast Cancer Mailing List. Contact ACOR at www.acor.org.

Cancer Hope Network is a national agency that provides free and confidential one-to-one emotional support by matching a cancer patient or family member with a volunteer who had a similar diagnosis. The volunteer visits over the phone or, when possible, in person. Contact the Cancer Hope Network at (877) 467-3638; info@cancerhopenetwork.org; www.cancer hope network.org; or 2 North Road, Suite A, Chester, NJ 07930.

The Cancer Wellness Center offers free emotional support to all cancer patients through its 24-hour hotline, support groups, relaxation/visualization groups, educational workshops, and library. Also offers support services to anyone affected by a cancer diagnosis. Contact the Cancer Wellness Center at (847) 509-9595 or (866) 292-9355; www.cancerwellness .org; or 215 Revere Drive, Northbrook, IL 60062.

Coping with Cancer Magazine covers issues helpful for cancer patients and survivors and encourages patients to assume greater responsibility in their treatment. Published bi-monthly. Yearly subscription costs $19.00. Contact Coping with Cancer at (615) 790-2400 (for subscription inquiries) or www.copingmag.com.

Gilda's Club Worldwide offers free support and networking groups, lectures, workshops, and social events in a nonresidential, homelike setting in thirty locations throughout the U.S. and Canada. Contact Gilda's Club Worldwide at (888) GILDA-4-U; www.gildasclub.org; or 322 Eighth Avenue, Suite 1402, New York, NY 10001.

The Humor Project, Inc. is a resource on the use of humor in coping with illness. A catalog is available. Contact the Humor Project at (518) 587-8770; www.humorproject.com; or 480 Broadway, Suite 210, Saratoga Springs, NY 12866.

Mamm Magazine covers issues helpful to women who have been diagnosed with breast and reproductive cancer, their partners and their families. Published ten times a year with up to three special issues. Yearly subscription costs $17.95. Contact MAMM Magazine at (877) 668-1800 or www.mamm.com.

Reach to Recovery is a program of the American Cancer Society. Trained volunteers who themselves have had breast cancer visit newly diagnosed patients and can offer information and support to the patient during the visit; services are appropriate after either mastectomy or lumpectomy. To request a visit, call the ACS at (800) ACS-2345.

Spinning Straw into Gold: Your Emotional Recovery from Breast Cancer by Ronnie Kaye, MFCC (Fireside, New York, NY, 1991, $13.00). Written by a psychotherapist who was diagnosed with breast cancer, this comprehensive guide to emotional recovery from the disease is based in part on her clients' stories. 224 pages. Bookstores or contact Simon and Schuster at (800) 223-2348 or www.simonsays.com.

Taking Time: Support for People with Cancer and the People Who Care About Them (National Cancer Institute, 2003). This booklet for people with cancer and their families addresses the feelings and concerns of others in similar situations and how they have coped. Contact the NCI's CIS at (800) 4-CANCER or https://cissecure.nci.nih.gov/ncipubs.

The Wellness Community offers extensive support and education programs that encourage emotional recovery and a feeling of wellness. To find a program near you, contact the national office at 919 18th Street, NW, Suite 54, Washington, D.C. 20006; (888) 793-WELL; www.thewellness community.org.

The Wellness Community Guide to Fighting for Recovery from Cancer by Harold H. Benjamin, PhD (JP Tarcher, New York, NY, Revised Edition—1995, $15.95). This revised and expanded edition describes over thirty practical methods that cancer patients can use to hasten recovery. 285 pages. Bookstores or contact the Penguin Putnam Publishing Group at (800) 788-6262 or www.penguinputnam.com.

After Breast Cancer: A Common Sense Guide to Life After Treatment by Hester Schnipper (Bantam, New York, NY, Updated Edition—2006, $16.00) A breast cancer survivor and oncology social worker, Schnipper helps prepare women for life after breast cancer by imparting information and advice in an intimate and direct manner. Bookstores or contact Bantam Dell at www.bantamdell.com.

SEXUALITY AND FERTILITY

Breast Cancer: Coping with Your Changing Feelings (CancerCare, Inc., 2007). This fact sheet gives women tips on how they can look and feel as good as possible while they are being treated for breast cancer. It advises those who are feeling completely disinterested in physical intimacy to discuss this issue with their doctor. Visit www.cancercare.org to read it online.

Fertile Hope is a nonprofit organization that offers support and information to cancer patients dealing with fertility issues. Contact Fertile Hope at (888) 994-HOPE or www.fertilehope.org.

No Less a Woman: Femininity, Sexuality and Breast Cancer by Deborah Kahane, MSW (Hunter House Publishers, Alameda, CA, Second Edition—2006, $14.95). This book, written by a breast cancer survivor, addresses the psychosocial and sexual impact that breast cancer has on the lives of women. Includes personal stories from several women and important resources. 320 pages. Bookstores or contact Hunter House Publishers at (800) 266-5592 or www.hunterhouse.com.

Sexuality and Cancer: For the Woman Who Has Cancer, and Her Partner (American Cancer Society, 2006). This book offers information about cancer, sexuality, and possible areas of concern for the patient and her partner. Includes a resource section. Also available in Spanish. Contact the ACS at (800) ACS-2345 if you would like to be sent a print version, or read it online at www.cancer.org.

Sexuality and Fertility After Cancer by Leslie R. Schover, PhD (John Wiley and Sons, New York, NY, 1997, $15.95). This book explains how treatment may emotionally and physically interfere with male and female sexual function and fertility. As a resource, it helps survivors and their partners learn to enjoy sex again and make informed choices about having children. 288 pages. Bookstores or contact John Wiley and Sons at (877) 762-2974 or www.wiley.com.

Sexuality and Intimacy (Susan G. Komen Breast Cancer Foundation, 2007). This one-page fact sheet in the Facts for Life series discusses basic issues related to sexuality and intimacy for breast cancer patients. Contact Komen at (877) SGK-SHOP or www.komen.org.

FAMILY SUPPORT

Cancer Caregivers: A Resource Guide by Karen Kirzner Adler and Rozlyn Forman Kleiman (Upstream Press, 2001, $17.95). This book offers resources and suggestions for the many questions that a caregiver for a person with cancer may face. 272 pages. Contact Upstream Press at (877) 401-9500 or www.upstreampress.com.

Caregiving: A Step-by-Step Resource for Caring for the Person with Cancer at Home by Peter S. Houts, PhD, and Julia A. Bucher, RN, PhD (American Cancer Society, 2003, $18.95). A comprehensive resource that offers practical solutions to the many conditions and situations that a caregiver caring for a person with cancer in the home may face. Includes a resource section. 304 pages. Contact the ACS at (800) ACS-2345 or www.cancer.org.

Caring for the Patient with Cancer at Home: A Guide for Patients and Families (American Cancer Society, 2007 Edition). A guidebook with detailed, helpful information on how to care for the patient at home. Contact the ACS at (800) ACS-2345 or visit www.cancer.org to read it online.

Handbook for Mothers Supporting Daughters with Breast Cancer (Mothers Supporting Daughters with Breast Cancer, 1999). This handbook offers practical advice and resources for mothers of women with breast cancer. Contact MSDBC at (410) 778-1982; www.mothersdaughters.org; or 25235 Fox Chase Drive, Chestertown, MD 21620-3409.

Caregiving for Your Loved One with Cancer (CancerCare, Inc., 2005). This booklet advises caregivers on how they can support and nurture themselves while providing all of the practical and emotional support that their loved one with cancer needs. Contact CancerCare at (800) 813-HOPE, info@cancercare.org, or read it online at www.cancercare.org/pdf/booklets/ccc_caregiver.pdf.

The National Family Caregivers Association offers information, education, support, public awareness, and advocacy to address the common needs of family caregivers. Contact the National Family Caregivers Association at 10400 Connecticut Avenue #500, Kensington, MD 20895-3944; (800) 896-3650; info@nfcacares.org; or www.nfcacares.org.

What's Happening to the Woman We Love? Families Coping with Breast Cancer (Susan G. Komen Breast Cancer Foundation, 2004). This booklet for families of a newly diagnosed woman offers suggestions of ways to be helpful and supportive. Includes a resource section. Also available in Spanish. Contact Komen at (877) SGK-SHOP or www.komen.org.

WEBSITES

www.caregiving.com is the website of the Center for Family Caregivers, which offers online support groups for new and seasoned caregivers, caregiving professionals, a subscription newsletter, and journal links. This site focuses on the caregivers of older adults.

www.caregiving.org is the website of the National Alliance for Caregiving, which offers resources for family caregivers.

www.cancerguide.com is a for-profit site that offers online support, assessment tools, and a toll-free number to reach someone who can help an individual who is overwhelmed with caregiving responsibilities. Contact www.cancerguide.com or (888) 389-8839.

INDEX

Note: Page numbers in *italics* indicate illustrations.

ABOUT THE AUTHORS

Yashar Hirshaut is a medical oncologist specializing in the treatment of breast cancer. A graduate of the Albert Einstein College of Medicine, he completed his oncology training at the National Cancer Institute in Bethesda, Maryland, and at the Memorial Sloan-Kettering Cancer Center in New York. From 1970 to 1986 he served as an attending physician at Memorial Sloan-Kettering on the Clinical Immunology Service and as associate professor of medicine at the Cornell University Medical College. He was also head of the Laboratory for Immunodiagnosis at Sloan-Kettering. In addition to being in private practice, he is currently associate clinical professor of medicine at the Weill Medical College of Cornell University, adjunct professor of biology at Yeshiva University, and an attending physician at the Mount Sinai Medical Center and Beth Israel and Lenox Hill Hospitals in New York City. Dr. Hirshaut was Editor-in-Chief of the professional journal *Cancer Investigation* from 1981 to 2006. He is chairman of the Israel Cancer Research Fund, which provides peer-reviewed funding for basic cancer research.

Peter I. Pressman is a surgical oncologist who specializes in the treatment of breast cancer. A graduate of Columbia College and the Columbia University College of Physicians and Surgeons, he trained at Presbyterian Hospital and the Columbia Division of Bellevue Hospital in New York City. Dr. Pressman has been in private practice in New York for more than thirty-five years and is Clinical Professor of Surgery at the Weill Medical College of Cornell University and Director of the Genetics Risk Assessment Program at the Breast Center. He was attending surgeon at Beth Israel Medical Center and Lenox Hill Hospital. He has been consultant to the Guttman Breast Diagnostic Institute and president of the New York Metropolitan Breast Cancer Group, as well as a member of the Board of Directors (New York City division) and the Breast Cancer Detection and Treatment Subcommittee (national) of the American Cancer Society. He has published widely in the medical literature and has been named by *American Health*, *Good Housekeeping*, *New York*, and *Town and Country* magazines as among the best breast cancer doctors in New York City and in the nation.